AF818049

Studies in Systems, Decision and Control

Volume 324

Series Editor

Janusz Kacprzyk, Systems Research Institute, Polish Academy of Sciences, Warsaw, Poland

The series "Studies in Systems, Decision and Control" (SSDC) covers both new developments and advances, as well as the state of the art, in the various areas of broadly perceived systems, decision making and control–quickly, up to date and with a high quality. The intent is to cover the theory, applications, and perspectives on the state of the art and future developments relevant to systems, decision making, control, complex processes and related areas, as embedded in the fields of engineering, computer science, physics, economics, social and life sciences, as well as the paradigms and methodologies behind them. The series contains monographs, textbooks, lecture notes and edited volumes in systems, decision making and control spanning the areas of Cyber-Physical Systems, Autonomous Systems, Sensor Networks, Control Systems, Energy Systems, Automotive Systems, Biological Systems, Vehicular Networking and Connected Vehicles, Aerospace Systems, Automation, Manufacturing, Smart Grids, Nonlinear Systems, Power Systems, Robotics, Social Systems, Economic Systems and other. Of particular value to both the contributors and the readership are the short publication timeframe and the world-wide distribution and exposure which enable both a wide and rapid dissemination of research output.

** Indexing: The books of this series are submitted to ISI, SCOPUS, DBLP, Ulrichs, MathSciNet, Current Mathematical Publications, Mathematical Reviews, Zentralblatt Math: MetaPress and Springerlink.

More information about this series at http://www.springer.com/series/13304

Fadi Al-Turjman • Ajantha Devi • Anand Nayyar
Editors

Emerging Technologies for Battling Covid-19

Applications and Innovations

Springer

Editors
Fadi Al-Turjman
Research Center for AI and IoT
Near East University, Nicosia,
via Mersin 10, Turkey

Ajantha Devi
Research Head
AP3 Solutions
Chennai, Tamil Nadu, India

Anand Nayyar
Graduate School
Faculty in Information Technology
Duy Tan University,
Da Nang, Vietnam

ISSN 2198-4182 ISSN 2198-4190 (electronic)
Studies in Systems, Decision and Control
ISBN 978-3-030-60038-9 ISBN 978-3-030-60039-6 (eBook)
https://doi.org/10.1007/978-3-030-60039-6

© The Editor(s) (if applicable) and The Author(s), under exclusive license to
Springer Nature Switzerland AG 2021
This work is subject to copyright. All rights are reserved by the Publisher, whether the whole or part of the material is concerned, specifically the rights of translation, reprinting, reuse of illustrations, recitation, broadcasting, reproduction on microfilms or in any other physical way, and transmission or information storage and retrieval, electronic adaptation, computer software, or by similar or dissimilar methodology now known or hereafter developed.
The use of general descriptive names, registered names, trademarks, service marks, etc. in this publication does not imply, even in the absence of a specific statement, that such names are exempt from the relevant protective laws and regulations and therefore free for general use.
The publisher, the authors, and the editors are safe to assume that the advice and information in this book are believed to be true and accurate at the date of publication. Neither the publisher nor the authors or the editors give a warranty, expressed or implied, with respect to the material contained herein or for any errors or omissions that may have been made. The publisher remains neutral with regard to jurisdictional claims in published maps and institutional affiliations.

This Springer imprint is published by the registered company Springer Nature Switzerland AG
The registered company address is: Gewerbestrasse 11, 6330 Cham, Switzerland

Preface

As the world faces health crisis, the healthcare industry is looking for new technologies to monitor and control the spread of COVID-19. It requires the support of new technologies like Artificial Intelligence (AI), Internet of Things (IoT), Big Data, and Deep Learning to fight and look ahead against new diseases. In the present situation, researchers, scientists, research and development professionals, and other industry professionals are struggling hard to combat the challenges owing to COVID-19. New practical and cost-effective solutions are sought to mitigate the challenges.

In this book, *Emerging Technologies for Battling COVID-19: Applications and Innovations*, we have made a strong attempt to present the advances in technologies that can assist the worldwide governments and healthcare specialists to come out with guidelines and design systems to manage the COVID-19 pandemic. The COVID-19 management is mainly based on (1) maintaining proper physical hygiene, (2) enforcing social distancing, (3) using face masks to protect against or limit the spread of COVID-19, (4) avoiding touching of the face, (5) contactless control of appliances to stop the spread of the virus, (6) self-isolation in case of suspicion, (7) contact tracing process, (8) home quarantine for patients, (9) screening and monitoring of individuals, and (10) mass screening and testing. The chapters in the book highlight various COVID-19 challenges faced by individuals and elaborate the benefits of latest technologies.

The objective of this book is to enlighten the reader about various technologies such as Artificial Intelligence, Drones, IoT, and Big Data on COVID-19 and study its impact and to provide solutions to overcome the real-time challenges.

The book has 17 chapters. Chapter 1 titled "Dynamic Models and Control Techniques for Drone Delivery of Medications and Other Healthcare Items in COVID-19 Hotspots" proposes a multi-constraint and multi-objective gain-based simulation-optimization approach for scheduling the linear and nonlinear dynamic and controllable drone-movement models. In addition, the performance of the proposed system is measured using performance and security metrics. Chapter 2 titled "Identification of COVID-19 in Human Bodies Using the Machine Learning Approach" utilizes Machine Learning approach on varied datasets available for prediction, detection, and stage identification of COVID-19. Chapter 3 titled

"COVID-19 Epidemic Analysis and Prediction Using Machine Learning Algorithm" applies ARIMA Model, Holt-Winter Mode, SARIMAX model, Polynomial Regression and LSTM on COVID-19 datasets on varied Datasets by John Hopkins CSSE, World meters, and Kaggle and concludes that the polynomial regression model shows better accuracy in prediction of affected cases and number of deaths. Chapter 4 titled "Big Data and Modern-Day Technologies in COVID-19 Pandemic: Opportunities, Challenges, and Future Avenues" aims to identify several use cases where the big medical data from the patients, epidemiological data, social media data, and environment-related data can be used to identify patterns, causes, and other growing factors of COVID-19 pandemic with a goal to mitigate the damages and contain further spread of the disease. The chapter also discusses the impact of a preferred mitigation measure of nationwide lockdown due to the increasing number of new novel coronavirus positive patients as well as the impact on the environment by analyzing the available data. In addition, challenges associated with handling the massive amount of data generated during such pandemics are presented. Chapter 5 titled "Applications of Artificial Intelligence and Internet of Things for Detection and Future Directions to Fight Against COVID-19" highlights the use of various AI and Machine Learning (ML) algorithms for detecting the most threatening symptoms and features of COVID-19. Chapter 6 titled "COVID-19 Under Origin and Transmission: A Data-Driven Analysis for India and Bangladesh" analyzes the COVID-19 outbreak situation considering confirmed cases, recoveries, and mortality rate percentages using data available for India and Bangladesh. Chapter 7 titled "Robotics and Drone-Based Solution for the Impact of COVID-19 Worldwide Using AI and IoT" discusses the various solutions based on drones and robots in the field of AI and IOT, such as drones being used for social distancing and robots for sanitization. In addition, analysis has been made about the total number of cases and deaths around the world and how it has affected humanity and what measures have been taken to control this deadly disease. Chapter 8 titled "Wearable Devices and COVID-19: State of the Art, Framework, and Challenges" highlights the impact of wearable devices for combating COVID-19 and also gives a detailed review of efficient techniques and algorithms for data analysis based on vital body signals obtained from wearable devices. In addition, the chapter addresses various challenges associated with wearable devices in COVID-19 scenario like real-time processing, heterogeneity, interoperability, security, and privacy. Chapter 9 titled "Effectiveness of Big Data in Early Prediction and Measure for COVID-19 Using Data Science" highlights the utility of Data Science for COVID-19 for early detection. Chapter 10 titled "COVID-19: Creating Paradigm Shift in Education System" reviews the educational challenges and opportunities posed by the unexpected outbreak of COVID-19 pandemic and explores the various platforms readily available for adopting digital/online learning, and some recommendations are made for future education system. Chapter 11 titled "Perspectives to Definition of Data Visualization: A Mapping Study and Discussion on Coronavirus Dataset" applies visualization techniques to comprehend the advancement of coronaviruses. Chapter 12 titled "Disaster Management Using Recent Technologies During COVID-19" studies the impact of lockdown pertaining to sectors like transportation, markets, shops, public gatherings, medical facilities, and identification of people suffering from coronavirus and addresses these issues using various technologies like drones for monitoring activity, AI, technology for planning and prediction in order to curtail the growth rate of people suffering from coronavirus using algorithms, etc. Chapter 13 titled "COVID-19 Impact on Education System Globally" studies the impact of COVID-19 on the educational system worldwide and the strategies that might be useful to fill the gap created by closure of schools during COVID-19. Chapter 14 titled "Mobile Technology Solutions for COVID-19" explores viable mobile big data solutions to combat this pandemic while adhering to principles of privacy and ethics. In addition to this, a novel tele-health solution is proposed for combating the coronavirus situation. Chapter 15 titled "Predictive Analysis of COVID-19 transmission: Mathematical Modeling Study" proposes a predictive model to identify the severity of this disease transmission and also find the topographical spread of the contagion. Chapter 16 titled "Analyzing the Economic Depression Post-COVID-19 Using Big Data Analytics" highlights the depression suffered by various sectors post-COVID-19 as a result of the lockdown effect along with various recent policies implemented. It also covers visualizing these issues with big data analytics perspective and how the concept of AI and other technologies are working across in order to solve these issues. It covers in brief how these upcoming technologies have been able to contribute to the healthcare sector while fighting against COVID-19 or uplifting the economy by helping the industry to build and design new models or plans to regain the cash inflow. Chapter 17 titled "Intrinsic and Extrinsic Motivation for Online Teaching in COVID-19: Applications, Issues, and Solutions" proposes an online Gamified education system to enhance the various intrinsic and extrinsic motivational factors which are directly proportional to high student engagement.

The book will be useful for students, healthcare professionals, engineers, or developers to have a strong understanding of the pandemic and what techniques in terms of technology can be used to combat this pandemic situation. All these aspects of the book are imperative for safeguarding the human race from more loss of resources and economies due to COVID-19. I hope this work might increase the interest in this field of research and that the reader will find it useful for their investigations, management, and clinical usage.

Mersin 10, Turkey — Fadi Al-Turjman
Chennai, Tamil Nadu, India — Ajantha Devi
Da Nang, Viet Nam — Anand Nayyar

Acknowledgments

This book was conceptualized considering the unprecedented pandemic of COVID-19 and to focus on various aspects of emerging technologies for battling COVID-19. All these aspects are imperative for safeguarding the human race from more loss of resources and economies due to COVID-19. To overcome these issues and fill the gap, we hope this book shall provide a readily available resource in this area. The aim of this book is to acknowledge the potential of COVID-19 and remedies to mitigate it.

We are grateful to all the contributors who trusted us and supported our work. I hope they will be proud like us on the release of this book. I would also like to thank Springer Nature Publisher and all team members to not only consider this book for publication but also publish in the shortest possible time, despite COVID-19 pandemic-associated international restrictions, lockdown, work from home, and several other limiting factors.

We would like to thank our colleagues, family members, and friends who provided a lot of encouragement and support during the work on this book.

Fadi Al-Turjman
Ajantha Devi
Anand Nayyar

Contents

About the Editors

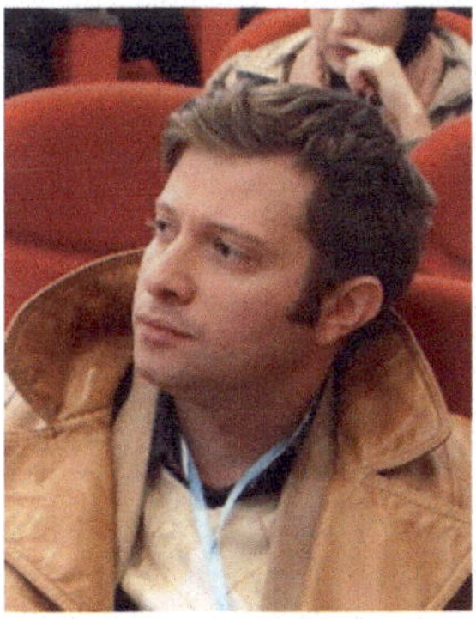

Fadi Al-Turjman received his Ph.D. in computer science from Queen's University, Kingston, Ontario, Canada, in 2011. He is a full professor and a research center director at Near East University, Nicosia, Cyprus. Prof. Al-Turjman is a leading authority in the areas of smart/intelligent, wireless, and mobile networks' architectures, protocols, deployments, and performance evaluation. His publication history spans over 250 publications in journals, conferences, patents, books, and book chapters, in addition to numerous keynotes and plenary talks at flagship venues. He has authored and edited more than 25 books about cognition, security, and wireless sensor networks' deployments in smart environments, published by Taylor and Francis, Elsevier, and Springer. He has received several recognitions and best papers' awards at top international conferences. He also received the prestigious Best Research Paper Award from Elsevier Computer Communications Journal for the period 2015-2018, in addition to the Top Researcher Award for 2018 at Antalya Bilim University, Turkey. Prof. Al-Turjman has led a number of international symposia and workshops in flagship communication society conferences. Currently, he servevs as an associate editor and the lead guest/associate editor for several well-reputed journals, including the IEEE Communications Surveys and Tutorials (IF 23.9) and the Elsevier Sustainable Cities and Society (IF 5.7).

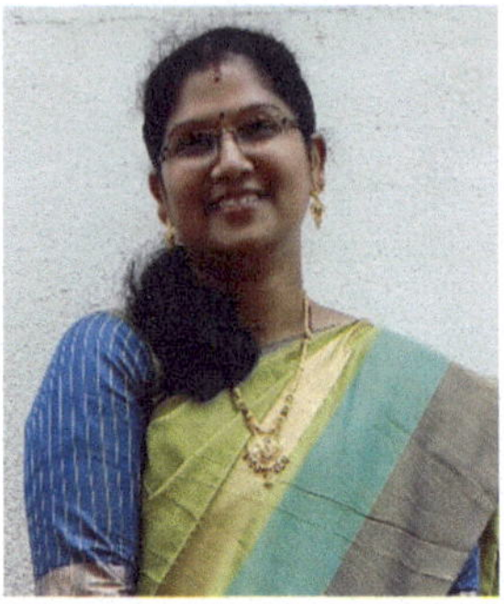

Ajantha Devi is working as a research head in AP3 Solutions, Chennai, Tamil Nadu, India. She received her PhD from the University of Madras in 2015. She has worked as Project Fellow under UGC Major Research Project. She has been certified as "Microsoft Certified Application Developer" (MCAD) and "Microsoft Certified Technical Specialist" (MCTS) from Microsoft Corp. She had published more than 30 papers in international journals and conference proceedings. Her work is based on artificial intelligence, machine learning and deep learning techniques under image processing, signal processing, pattern matching, and natural language processing. She has received a number of best paper presentation awards.

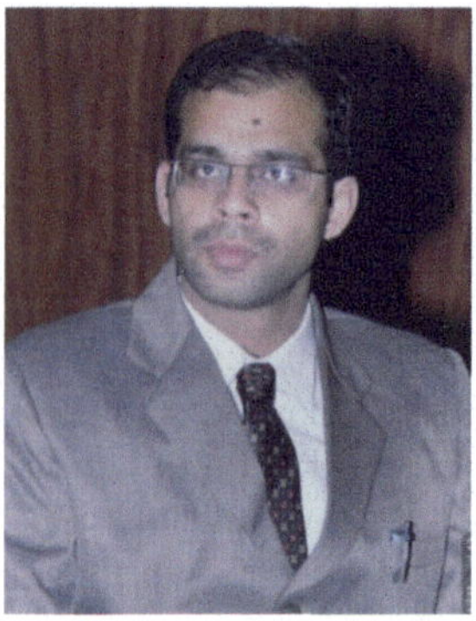

Anand Nayyar received his Ph.D. (Computer Science) from Desh Bhagat University in 2017 in the area of Wireless Sensor Networks. He is currently working in Graduate School, Duy Tan University, Da Nang, Viet Nam. He is a certified professional with more than 75 professional certificates from CISCO, Microsoft, Oracle, Google, Beingcert, EXIN, GAQM, Cyberoam, and many more. He has published more than 300 research papers in various national and international conferences and international journals (Scopus/SCI/SCIE/SSCI Indexed). He is a member of more than 50+ associations as Senior and Life Member and also acts as ACM Distinguished Speaker. He has authored/coauthored and edited 25 books in the field of computer science. He served for more than 400 international conferences as program committee/advisory board/review board member. He has Five Australian Patents to his credit in the domain of Wireless Communications, Artificial Intelligence and Image Processing. He is currently working in the area of Wireless Sensor Networks, MANETS, Swarm Intelligence, Cloud Computing, Internet of Things, Blockchain, Machine Learning, Deep Learning, Cyber Security, Network Simulation, and Wireless Communications. He was awarded 30+ awards for teaching and research—Young Scientist, Best Scientist, Young Researcher Award, Outstanding Researcher Award. He is the Editor-in-Chief of IGI-Global, USA Journal titled *International Journal of Smart Vehicles and Smart Transportation (IJSVST).*

Chapter 1
Dynamic Models and Control Techniques for Drone Delivery of Medications and Other Healthcare Items in COVID-19 Hotspots

Kriti Sharma, Harvinder Singh, Deepak Kumar Sharma, Adarsh Kumar, Anand Nayyar, and Rajalakshmi Krishnamurthi

Abstract Drone-based dynamic model and control techniques vary from classical linear proportional integral derivative (CPID) to complex nonlinear multiconstrained and multi-objective schemes such as backstepping, sliding window mode, size-based models, and operation-based models, among others. These approaches can be classified as per their usage. Thus, some will be efficient for indoor operations, and others will be useful for outdoor operations. The performance of both types of drone-based smart healthcare systems can be measured in terms of stabilizing the

K. Sharma
Department of Systemics, School of Computer Science, University of Petroleum and Energy Studies, Dehradun, Uttrakhand, India

Department of Computer Science Engineering and Information Technology, K R Manglam University, Gurgaon, Haryana, India
e-mail: kriti.s@krmangalam.edu.in

H. Singh
Department of Virtualization, School of Computer Science, University of Petroleum and Energy Studies, Dehradun, Uttrakhand, India
e-mail: hsingh@ddn.upes.ac.in

D. K. Sharma
Department of Informatics, School of Computer Science, University of Petroleum and Energy Studies, Dehradun, Uttrakhand, India
e-mail: dksharma@ddn.upes.ac.in

A. Kumar (✉)
Department of Systemics, School of Computer Science, University of Petroleum and Energy Studies, Dehradun, Uttrakhand, India
e-mail: adarsh.kumar@ddn.upes.ac.in

© The Author(s), under exclusive license to Springer Nature Switzerland AG 2021

F. Al-Turjman et al. (eds.), *Emerging Technologies for Battling Covid-19*,
Studies in Systems, Decision and Control 324,
https://doi.org/10.1007/978-3-030-60039-6_1

attitude for both indoor and outdoor operations as per requirements. Further, gain-based drone scheduling is commonly used in flight controllers. In COVID-19 pandemic situations, the gains can be measured using an alternative way. Here, different parameters like medication advantage to COVID-19 pandemic areas, identifying the COVID-19 hotspots, sanitizing requirements and potentials, finding the COVID-19 chain, etc., could be considered in gain measurement for the deployment of drone-based COVID-19's smart healthcare. This work proposes a multi-constraint and multi-objective gain-based simulation-optimization approach for scheduling the linear and nonlinear dynamic and controllable drone movement models. The proposed model considered the identity-based lower and upper limits of control interface. Further, this interface is having the provision to include some human factors in its execution. The performance of the overall system is measured using performance and security metrics. In performance, drone-based smart healthcare systems' efficiency, accuracy, and effectiveness are measured. The measurements are analyzed by varying optimization parameters. In the security, lightweight cryptography primitives and protocols are analyzed for performance measurements. These lightweight cryptography primitives and protocols ensure secure data storage, transmission, and processing at any device. Further, the scope of centralized and distributed systems of drone cooperations for COVID-19 monitoring, sanitization, cleaning, and control room will be explored to have time-saving and autonomous drone-based smart healthcare systems.

Keywords COVID-19 · Dynamic models · Industry 4.0 · Simulation · Healthcare 4.0 · Pandemic

1.1 Introduction

This section explains the drone-based systems, its features, and applications (specifically in the healthcare section). Details are given as follows.

A. Nayyar
Graduate School, Faculty of Information Technology, Duy Tan University, Da Nang, Vietnam
e-mail: anandnayyar@duytan.edu.vn

R. Krishnamurthi
Department of Computer Science and Engineering, Jaypee Institute of Information Technology, Noida, India
e-mail: k.rajalakshmi@ddn.upes.ac.in

1.1.1 *What Is Smart Healthcare System and COVID-19 Pandemics*

The latest technology like big data, IoT, data analytics, cloud computing, and many others has revolutionized the traditional healthcare system into a smart healthcare system. In a smart healthcare system, a patient's biological and psychological data (in form of signals) is collected, recorded, analyzed, stored (as a "history" for future consultation), and transmitted to doctors and healthcare units [1]. This enables continuous, prompt, and regular checkup of blood pressure, diabetes, and heart rate of patients. ICT is one of the components of a successful smart healthcare system as being connected to smart devices, there are regular and immediate follow-ups between patient and doctors. Features like self-monitoring and auto-reporting have encouraged players to foresee the APAC and EMEA sector to reach new heights of USD 251 billion by 2022 [2].

Reasons for such expanding popularity of smart healthcare system are as follows:

- Digitizing and central storage of patients' records, known as electronic health records (EHR), have reduced intermediate paper mess at patient's and hospital's end. No matter even if the patient forgets to give some health-related input to the medical practitioner, it will be visible at the time of examination because of EHR.
- Alarming abnormality about patient's condition to doctor or hospital treating him through telemedicine gives a sense of personal touch and care.
- In remote areas where medical facilities are not up to the mark, smart healthcare is boon to such a section of society by providing remote diagnosis and prescribing ad delivering medicines.
- Improvement in computational power concerning lesser time lag and accurate result with low power consumption and well connected to the Internet network.
- The patient can view their reports on supporting portable digital assistant in 2D or 3D result set.
- Wait time between patients and doctor's interaction is reduced to quite an extent.
- Quick response time of diagnosis and prescription increases adoption of this changing trend in the healthcare sector.
- Remote facilities related to health have shown a downfall in footfall of patients to hospitals and clinics.
- Hospitals with smart healthcare facilities may include radio-frequency identification technology (through sensors) responding to inventory or live location of medical equipment and resources [3].
- Follow-up between insurance policyholder and the insurance company will be transparent for patient's personal and medical data collection, health updates, risk analysis, claim processing, and fraud detection.

High-end technology in smart healthcare systems has shown an effective result in various ways:

- It reduces efforts and expenditures. For example, costs of health clinic visits can be reduced by wearing a portable medical equipment when patient is under observation of a doctor or any family member.
- Usually, it is normal practice that a patient visits a doctor after an abnormality has occurred (maybe unaware or careless); thus, smart healthcare helps to predict an epidemic by seeing sprouting symptoms at the initial stage.
- Immediate response action has improved and saved many lives by providing immediate first aid or similar assistance to patients.

The smart healthcare system is scalable, cost-effective, efficient, and hard real-time responsive, making it adoptable by an aging population, disabled individuals, population at remote sites, and people living alone. Although smart healthcare has all features to fit in society, on other side, few challenges as mentioned below exist:

- Electronic health records (EHRs) are centrally stored and thus very helpful for data sharing, while it is vulnerable to hacking at a point if security is compromised at any point.
- The IoT environment is a costly affair, and the camera needs funds in implementing and maintenance of sensors, monitors, and detectors.
- Technological drift from traditional work style often leads to a lack of coordination (communication gap and technology knowledge are few to mention) from either of the participating entity.
- High-speed data transformation from analog to digital signals for processing should not be compromised with data loss or inaccurate results. High precision needs to be maintained by analytics to generate instant results (most of the times).
- Sudden power cutoff may lead to incomplete and dangerous consequences to the patient.

Despite the abovementioned challenges, smart healthcare systems have explosively shown its capability to serve the society since late 2019. The World Health Organization (WHO) announced an infectious disease caused by acute respiratory syndrome virus (in Wuhan (China) in December 2019) called coronavirus disease 2019 or COVID-19 (survival span is 72 h) [4]. A person suffering fever, lethargy, dry cough with a runny nose, sore throat, and ache may be suspected to be infected with coronavirus. It is considered to be pandemic because of its spreading pattern in chain reaction format with no demographic boundary limits. The spread of coronavirus is vital as no vaccine against it is yet announced by any nation across the world [4]. Thus, the WHO has shared guidelines as preventive measures to be taken across the nations, like social awareness, sanitizing, enhancing emergency response mechanisms, contact tracing, treating the infected patient, and encouraging social distancing. The smart healthcare system has shown its superlative ability during the outbreak of pandemic ranging from recording human health status to sanitization, telemedicine, and diagnosis of the infected patient from the mass of the population.

1.1.2 Importance of Drone-Based Systems in Smart Healthcare System

Unmanned aerial vehicles (UAV) or drones are innovations of technology which are operated by a remotely located pilot (under guidelines framed by the Ministry of Civil Aviation) to fly in airspace. Drones are facilitators to the smart healthcare sector as they are not restricted by traffic, site connectivity, a span of the day, weather, and demographic boundaries. There was a shift from prolonged admission of aged people in hospitals to nursing care at home. In this model, nurses were assigned to take care of patients as and when they needed it. This may lead to many long hours in a day where nurses have nothing critical to attend regarding patients. This refers to a situation where a resource from the hospital (nurse) is occupied for extra time and also increases the cost of the patient's treatment. Also, in war sites and areas affected by flood and drought, where basic amenities for survival are not available, drones have proven quite helpful by delivering essential medical and food supplies. In such situations, due to its aerial view capability, global positioning system, and high transmission speed, drones are in huge demand to deliver vaccines, drugs, blood, and food packets and to collect samples for testing [5–7]. Drones are used from surveillance to first aid transmission as the need arises. In situations where delay in supply of lifesaving drugs, medical aid, or support is not acceptable and the area is inaccessible (because of natural disaster, remote areas, or poor access to road connectivity), drones have come to the rescue. The major loss was avoided by providing timely assistance of survey and relief measures to the site hit by Typhoon Haiyan in the Philippines [8]. The photogrammetry feature of drones has made detection of an increasing level of particular constituent possible (e.g., tumor detection in the human body) leading to timely treatment or taking precautionary measures [9, 10]. In Rwanda, blood and vaccines were delivered to its citizens via drones [11]. It is estimated that delivering drugs and samples and other support via drones are efficient and taking one-fourth of the time taken by road commuters [12]. Drones not only save lives by transmitting aids and lifesaving supplements like vaccines or blood but also reduce the chances of collision and thus save lives on the road. Vehicles carrying such assistance over road run at high speed and thus may be dangerous for the life of the driver or the people on road.

1.1.3 Indoor and Outdoor Drone-Based Systems for Medication and Monitoring in Smart Healthcare

UAVs were built to carry out those tasks and operations where humans had certain limitations like environmental challenges or to automate and make existing operations more efficient. UAV is a significant result of the Internet of Things that builds up an application for remote regulation and viewing using sensors and transceivers

[13]. As per application and usability, drones can be used in a closed environment (indoor drones) or under the open sky (outdoor). UAVs used outdoor are more common, and they serve several purposes like surveillance for defense organizations, rescue and emergency response operations, monitoring wildlife conservation, agriculture purposes, weather forecasting, and many more. In most of the use cases mentioned above, there are regulatory clearances that are required for a drone manufacturer and drone customer that they need to obtain from the concerned authorities before they can start using drones commercially. Such drones play a very critical role in the healthcare domain when they are used for delivering life care medications and supplies in battlefields or disaster-struck areas. Outdoor drones are usually bigger having higher payload capacities of up to 8–10 kg and higher flight time as they may need to fly several kilometers in remote areas for surveillance or relief measures. Outdoor drones need a Global Positioning System (GPS) for navigation and tracking purposes, and they are controlled by a control circuit box. Due to higher specifications and high-grade sensors being used, the overall cost of outdoor drones is higher as compared to that of indoor drones.

The applicability of a UAV is not limited to only outdoor applications, but it can also be used in indoor environments such as in the manufacturing and services industries. In situations where a bounded premise (hospitals, production, home, warehouse, and many others) needs to be under supervision, an indoor drone-based system is a good option. Such a UAV needs no clearance pass from aviation centers during a flight in most of the cases. The patients could get aid or medicines inside their homes without stepping out of their homes [7, 11]. This is very beneficial for bedridden patients or in a lockdown situation. Indoor drones can also be used for inspection of machines inside an industrial facility with predetermined flight paths avoiding collisions. As outdoor drones use GPS for navigation, indoor drones use indoor positioning system (IPS) or Bluetooth technology for safe navigation and to avoid collision [4, 5, 14–25]. Indoor drones are controlled by an intelligent flight control system (IFCS), and flight of indoor drone is marked safe by protecting propeller using guards and avoiding curtains in their path of flight. While using drone inside closed premises, a drone's flight path, orientation, and ground clearance level of flight should be well programmed over an integrated circuit. Although payload attached to such drones is not bulky but lighter commands like carrying laundry to the washing area, calling for a medicine from a room and others is a big help to the aged population or persons in need (like a person with plastered leg). Indoor drones are small in size, and the battery life is comparatively fit for local movement between points visible through the naked eyes over line of sight (LOS). In contrast to outdoor drones, indoor drones are agile, compact, and lightweight, and sensors like GPS (add-on to the cost of a drone) are not required which lowers down the cost.

1.1.4 *Research Challenges in Designing and Developing Drone-Based Smart Healthcare Systems*

All the applications and case studies discussed in this research and many other similar researches tell us that usability of drones in healthcare has effectively reduced response time and surpassed natural restrictions. Still while designing and creating a drone-based smart healthcare system, it is important to think holistically about the problem to be solved, the users—patients, medical professionals, record keepers, and drone manufacturers. Research challenges also include setting up parameters to evaluate the performance of the drones. The performance should be measured in terms of technical performance, usability, acceptance of the system by the user, and efficacy of the system. Overall acceptance for general everyday use even in healthcare is still very low. There are several challenges to overcome, and they are not just limited to technology but also regulatory aspects.

While transmitting health-related aid or services via an aerial channel through drones, a highly accurate navigation system is required. UAV should in hard real-time synchronization with ground control unit be operated by a pilot who is monitoring the movement of the drone to the target for the intended purpose by integrating ground controls with aerospace allocated for drone flights. As drones carry medicines or samples to-and-fro between target site to ground site, APM control board should be capable enough to hold payload during flight [15]. In usual case, if payload overshoots threshold of APM, it won't allow the drone to fly. After attending remote target site, the drones are pre-commanded to return to the base location. This concept of the drone is called a return to home (RTH) feature. Drones have home GPS location with exact longitude and latitude, and this helps RTH feature to be active and well addressed for safe and on-site landing. Communicating medium between the pilot and receiver (similar to IoT-enabled unit) should be error- and disturbance-free during signal transmission [16]. Any disturbance in signal transmission during the telemedicine process may result in fatal consequences. Thus, to counter such an unaffordable situation, highly efficient and dedicated air to ground channel is required to work against a blockage, elevation, and weather conditions also. In the healthcare system, using aerial technology like drones needs multiple participating technologies to synchronize on a common platform to achieve a common objective. Drone in healthcare uses multiple technology coordinates to accomplish accurate results by securing functionalities of sensors and networks along with data of patients [13]. Drones fly to unseen remote sites by path drawn by the pilot. A specific predesigned algorithm may not work all the time or in all situations. An algorithm to select optimal flight paths among all possible navigation paths is complicated and critical as it overall reflects the functionality of drone in rescue or assisting action. Drones are fully or partially automated with reflexes in case of an unexpected situation or conditions like low power mode or encountering an obstacle. Such sensitivity of drones increases designing complexity and needs highly sensitive sensors along with add-ons related to guarding dedicated components of drones under such conditions.

Details of people being attended by drones are recorded and used by medical authorities for treatment and cure in the form of electronic health records (EHRs). These EHRs need to be uniform at the patient's end and to the hospital/doctor in charge, and also data should transmit between intended end users. Data should not get compromised with its confidentiality or integrity aspect. Attackers will make every possible attempt of spoofing, traffic analysis, masquerading, phishing, or non-repudiation using IPsec to extract data from IoT-embedded devices (patient or payload) or the network. Healthcare services provide two-way authentication and added encryption of data which is time-consuming and disturbing phase for many non-technical users especially at the time of emergency. Multilevel authentication and encryption phase result in a time-consuming and disturbing phase at the time of emergency [4]. Firewall and intrusion detection and prevention system (IDPS) counter routing attack at the network layer of the OSI reference model. This enables us to keep a check on incoming or outgoing data, and in return authentication is maintained. A challenge was recorded as data authentication was disturbed by denial of service attack. Attackers fly self-governed own drones in shared airspace and send multiple signals to the targeted genuine drone. The targeted genuine drone mixes up with the original signal and loses real informative signals because of modified or overflooded incoming signals to the genuine drone in the communication network [5].

1.1.5 Organization of Work

This work is organized in a systematic manner where Sect. 1.1 introduces the smart healthcare system and its significance in the COVID-19 pandemic. It includes functionalities of smart healthcare like remote examination of patients and assistance by indoor and outdoor drones and challenges faced while designing and developing the systems. COVID-19 hotspots are discussed in Sect. 1.2, which further explains adopted preventive and alert methods along with its impact on social and economic sectors. Further, rules, regulations, policies, and procedures of COVID-19 monitoring and control rooms are discussed. In Sect. 1.3, a literature survey of recently developed drone-based systems (agriculture, mining sites, defense, and healthcare are few to mention), COVID-19 hotspots, and drone movement for monitoring and data analysis over such areas along with drone-based systems for smart healthcare systems in other pandemic situations is discussed. Drone-based frameworks for smart healthcare systems using Industry 4.0 trends in COVID-19 hotspots are discussed in Sect. 1.3. Section 1.4 deals with a real-time drone-based system for COVID-19 along with its benefits and limitations. Section 1.5 is about drone-based simulation done for COVID-19 hotspot tracking (monitoring, analysis, control room positioning). In Sect. 1.6, outdoor COVID-19 hotspot tracking, monitoring, analysis, and control room positioning are discussed. Conclusion and future scope of work constitute Sect. 1.7.

1.2 COVID-19 Hotpots

This section introduces COVID-19 hotspot, positions and statistics, prevention and alert methods, effects over social and economic sectors, and rules and regulations.

1.2.1 What Is COVID-19 Hotspot

On 11 March 2020, after spreading to more than 100 countries and report of thousands of cases within a few months, the World Health Organization declared the outbreak as "pandemic" resulting in a socioeconomic crisis of an unprecedented scale. Most of the nations focusing on identifying critical regions and strategies to avoid the spread of the virus. A hotspot is a region where a comparatively higher number of confirmed COVID-19 cases are reported [17]. The confirmed cases may not be from the same family, thereby increasing the chances of community transmission of the virus in such regions. To avoid spreading it further, governing bodies sealed off such regions to stop people from coming out of their home. These regions can vary in the geographical area from a small society of people to a city or a district in some countries.

1.2.2 Worldwide COVID-19 Hotspot Positions and Statistics

On 31 December 2019, the first case of pneumonia of unknown cause was detected in Wuhan City, China [18]. From the data provided by the World Health Organization [19], Fig. 1.1 shows a timeline of how rapidly it spread to the majority of the countries worldwide starting from the first case reported outside of China in Thailand (8 January 2020) followed by Japan (14 January 2020) and the Republic of Korea (19 January 2020). On 20 January 2020, the USA reported its first case and was the

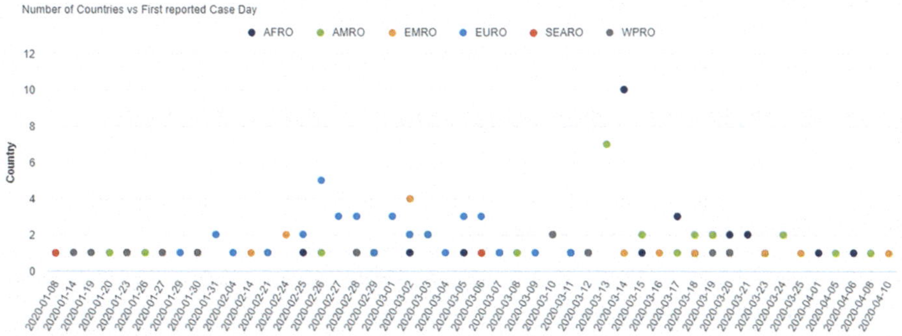

Fig. 1.1 Number of countries and first reported COVID-19 case day

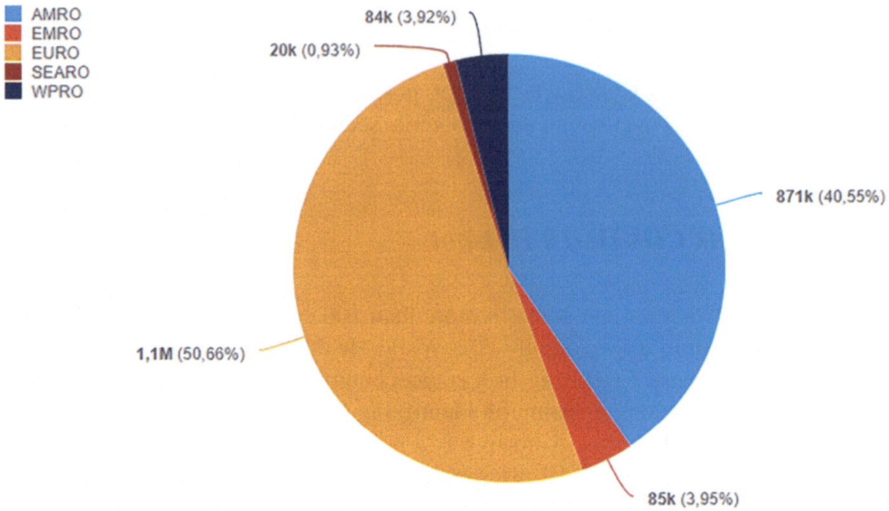

Fig. 1.2 Region-wise confirmed cases distribution as of 22 April 2020

most affected country with more than 38,000 deaths as of 22 April 2020 [20]. On 10 April 2020, the latest country to report COVID-19 case was Yemen.

Figure 1.1 shows timeline of several countries reporting their first confirmed case from six regions divided by the World Health Organization: Africa (AFRO), America (AMRO), Eastern Mediterranean (EMRO), Europe (EURO), Southeast Asia (SEARO), and Western Pacific (WPRO) [21].

As of 22 April 2020, the totally confirmed cases of COVID-19 are 2,471,136, and 169,006 deaths have been reported by the WHO [19, 20]. As shown in Fig. 1.2, the European region and the region of America are the most affected regions with more than 90% of the worldwide cases. To understand the worldwide position, Fig. 1.3 shows the number of COVID-19 confirmed cases in the top 20 affected countries. Figure 1.4 shows several deaths due to COVID-19 in the top 20 affected countries.

1.2.3 COVID-19 Pandemic Prevention and Alert Methods

To reduce the spread of the virus, the following preventive measures are suggested by the WHO and other concerned agencies:

- Clean your hands with alcohol-based hand sanitizer or wash it regularly with soap and water to kill viruses.
- Avoid touching the face as the virus can enter your body through the nose, mouth, and eyes.

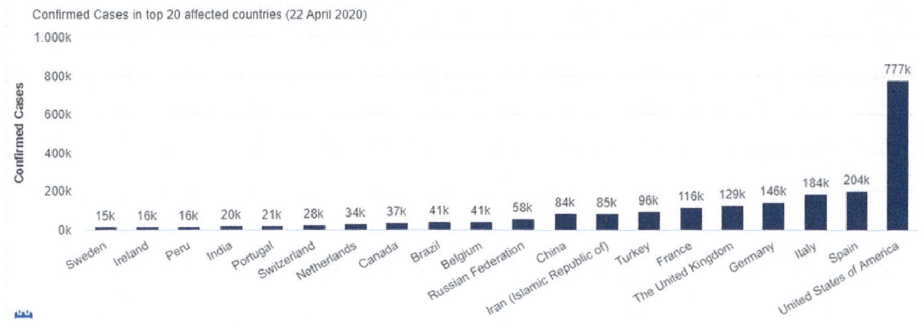

Fig. 1.3 COVID-19 confirmed cases in the top 20 affected countries till 22 April 2020

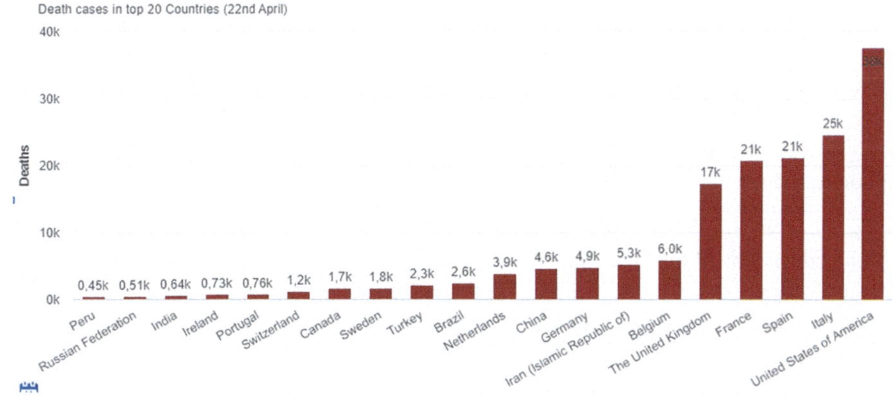

Fig. 1.4 Number of deaths in the top 20 affected countries as of 22 April 2020

- Maintain good respiratory hygiene. Use tissue paper or bent elbow to cover your mouth and nose and then dispose of used tissue immediately. Droplet is one of the carriers of the virus, and this will ensure fewer droplets in the environment.
- If you are feeling unwell, then you need to stay at home. If symptoms are cough, fever, and breathing issues, then immediately consult the doctor. This will ensure timely treatment.
- Maintain a minimum of 3 ft. distance between yourself and another person. Avoid handshakes or other physical contacts.
- Keep yourself up to date with the latest hotspots and avoid traveling to such hotspots.

In case of any pandemic situation like COVID-19, the government must alert the following:

- Airports for screening passengers who have travel history from affected areas.
- Educational institutes need to follow preventive measures.

- Health organizations to keep the preparation for handing the patients. Health organizations should give proper training to all health workers to deal with the situation.
- Law enforcement agencies for strict implementation of lockdown.
- All essential service providers.

1.2.4 COVID-19 Pandemic Effects in Social and Economic Sectors

The COVID-19 pandemic has already affected the lives of many people by restricting their movements. On 18 March 2020, the WHO issued a report to address mental health and psychosocial issues of the general public, healthcare workers, team leaders or managers in health facilities, guardians of children, old people, and people with underlying health conditions [24]. Many people are now hesitating to keep their pets as they may pass on the coronavirus to them [25]. Millions of people may lose jobs worldwide, thereby increasing unemployment and poverty. The effect of a pandemic situation can be seen in these sectors:

- *Education sector*: Most of the educational institutes worldwide are temporarily closed to control the spread of the virus. According to data released by UNESCO on 18 Apr 2020, 91.3% (1,575,270,054) of the total enrolled learners from 191 nations are affected [14]. Children from poor sections may drop out of school permanently [15].
- *Religious sector*: Temples, churches, mosques, and other religious places have started offering services online for the devotees [16].
- *Sports sector*: The majority of international sports events are either called off or rescheduled [26].
- *Entertainment industry*: Most of the media events are now canceled or delayed [27]. The demand of online digital media platforms like Netflix, Amazon Prime, etc., has increased.
- *Aviation industry*: Due to the cancellation of flights, few airlines have sent their employees on leave without salary on a rotational basis [24].
- *Tourism industry*: Countries with high earnings from tourism are greatly affected. Hotels and restaurants are closed temporarily.
- *Transportation sector*: All local transportations are closed or have restricted access.
- *Science and technology sector*: Various organizations have asked their employees to work from home. Leading space agencies like NASA have halted their space and technology projects.

Worldwide border seal has affected international trade of various goods and commodities. Various industries have stopped their production. Financial markets have collapsed. Manufacturing industries are seeing a large drop in the demand.

1.2.5 Rules, Regulations, Policies, and Procedures for COVID-19 Monitoring and Control Room

To deal with the pandemic situation, strong measures are required for effective containment of COVID-19. The worldwide focus has been to upgrade health infrastructure by providing COVID-19-dedicated hospitals and other medical equipment. The public is advised to follow social distancing, and, in some places, the government has forced complete lockdown to reduce further spread of COVID-19.

On 25 March 2020, the WHO has released guidelines: "operational guidance for maintaining essential health services during an outbreak" [28]. The report focuses on building coordination mechanisms to help response teams, determining essential services and optimization of delivery platforms, setting up the efficient flow of patients, managing health workers, and identifying mechanisms to keep track of essential medications, equipment, and supplies.

Some of the important containment policies and procedures are as follows [17, 22]:

- Social distancing while interacting in public places.
- Quarantine people if found any contact history or travel record from the affected area.
- Active surveillance in all possible hotspot zones.
- Testing maximum possible suspected cases.
- Isolation of all COVID-19-positive cases and providing suitable medical care.
- Mass awareness of preventive public health measures through all possible channels.
- In the hotspot regions special teams to be formed to search for new cases and do contact tracing.
- Expanding laboratory capacity for testing a higher number of cases.
- The government should review the existing legal instruments that provide legal support to implement the containment plan.

For information management, the control room has to be set up at state and district levels. A control room for the team at hotspot zones can also be set up depending on the number of cases. Data managers at the state level will compile data from various districts and update the total number of suspects, confirmed, critical, deaths, and contacts under surveillance with a centralized control room [22].

1.3 Literature Survey

This section presents the literature survey over drone-based systems in various applications. Further, drone-based usage in COVID-19 pandemic, hotspot identification, monitoring, sanitization, etc., are explored. The details are presented as follows.

1.3.1 Literature over Recently Developed Drone-Based Systems

In recent past years, drone technology has been used by government organizations, defense organizations, and private companies for both humanitarian causes and commercial purposes. The technology and types of drones have also evolved, and still a lot of research is being done to improve the performance and save time and costs by using drones in the areas where humans or other machines either take more time or cannot reach easily. Table 1.1 shows the areas where drone manufacturers are harnessing the technology for both social and commercial purposes.

Drones in Healthcare Conventional healthcare ecosystem requires a lot of human intervention starting from examining the patients to the distributing and transporting of medical supplies. Timely delivery of medicines, blood, and other supplies is very important in healthcare. The location of distribution can be difficult to access via vehicles due to poor infrastructure, remote areas, accidents, or traffic congestion. In metro cities, traffic can cause huge problems in delivery at peak hours. Since a drone can fly over the roads and inaccessible routes or areas, the healthcare organizations have started using drones to provide healthcare facilities.

Delivery of Medical Supplies, Blood, Lifesaving Equipment, and Sample Transportation Drones have been used in many social and humanitarian causes to deliver emergency aid medical supplies and other aid packages in different countries during natural disasters. Drones are also helping elderly people who need regular checkups and medical facilities, but due to the lack of transportation, they miss appointments as they might be living in rural areas or areas which are not easily accessible. In such situations, drone-based systems help deliver routine test kits and refills of medicines and pick up test reports from the home location of elderly people, thereby reducing the workload of medical teams (doctors and nurses) and reducing travel time for the patients. An interesting application of drones can be in the delivery of AEDs (automated external defibrillators). In case of heart attacks, the survival rate is low, and the patient needs to be given a shock with a defibrillator within minutes of the attack. Survival chance reduces as the time expires to use a defibrillator (74% chances of survival in the first 3 min and 50% after 5 min). Conventionally, AEDs are carried via ambulance, and in a study done in Stockholm, it takes around 13 min on average for an ambulance to reach a patient. If drones are to be used, then AEDs might reach faster than ambulance (>80% of the times) in seven out of ten places researched [45, 46].

Tracking and Monitoring Adversely Affected Areas Drones have proved very useful in tracking, monitoring, and gathering data from areas that get affected by a natural disaster or by a pandemic (a recent example being COVID-19). When there is a natural calamity or a pandemic situation, the affected areas could become inaccessible using UAVs that can be remotely controlled and can fly over such areas hit by disasters like the earthquake in Haiti (2010), Hurricane Sandy (the USA, Canada, and the Caribbean, 2012), Typhoon Haiyan in the Philippines (2013), and the

Table 1.1 Application of drone in various areas

Area	Usage	Consumer(s)	Manufacturer(s)	Type of UAV
Defense	Surveillance	US Marines [26], British Army [27], Australian Army [24], the Netherland's Army [25], Indian National Security Guard [29]	Prox Dynamics (acquired by FLIR Systems)	Micro (The Black Hornet Nano)
Rescue and emergency response	Affected areas and victim identification	Fire Department of Los Angeles [30], European Emergency Number Association (EENA) [31]	DJI, USA	Hybrid (Matrice 200 series, Matrice 600 series, Phantom 4 Pro)
Wildlife conservation	Track animals and mammals and collect samples	The Ocean Alliance [32]	DJI, USA	Hybrid
Healthcare	Delivery of medical supplies, collection of samples and reports	Government of Rwanda [33], Government of Malawi [34]	Zipline, USA Matternet, USA	Small and large drones
Agriculture	Analytics, seed planting, plant health monitoring [35]	Deveron UAS Corp [36], state governments, the USA [37]	Raptor Maps, USA DroneSeed, USA	Large drones (up to 57 kg payload)
Weather forecasting	Data collection, imagery	Australian Government [38]	Saildrone	Drone: 7 m in length and 4 m in height
Mining	3D mine mapping, site planning	Mining companies in the USA, Israel, Australia [39]	Airobotics, USA Terra Drone, Japan	Multi-rotor drones
Infrastructure and construction	Site survey, goods transportation, aerial photography	Microsoft [40]	Skycatch, USA	Unknown
Retail and logistics	Last mile delivery, Warehouse operations	Amazon [41]	Amazon, USA	Hybrid (fly range 15 miles, payload up to 5 lb)
Sports	Live broadcasting, video recording	Fox Sports [42], ESPN		
Entertainment	Cinematography, aerial live shows	Hollywood, Universal Studios [43]		
Telecommunication	Radio tower inspection	AT&T, Verizon [44]	Skyward, USA	

earthquake in Nepal (2015) [47]. During the recent COVID-19 pandemic situation, different countries have used drones to track people's movements so that they maintain social distancing, to monitor the health and record temperatures from a distance in highly populated and remote areas, and also to carry samples and test reports between healthcare centers and affected areas [48, 49].

Medical Evacuation The unique design and ability of a UAV to fly in inaccessible terrain have been used to locate and rescue a lot of victims. In a recent case of a mishap during rappelling, it was reported how a person was located using a UAV [50]. Another study conducted by researchers in Turkey highlights the usage of drones in searching for injured or missing skiers on mountain slopes [51]. Table 1.2 shows the other applications of drones in the healthcare system.

1.3.2 Literature over COVID-19 Hotpots

Coronavirus (CoV) is a single-stranded RNA virus that affects the respiratory and intestinal system of human beings and animals. Out of seven human coronaviruses (HCoVs) having varying degrees of impact over respiration pattern, severe acute respiratory syndrome CoV (SARS-CoV), Middle East respiratory syndrome CoV (MERS-CoV), and SARS-CoV-2 (COVID-19) result in more deaths as compared to the other four. High transmission rate makes COVID-19 as highly contagious which has resulted in 1,133,758 reported cases globally, out of which 3374 confirmed cases are in India, while the count of death is 62,784 (globally) and 77 (India) according to the report generated on 5 April 2020 by the World Health Organization [57]. During the initial phase of COVD-19 when it started spreading from China, people with cough and cold were asked to quarantine themselves or were quarantined forcefully. As it started spreading to other countries like Thailand, South Korea, Vietnam, Italy, Iran, and the USA, the travel history of people was being checked, and anyone who traveled to these countries in the last 14 days was also examined for the symptoms. As symptoms are visible after a time gap of 10–14 days, unknowingly patients or carriers infected numerous other people by providing hosts to the novel virus. It led to a chain reaction, and the virus grew exponentially, creating some areas in a particular city where more people got affected in a very short period. Areas where a relatively higher number of positive COVID-19 cases are reported come under the category of "hotspot." In Delhi and Uttar Pradesh, areas with more than six positive confirmed cases (irrespective of the area of the site) were declared as hotspots or "Red Zones" [58].

In areas where transmission happened rapidly and virus carriers were difficult to control, extra precautionary measures were taken to monitor the movement of people, and quarantine zones were created where no entry or exit was allowed. As the virus spread to most of the countries, on 11 March 2020, the WHO declared it a pandemic. By that time many countries have enforced nationwide lockdown already, and the concept of social distancing was being promoted aggressively in the media

Table 1.2 Application of drone in the healthcare system

Year	Country	Manufacturer	Type of UAV	Applications/purpose	Supporter(s)
2007	South Africa	Custom-built (e-Juba or electronic pigeon project)	Hybrid	Facilitate transportation of microbiological test samples up to 500 g of payload [52]	NHLS and Denel Dynamics (UAV Division)
2014	Bhutan	Matternet, USA	Hybrid (fixed wing and quadcopter)	Delivering medical supplies via drones to remote hospitals [53]	The WHO and Bhutan's Ministry of Health
2016	Ghana	Unknown	Unknown	Delivering contraceptives and other medical supplies to remote villages; delivery times reduced from 2 days to 30 min at a reasonable price of $15/flight [54]	The United Nations Population Fund and the Dutch government
2017	Malawi	Matternet, USA	Hybrid (fixed wing and quadcopter)	Collection of medical samples (TB and HIV diagnosis) and delivery of medication [55]	Government of Malawi and UNICEF
2018	Tanzania	Wingcopter, Germany	Hybrid (fixed wing and quadcopter)	Delivery of medicines to a remote island in Lake Victoria; reduced delivery time from 6 h (road/ferry) to 40 min [56]	DHL and Deutsche GIZ
2016–2018	Madagascar	Technology Delta Quad	Hybrid (fixed wing and quadcopter)	Sputum and medication transport for diagnosis and treatment of tuberculosis [55]	Government of Madagascar
2017	Senegal	Vayu	Hybrid (fixed wing and quadcopter)	Delivering urgent medicines and collection of samples [55]	BMGF, Senegal Government

to spread awareness. India announced its first nationwide lockdown on 24 March 2020, of 21 days, and issued the guidelines for the citizens and different organizations to be followed. COVID-19 tests started to happen, and a list of hotspots was released which used to be updated every day as more and more tests were conducted all over the country. No movement is allowed in hotspots, and people cannot step out of their homes even for groceries or medicines. The government ensures door-step deliveries of limited essential items including groceries and medicines. Strict monitoring is done by the police force inside and on the perimeter of all hotspots. Testing of the population inside hotspots is intensified, and state governments start "pool testing." It is carried out by collecting several samples in a tube and testing them together for COVID-19. If the result is negative, then all people are considered unaffected, and if the result is positive, then every person is tested individually [59]. Government agencies took measures to spread awareness among people about social distancing and surveillance and requested citizens to help medical professionals in carrying out tests. Regular preventive health measures like sanitization of societies, regular checkups, and surveying to gather information on recent travel history (even house-to-house survey) were taken by healthcare organizations in COVID-19 hotspot zones. Social media and technology played a significant role to help people as in many societies under quarantine, people started using WhatsApp (social networking application) and Google sheets to create and share grocery and medicine needs. The lists were accessed by shop owners, and then required items were ultimately delivered to the doorsteps. Table 1.3 shows the list of COVID-19 hotspots.

1.3.3 Literature over Drone-Based Movement Tracing, Monitoring, and Data Analysis for COVID-19 Hotspots

UAV/Drones for Commercial Purposes Near the Mediterranean Sea, it is always more difficult to maintain a golf course. For such kind of difficult terrains, drone technology is used for the maintenance of the golf course. The data collected from the drones gives a lot of agronomical information to increase productivity. A UAV is a device used by the greenkeeper of the golf course for making decisions regarding the maintenance of the golf course. Drones can help with early detection of turf deterioration and illustration of irrigation throw and uniformity. It can help in analyzing turf textures, diseases, and weeds. It can be used for optimal golf course irrigation design. It can help optimize irrigation scheduling to prevent water wastage. Drones can easily detect poor irrigation coverage and uneven turf growth. Their multi-spectral cameras identify a specific compound as nitrates found in fertilizer or type of grass. UAV/drone surveying and mapping operations help in preparing 3D modeling for golf resort development and reconstruction. Drones can create GIS-based tree management plans and generate 3D models showing investors what the resort will look like [35].

UAV/Drones for Military Purposes The US Army's future frontline fighters may have an interesting new use for their grenade launchers. The idea is to shoot tiny camera drones into the sky which can then survey the vicinity for enemy threats. Army Research Lab scientists are developing micro-drones the same size as the Army's 40 mm grenade, which are meant to be fired by the service's standard M203 grenade launchers. They have dubbed the new drones Grenade Launched Unmanned Aerial Systems, or GLUAS. This is probably a one-of-a-kind experiment anywhere in the world and holds a lot of promise. Infantrymen often find themselves in a situation where they can see the enemy from their location as they may be behind a natural or man-made barrier. In this situation, it is very useful if they can in some

Table 1.3 List of COVID-19 hotspots [60]

State	District/city
Andhra Pradesh	Kurnool, Guntur, Nellore, Prakasam, Krishna, YSR, West Godavari, Chittoor, Visakhapatnam, East Godavari, Anantapur
Bihar	Gaya, Begusarai, Munger, Siwan
Chandigarh	Chandigarh
Delhi	North West Delhi, South Delhi, Shahdara, South East Delhi, West Delhi, North Delhi, Central Delhi, East Delhi, New Delhi, South West Delhi
Gujarat	Patan, Ahmedabad, Vadodara, Surat, Bhavnagar, Rajkot
Haryana	Ambala, Karnal, Nuh, Gurgaon, Faridabad, Palwal
Jammu and Kashmir	Shopian, Rajouri, Srinagar, Bandipora, Baramulla, Jammu, Udhampur, Kupwara
Karnataka	Dakshina Kannada, Bidar, Kalaburagi, Bagalkot, Dharwad, Bengaluru Urban, Mysuru, Belagavi
Kerala	Wayanad, Kasaragod, Kannur, Ernakulam, Malappuram, Thiruvananthapuram, Pathanamthitta
Madhya Pradesh	Morena, Indore, Bhopal, Khargone, Ujjain, Hoshangabad
Maharashtra	Kolhapur, Amravati, Palghar, Mumbai, Pune, Thane, Nagpur, Sangli, Ahmednagar, Yavatmal, Aurangabad, Buldhana, Mumbai Suburban, Nashik
Odisha	Bhadrak, Khordha
Punjab	Amritsar, Mansa, Ludhiana, Moga, SAS Nagar, SBS Nagar, Jalandhar, Pathankot
Rajasthan	Udaipur, Jaipur, Tonk, Jodhpur, Banswara, Kota, Jhunjhunu, Bhilwara, Jaisalmer, Bikaner, Jhalawar, Bharatpur
Tamil Nadu	Chennai, Tiruchirappalli, Coimbatore, Erode, Tirunelveli, Dindigul, Villuppuram, Namakkal, Theni, Chengalpattu, Tiruppur, Vellore, Madurai, Tuticorin, Karur, Virudhunagar, Kanyakumari, Cuddalore, Tiruvallur, Tiruvarur, Salem, Nagapattinam
Telangana	Nalgonda, Hyderabad, Nizamabad, Warangal Urban, Ranga Reddy, Jogulamba Gadwal, Medchal-Malkajgiri, Karimnagar, Nirmal
Uttarakhand	Nainital, Udham Singh Nagar, Dehradun
West Bengal	Kolkata, Howrah, Purba Medinipur, North 24 Paraganas
Andaman and Nicobar	South Andaman
Assam	Golaghat, Morigaon, Nalbari, Goalpara, Dhubri
Himachal Pradesh	Solan, Una, Sirmaur, Chamba, Kangra
Jharkhand	Ranchi, Bokaro

way get an eye on the enemy and able to observe their movements remotely. Soldiers under attack from an unseen enemy could fire the GLAUS and almost instantly receive a "bird's eye view" of the battlefield. GLAUS thus provides an autonomy and intelligence platform to help soldiers perform useful missions while having a lookout from hundreds of feet in the air. Since the drones are similar in size, weight, and shape to the US Army's standard grenades, they would most likely fit into the standard kit combat soldiers carry. Once launched, the drones spread their wings, and their motor takes over allowing soldiers to control them using a joystick or other handheld device. The camera sends live video feedback to the soldiers on the ground and adds GPS receivers to the drones, allowing soldiers to identify the exact location of objects or persons observed from the air. Information is key in the modern battlefield. Ability to quickly perform a recon and analyze the situation can be the difference between life and death [61].

UAV/Drones for Animal Tracking Animal tracking and sensor technology programs for beef sustainability are related to animal health welfare. GPS collars were typically designed with wildlife in mind, and so they put in sensors such as mortality sensors that would notify the researcher when the animal was dead, or they would incorporate a very high-frequency transmitter that tracks and recovers the animal even if the GPS unit failed. There are a couple of sensors that would be common to both wildlife and domestic livestock; they have temperature sensors built in and have activity sensors that will help in monitoring the behavior of the species. Additionally, drones equipped with high-resolution cameras are used for tracking and monitoring every activity of the animal under surveillance.

UAV/Drones for Personal/Community Surveillance Nowadays drones are used in various applications. The challenge is how they can be used, where they can be used, and for what purposes. They were used extensively in application areas like assessing damage in a flood or in an insurance-related loss [62]. Surveillance refers to the sneaking in the personal life of an individual for getting private information about him without being caught [17]. New laws are coming down from the authorities that require people flying drones for commercial use to have license [34]. So if you are going to use a drone to conduct an investigation or surveillance, you have to follow the legal parameters of the law, and the evidence and information that you obtain will be admissible and usable.

1.3.4 Literature over Drone-Based System for Smart Healthcare Systems and Other Pandemic Situations

In recent times, researchers and scientists are doing their best in the containment of the spread of the COVID-19 virus. A surgeon and his team have developed a drone to use for organ transplant transportation for the patients affected by the COVID-19 virus. Apart from this, it is amazing seeing something as useful as a drone being used for so many different applications. Scientists and researchers are building big-enough drones where they can be attached to fire-retardant stuff. The drones can fly up in the air and shoot the flame with the retardant stuff through the window of a burning 20-story building [15]. Amazon is going to start delivering stuff to customers via drones [30].

For detecting the symptoms of COVID-19 in a patient, nowadays, research scientists have outfitted the drones with coolers and biosensors that can monitor the health of the organ of a probable patient throughout its whole aerial journey. On the drone, a human organ-monitoring apparatus travelling for long distance measures all the biophysical properties like temperature, pressure, vibration, and altitude of the organ of an individual. Further, an android application is developed where a health worker can watch it and suggest preventive and precautionary measures to be taken in this regard [20].

When the number of COVID-19 patients is increasing exponentially, a fast and reliable organ transportation system is required. The drones can be used as a transportation device for short-distance travel like within a city, i.e., between two hospitals that are close to one another [5]. Drones are helping in the organ transportation between hospitals with a huge reduction in transportation time without having to deal with issues of security of the driver and vehicle, traffic on the roads, and police escorts requirements. Before the usage of drones for organ transportation, the organs are transported from hospital to hospital in transportation vans. So whatever type of traffic, the carriers are supposed to get on the road, and they can be stuck in that just like anybody else.

Nowadays, for transportation of organ using a drone, what hospital authorities have to do is just pop this organ onto a drone, send it into the air, and have it fly across the sky to its destination at another hospital. There would be a significant reduction in travel time. As soon as an organ leaves its donor body, that organ is made to reach the recipient's body. This increases the success rate of the surgeries in the hospitals which is significantly reducing the COVID-19 mortality rates. Drones are started to be considered as the most favorable aerial technology for transportation in the healthcare system.

1.4 Case Study 1: Drone-Based Real-Time System for COVID-19 Hotspots

This section explains the real-time drone system designed and used for the COVID-19 system. The details are presented as follows.

1.4.1 Real-Time Drone-Based System Description, Work, and Results in India

A drone is used in real life and has many applications like environmental study, commercial purposes, military services, and a whole gamut of other areas. There have been many technological advancements in developing UAVs to increase usage and adoption in different areas. Under a situation where the whole world is fighting a pandemic caused by a novel virus disease, COVID-19, the World Health Organization has proposed guidelines to be followed as precautionary measures like regular sanitization of hands, usage of face masks, and maintaining social distancing. The WHO is closely working with countries and their respective health organizations to conduct checkups and do tests of people in a phased manner. Since this virus spreads from human contact, the tests have to be conducted in a very controlled and regulated environment. Drones are proving to be of great help under these conditions to keep a regulatory check over health status, assistance to maintain social hygiene, and to spread awareness about government policies and social distancing. Developed countries like China, the USA, Italy, France, Australia, and few others where a large number of cities are under surveillance round the clock to restrict the transmission of the virus in every possible manner are already using drone technology. India has also developed an indigenous drone called Thermal Corona Combat Drone (TCCD), a project developed by the Indian Robotics Solution (IRS), India. IRS used an in-house designed PCB coded for thermal imaging, geothermal sensing, GPS tracking, photo and videography, and compaction.

The team from the Indian Robotics Solution has come up with an all-in-one multirotor drone to fight against COVID-19 spread. This thermal drone includes 6 propellers that help to take off vertically and fly at a height of 20 m using 1 set of lithium polymer batteries (200 cycles) as a source of power. The frame of TCCD is made up of a carbon fiber sheet and tube. TCCD is remotely operated, and it works at frequencies of 2.4 and 5.8 GHz. It supports three flight modes – autonomous mode using waypoint, manual mode, and hovering. High-definition cameras with optical zoom features provide clear images and features of video recording during the day and night span. TCCD is also equipped with an RGB camera with a spotlight feature for night vision. A three-axis gimbal has also been used for camera movement. Some of the tools used to develop this done are computer numerical control (CNC), waterjet, 3D printer, metal molder, and some other R&D software tools. Different machinery is used for sanitization. It has a built-in brushless pump having four nozzles and a sanitizer tank of 10 L (maximum payload capacity) that consists of a sanitizing solution which is sprayed in the form of droplets over the supervised area.

TCCD is helping medical officers by conducting surveillance in different areas. Surveillance is conducted to record the temperature of the people of those areas after getting approval from the concerned government agencies. People are requested to come to open areas (like rooftops or balconies) of their homes where the drone can conduct the scanning. Thermal scanning and thermal imaging techniques have been used to record human body temperature using two cameras as a part of the payload of the drone. An alarm attached to a drone beeps when the body temperature of an individual is found (using a spotlight feature of the attached camera) to be greater than normal body temperature (37 °C). If the alarm beeps, then either that individual is asked to come out of its premises or an official from the medical team goes inside the home for further checkups. Clusters of 60 satellites help in the global positioning of a person, and thus the exact location can be traced. Thermal image sensors enable a live view of an area over connected digital assistants like mobile phones, iPad, tablets, or others. Another feature of TCCD is it helps in carrying and delivering medical aid supplies to a location. It can cover an area of up to 1.5 km if the flight path is unidirectional, while for a flight path where the line of motion changes often, then it covers an area of 200 m^2 (on an average) within 30–45 min (only thermal imaging is used) and 10–12 min (if both thermal imaging and sanitization are used). TCCD successfully surveyed 15 densely populated areas in Delhi with a population strength of 10 lakhs. Figures 1.5 and 1.6 show pictures of TCCD and thermal imaging scanned results of the surveyed areas.

1.4.2 Real-Time Drone-Based System Advantages and Disadvantages

Drone technology is improving continuously as it is being explored day-by-day to greater depths. Humans are trying to overcome the limitations and improve existing processes or system efficiencies using drones. Some of the benefits of using a real-time drone-based system are as follows:

- Provides access to inaccessible areas like poor infrastructure, remote locations, natural calamities near hilly areas, or areas near huge water bodies.
- Faster response time as compared to conventional methods—Drones can reach faster than ambulances in a short period especially when an ambulance is not present nearby or there is an accident on the road or traffic congestion.
- Provides access to areas where human surveillance is not possible—Conducting the medical examination in containment zones during COVID-19 or areas where dangerous gas leakage may occur.
- Provides feasibility to track and monitor small areas—For public safety and security, the government needs to have an aerial view and real-time live recording of some areas of the city.
- Works under adverse environmental conditions—Serves continuously for long hours until the power supply lasts without any limitations of rain, humidity, or temperature variations.
- Highly accurate and precise—In agriculture, planting seeds with a uniform distribution in the field or spraying pesticides has been made possible as drones are pre-programmed to maintain a high degree of accuracy and precision.
- Real-time reporting and responsiveness helps in quick data processing.

Despite having so many benefits, drone-based systems also face challenges and have some disadvantages and concerns that need to be addressed for further advancements. Here are some of the disadvantages of a real-time drone-based system:

- Privacy concerns—People have expressed concerns over the usage and surveillance conducted, and the collected data is used for inappropriate purposes.

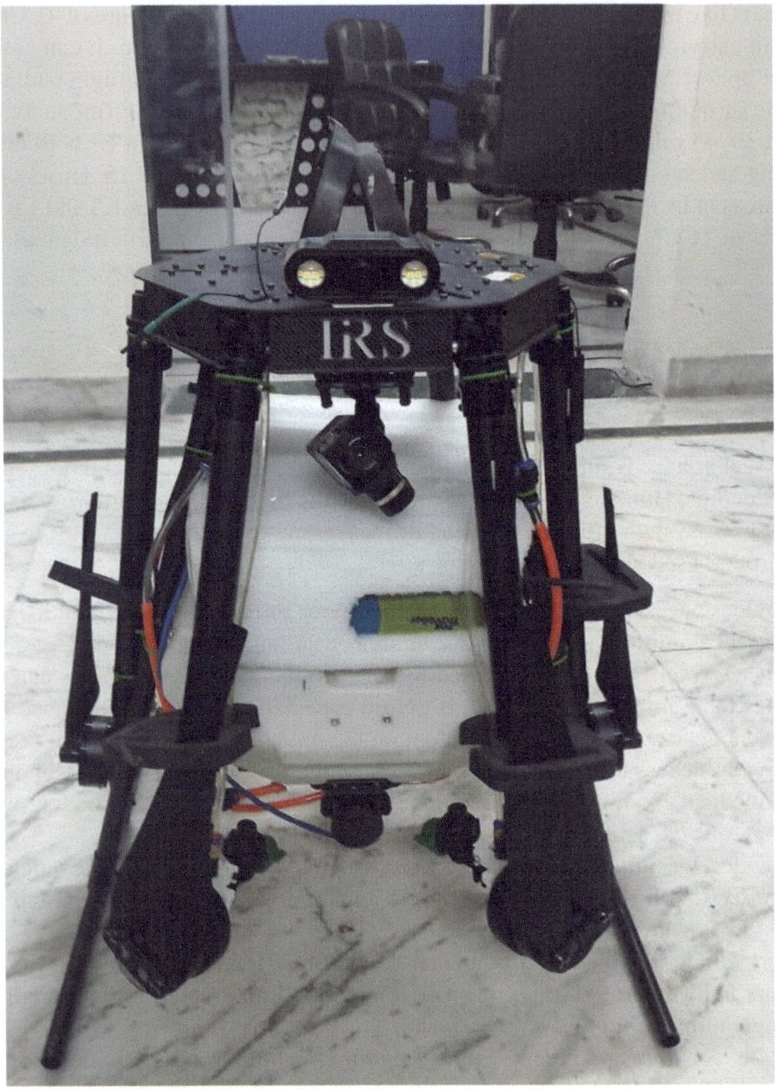

Fig. 1.5 Combat COVID-19 drone (in design)

- Not so cost-efficient—Developing and deploying drone-based systems is still a costlier affair as compared to other conventional methods (although they may be less effective).
- Regulatory issues—Flight clearance license from authorized agencies need to be issued before each flight, and this often feels like overhead in case of emergency.
- Suboptimal performance when fully automated—Optimal path finding for fully automated pilot drone need high precision and artificial intelligence as obstacles may change anytime during the flight in real time.

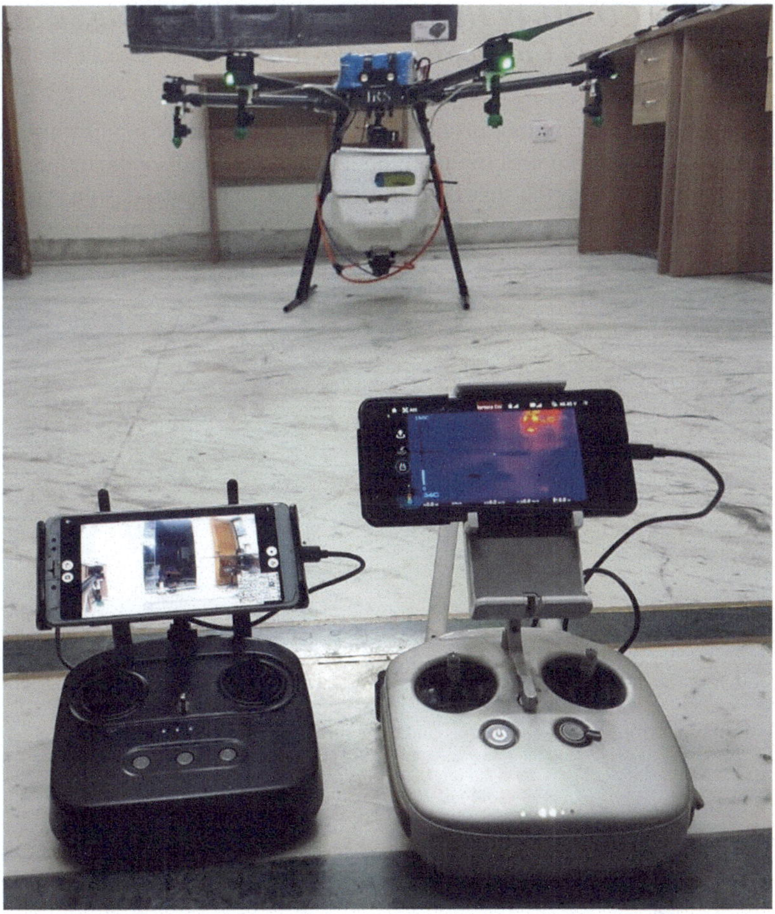

Fig. 1.6 Complete Combat COVID-19 design by the Indian Robotics Solution

1.5 Case Study 2: Drone-Based Simulation for COVID-19 Hotspot Tracking, Monitoring, Analysis, and Control Room Positioning

This section explains the indoor and outdoor drone-based activities. In this work, these activities include COVID-19 hotspot tracking, monitoring, analysis, and statistics for the control room. Both indoor and outdoor operations are explained as follows.

1.5.1 *Indoor COVID-19 Hotspot Tracking, Monitoring, Analysis, and Control Room Positioning*

This section explains the indoor drone-based hotspot detection, monitoring, analysis, and statistics for the control room. To understand and analyze the indoor drone-based system activities for the smart healthcare system, a hospital design is prepared as shown in Fig. 1.7. Figure 1.8 shows the 2D views of the proposed design and

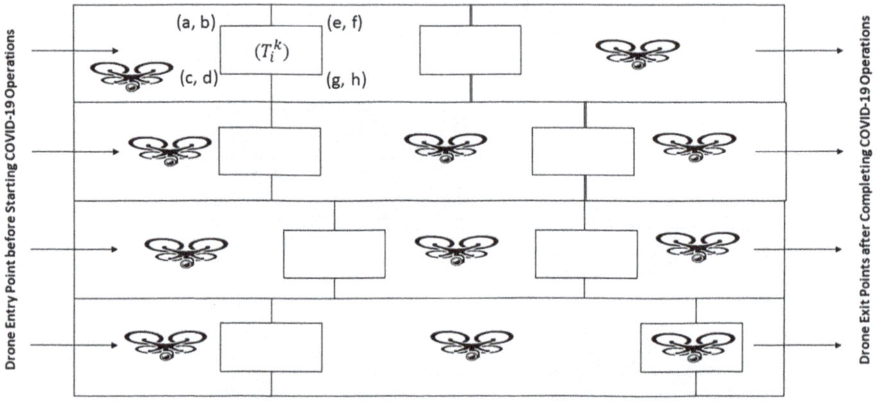

Fig. 1.7 Proposed drone's zones strategies and their movements

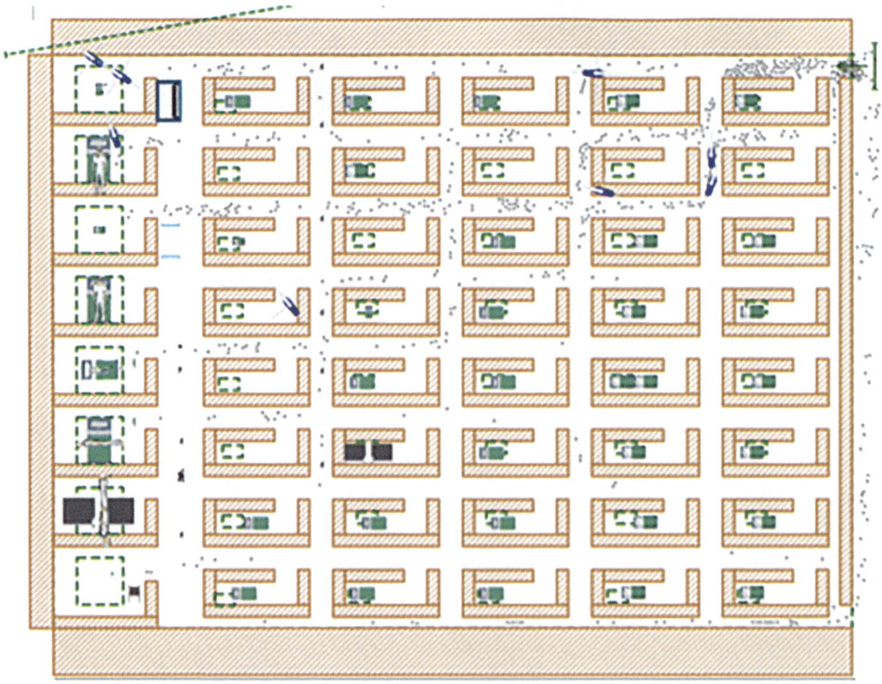

Fig. 1.8 Indoor hospital activities in execution (2D view)

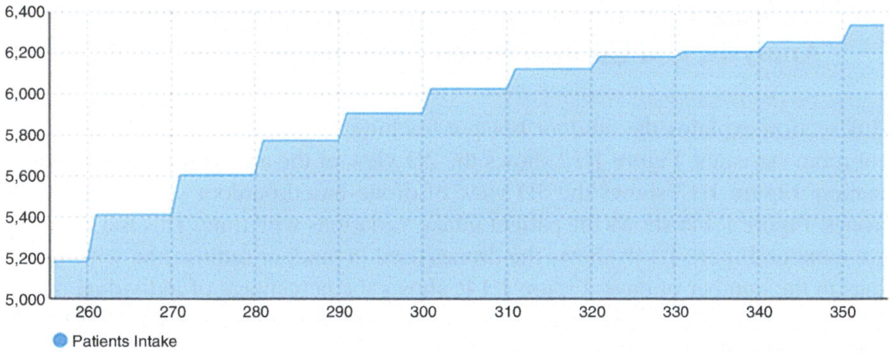

Fig. 1.9 Drone-based indoor hospital statistics 1 for control room

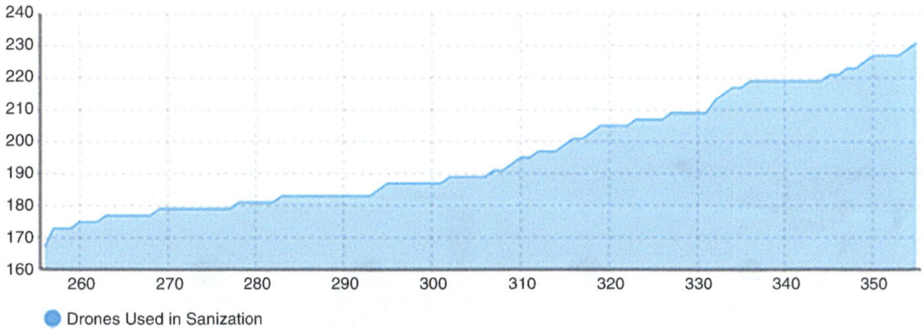

Fig. 1.10 Drone-based indoor hospital statistics 2 for control room

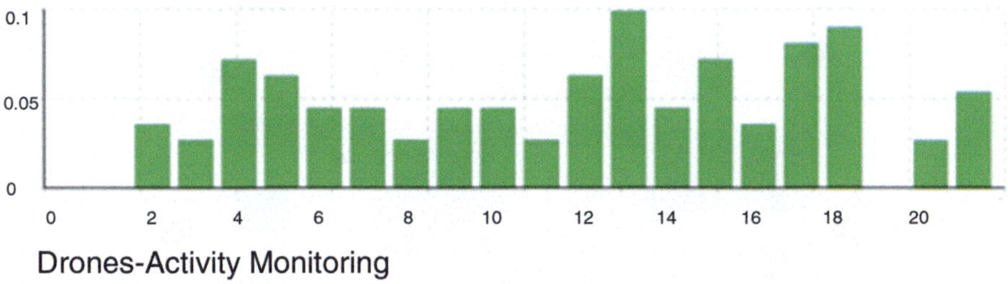

Fig. 1.11 Drone-based indoor hospital statistics 3 for control room

system execution. Figure 1.9 shows the patient's intake in the hospital with time. Figure 1.10 shows the number of drones used in hospital function with variations in the number of days. Figure 1.11 shows the percentage of individual drone utilization.

1.6 Outdoor COVID-19 Hotspot Tracking, Monitoring, Analysis, and Control Room Positioning

This section explains the outdoor hotspot tracking, monitoring, analysis, and control room statistics. Figure 1.12 shows the 2D view of the area considered for sanitization. Figure 1.13 shows the 3D view of drone-based outdoor sanitization with drones. Figure 1.14a shows the patient intake variations with time. This is a cumulative number. Figure 1.14b shows the drones used in outdoor sanitization with variations in the number of days. Figure 1.14c shows the percentage of individual drone utilization. Figure 1.14d shows the generation of thermal images for the COVID-19 hotspot. Overall, Fig. 1.14 presents the drone-based outdoor COVID-19 hotspot tracking, monitoring, analysis, and control room positioning.

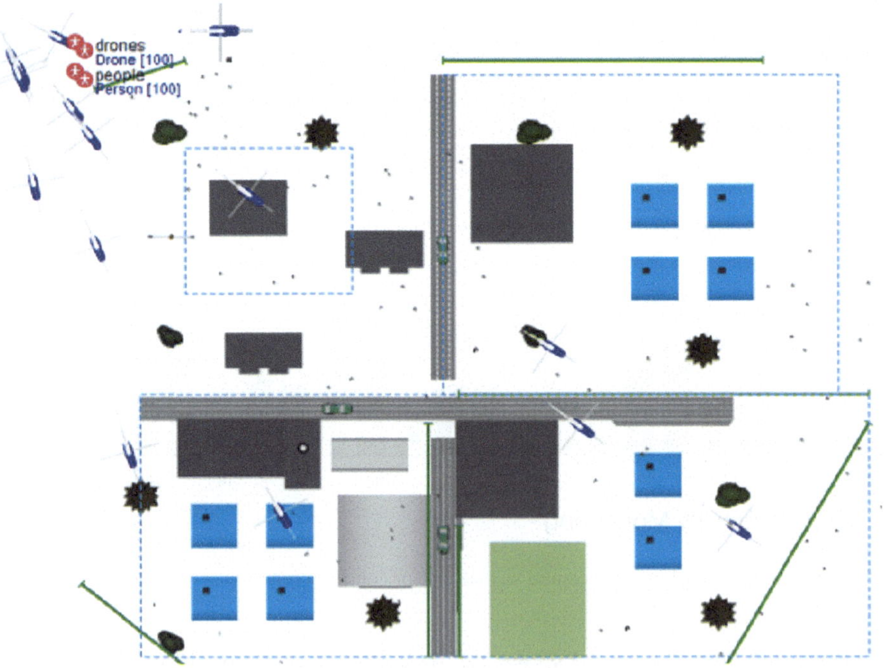

Fig. 1.12 Outdoor area considered forsanitization (2D view)

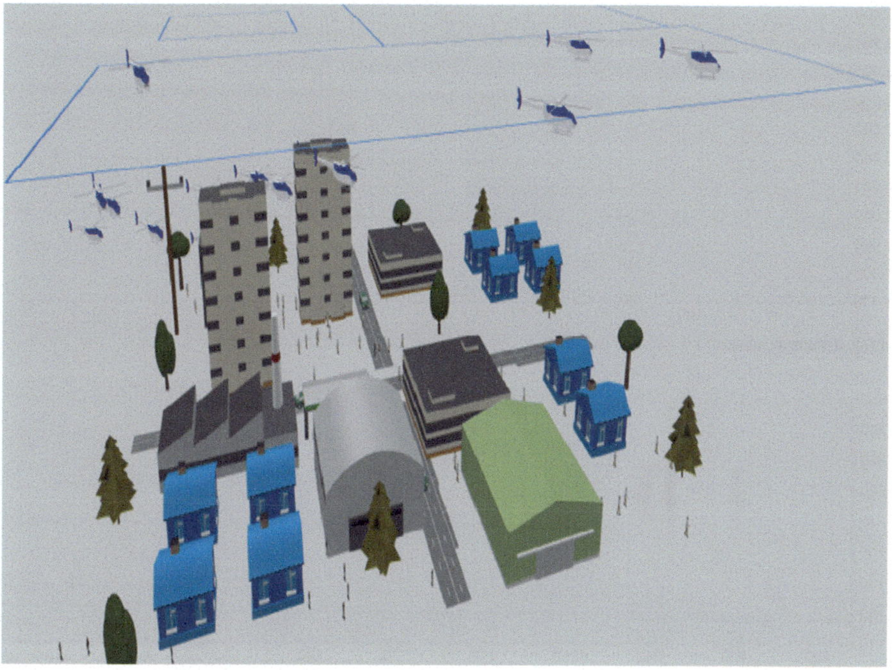

Fig. 1.13 Drone-based outdoor sanitization (3D view)

1.7 Conclusion and Future Scope

The present COVID-19 pandemic situation forces to propose methods of accurate and timely sharing of disease, its varying effects, causes, and treatment-related information. The pervasive internet connectivity helps to have presence of various types of equipments (such as drones, IoT, thermal imaging, IRS cameras, etc.) for collecting and sharing the required information as and when required. This work started with an overview of COVID-19, hotspots identification, monitoring, and effects over social and economic sectors. Further, drone-based approaches are explored for the COVID-19 pandemic. Here, drone-based indoor and outdoor COVID-19 operations (including sanitization, monitoring, data collection, and sharing) are explored. The real-time drone used for COVID-19 operation in a real scenario is discussed as well. In results and analysis, the number of patient intake, number of drones used, and percentage of individual drone utilization are evaluated and discussed.

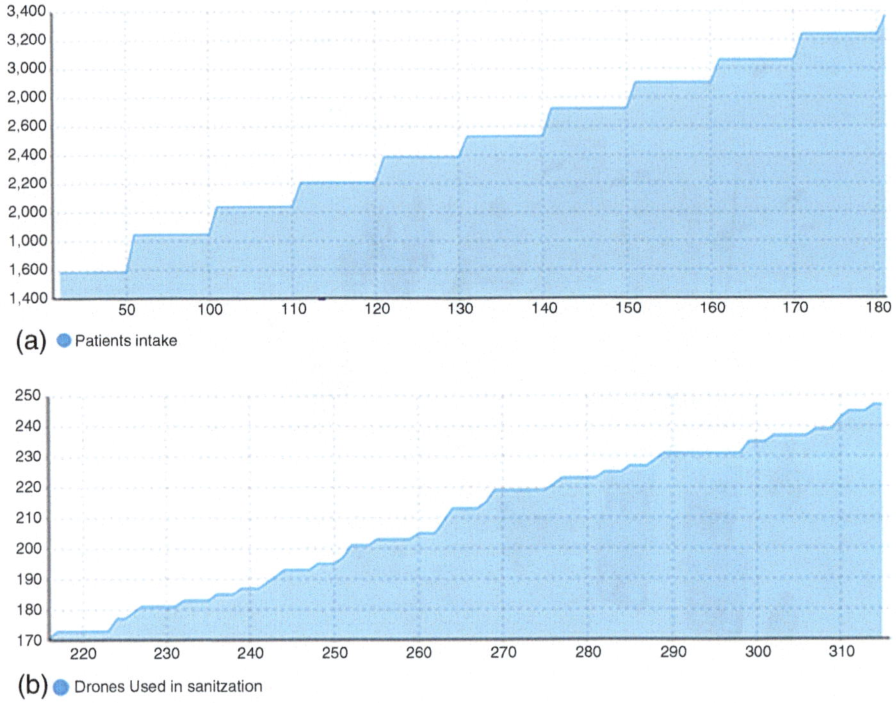

Fig. 1.14 Drone-based outdoor COVID-19 hotspot tracking, monitoring, analysis, and control room positioning. (**a**) Drone-based outdoor area statistics 1 for control room. (**b**) Drone-based outdoor area statistics 2 for control room. (**c**) Drone-based outdoor area statistics 3 for control room. (**d**) Drone-based outdoor COVID-19 hotspot detection

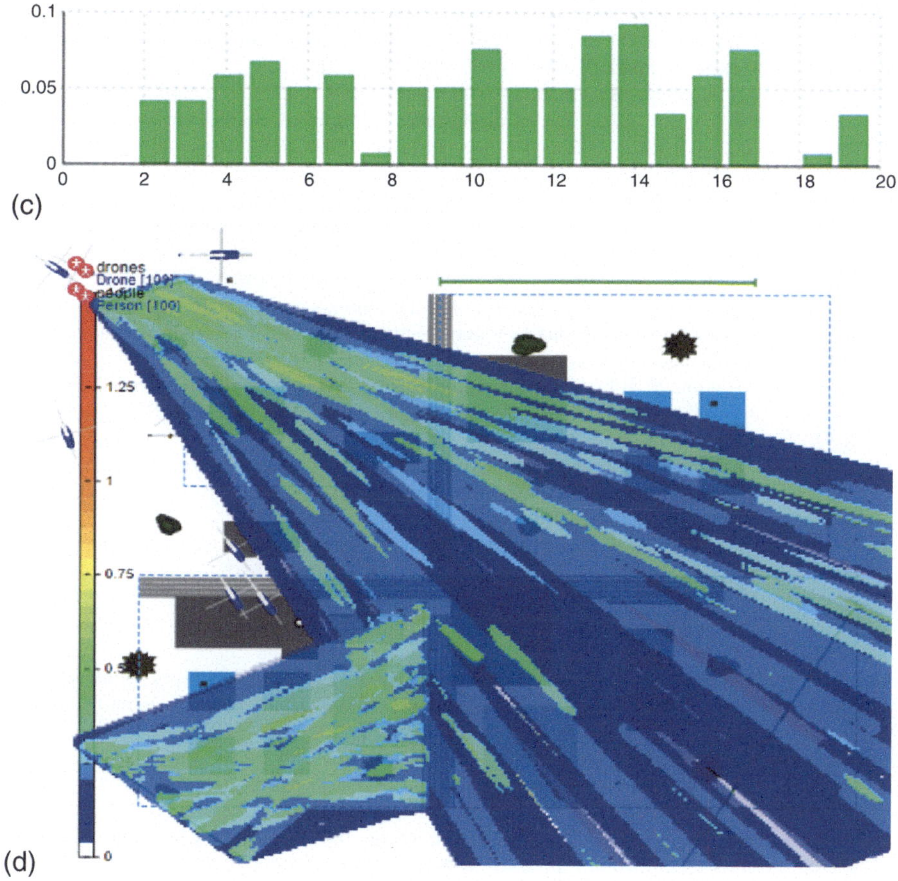

Fig. 1.14 (continued)

References

1. Yin, H., et al.: Smart healthcare. Found. Trends R Electron. Des. Autom. **2**(14), 1–67 (2018)
2. Smart Healthcare Market | Size, Share, Trends | Industry Analysis | Forecast 2023 | Technavio. https://www.technavio.com/report/global-smart-healthcare-market-analysis-share-2018?pk_vid=93ef3a154eacc0b71587065191fdca06&tnplus. Accessed 17 Apr 2020
3. IoT in Healthcare Industry | IoT Applications in Healthcare—Wipro. https://www.wipro.com/business-process/what-can-iot-do-for-healthcare-/. Accessed 18 Apr 2020
4. Coronavirus. https://www.who.int/health-topics/coronavirus#tab=tab_1. Accessed 18 Apr 2020
5. Haidari, L.A., et al.: The economic and operational value of using drones to transport vaccines. Vaccine. **34**(34), 4062–4067 (2016)
6. Thiels, C.A., Aho, J.M., Zietlow, S.P., Jenkins, D.H.: Use of unmanned aerial vehicles for medical product transport. Air Med. J. **34**(2), 104–108 (2015)
7. Van de Voorde, P., Gautama, S., Momont, A., Ionescu, C.M., De Paepe, P., Fraeyman, N.: The drone ambulance [A-UAS]: golden bullet or just a blank? Resuscitation. **116**, 46–48 (2017)

8. Drones: a force for good when flying in the face of disaster | Global development | The Guardian. https://www.theguardian.com/global-development/2015/jul/28/drones-flying-in-the-face-of-disaster-humanitarian-response. Accessed 15 Apr 2020
9. Capolupo, A., Pindozzi, S., Okello, C., Fiorentino, N., Boccia, L.: Photogrammetry for environmental monitoring: the use of drones and hydrological models for detection of soil contaminated by copper. Sci. Total Environ. **514**, 298–306 (2015). https://doi.org/10.1016/j.scitotenv.2015.01.109
10. Brady, J.M., Stokes, M.D., Bonnardel, J., Bertram, T.H.: Characterization of a quadrotor unmanned aircraft system for aerosol-particle-concentration measurements. Environ. Sci. Technol. **50**(3), 1376–1383 (2016). https://doi.org/10.1021/acs.est.5b05320
11. Drones in HealthCare. https://www.dronesinhealthcare.com/. Accessed 24 Apr 2020
12. Papua New Guinea: innovating to reach remote TB patients and improve access to treatment | MSF. https://www.msf.org/papua-new-guinea-innovating-reach-remote-tb-patients-and-improve-access-treatment. Accessed 22 Apr 2020
13. Lagkas, T., Argyriou, V., Bibi, S., Sarigiannidis, P.: UAV IoT framework views and challenges: towards protecting drones as 'things,'. Sensors (Switzerland). **18**(11), 1–21 (2018). https://doi.org/10.3390/s18114015
14. Poza-Luján, J.-L., Posadas-Yagüe, J.-L., Cristóbal, A., Rosa, M.: Indoor drones for the creative industries: distinctive features/opportunities in safety navigation. In: Drones and the Creative Industry, pp. 129–141. Springer, Heidelberg (2018)
15. Nithyavathy, N., Pavithra, S., Naveen, M., Logesh, B., James, T.: Design and development of drone for healthcare. Int. J. Sci. Technol. Res. **9**(1), 2676–2680 (2020)
16. Mozaffari, M., Saad, W., Bennis, M., Nam, Y.H., Debbah, M.: A tutorial on UAVs for wireless networks: applications, challenges, and open problems. IEEE Commun. Surv. Tutorials. **21**(3), 2334–2360 (2019)
17. Enabling delivery of essential health services during the COVID 19 outbreak: guidance note background. Available: https://www.who.int/publications-detail/covid-19-operational-guidance-for-maintaining-essential-health-. Accessed 20 Apr 2020
18. Coronavirus (COVID-19) events as they happen. https://www.who.int/emergencies/diseases/novel-coronavirus-2019/events-as-they-happen. Accessed 17 Apr 2020
19. WHO COVID-19 Dashboard. https://covid19.who.int/. Accessed 22 Apr 2020
20. Coronavirus disease 2019 (COVID-19) Situation Report–93. https://www.who.int/docs/default-source/coronaviruse/situation-reports/20200422-sitrep-93-covid-19.pdf?sfvrsn=35cf80d7_4. Accessed 22 Apr 2020
21. WHO | WHO Regional Offices. https://www.who.int/classifications/network/ro/en/. Accessed 22 Apr 2020
22. Containment Plan for Large Outbreaks Ministry of Health and Family Welfare Government of India. Accessed 20 Apr 2020
23. Administrator. Key messages and actions for COVID-19 prevention and control in schools, 2020. Accessed 20 Apr 2020
24. Australian Army tests out drones for surveillance—Hardware—Security—iTnews. https://www.itnews.com.au/news/australian-army-tests-out-drones-for-surveillance-406069. Accessed 20 Apr 2020
25. Netherlands procures Black Hornet micro UAVs | Jane's 360. https://web.archive.org/web/20180505131538/http://www.janes.com/article/79816/netherlands-procures-black-hornet-micro-uavs. Accessed 20 Apr 2020
26. Marines get a closer look at Black Hornet micro drone. https://www.marinecorpstimes.com/news/your-marine-corps/2015/09/22/marines-get-a-closer-look-at-black-hornet-micro-drone/. Accessed 20 Apr 2020
27. This notice in TED website. http://ted.europa.eu/udl?uri=TED:NOTICE:18214-2015:TEXT:EN:HTML. pp. 1–5 (2015)

28. COVID-19: operational guidance for maintaining essential health services during an outbreak. https://www.who.int/publications-detail/covid-19-operational-guidance-for-maintaining-essential-health-services-during-an-outbreak. Accessed 20 Apr 2020
29. Eye in the sky: NSG acquires Black Hornet Nano—world's smallest spy cam UAV | India News. https://www.timesnownews.com/india/article/eye-in-the-sky-nsg-acquires-black-hornet-nano-worlds-smallest-spy-cam-uav/300812. Accessed 20 Apr 2020
30. Los Angeles Fire Department And DJI Collaborate To Advance Drone Technology For Public Safety Applications. https://www.dji.com/newsroom/news/lafd-dji-collaborate-to-advance-drone-technology-for-public-safety-applications. Accessed 20 Apr 2020
31. DJI and EENA bring aerial technology to emergency providers. https://enterprise.dji.com/news/detail/dji-and-eena-bring-aerial-technology-to-emergency-providers-1. Accessed 20 Apr 2020
32. Ocean Alliance SnotBot and EarBot Drones Featured on BBC's Blue Planet Live—DRONELIFE. https://dronelife.com/2019/04/01/ocean-alliance-snotbot-earbot-drones-bbc-blue-planet/. Accessed 20 Apr 2020
33. The Lancet Haematology: Look! Up in the sky! It's a bird. It's a plane. It's a medical drone! Lancet Haematol. **4**(2), e56 (2017). https://doi.org/10.1016/S2352-3026(17)30004-2
34. Malawi tests first unmanned aerial vehicle flights for HIV early infant diagnosis. Press Centre, UNICEF. https://www.unicef.org/media/media_90462.html. Accessed 20 Apr 2020
35. Buters, T., Belton, D., Cross, A.: Seed and seedling detection using unmanned aerial vehicles and automated image classification in the monitoring of ecological recovery. Drones. **3**(3), 53 (2019). https://doi.org/10.3390/drones3030053
36. Case study: identifying pumpkins with drones and machine learning—raptor maps. https://raptormaps.com/case-study-identifying-pumpkins-drones-machine-learning/. Accessed 20 Apr 2020
37. Drones, seeds, & fires: how drone seed plants trees from the sky. CleanTechnica. https://cleantechnica.com/2019/02/08/drones-seeds-fires-how-droneseed-plants-trees-from-the-sky/. Accessed 20 Apr 2020
38. Home—Saildrone. https://research.csiro.au/saildrone/. Accessed 20 Apr 2020
39. Table of contents 目次. JLTA J. Kiyo **10**, p. Toc1 (2007). https://doi.org/10.20622/jltaj.10.0_toc1
40. On New Microsoft Campus, Skycatch Monitors construction with precision. https://blog.skycatch.com/on-new-microsoft-campus-skycatch-monitors-construction-with-precision. Accessed 20 Apr 2020
41. Holland Michel, A.: Amazon's Drone Patents (2017)
42. Eye in the sky: Fox Sports is bringing drones to sporting events—Digiday. https://digiday.com/media/eye-sky-fox-sports-bringing-drones-sporting-events/. Accessed 20 Apr 2020
43. 38 Ways drones/UAVs impact society: war to forecasting weather. CB Insights. https://www.cbinsights.com/research/drone-impact-society-uav/. Accessed 20 Apr 2020
44. The role of drones in in telecommunications tower inspection. https://www.rcrwireless.com/20170221/cell-tower-news/drones-telecommunications-tower-inspection-tag23-tag99. Accessed 20 Apr 2020
45. Sokullu, R., Balcı, A., Demir, E.: Drones and their application in ambient assisted living. International Conference on Engineering Technology (ICENTE'18), Konya, Turkey, Oct. 26–28, 2018.
46. Lennartsson, J.: Strategic Placement of Ambulance Drones for Delivering Defibrillators to Out of Hospital Cardiac Arrest Victims. KTH Royal Institute of Technology, Stockholm (2015)
47. Estrada, M.A.R., Ndoma, A.: The uses of unmanned aerial vehicles -UAV's- (or drones) in social logistic: natural disasters response and humanitarian relief aid. Procedia Comput. Sci. **149**, 375–383 (2019). https://doi.org/10.1016/j.procs.2019.01.151
48. Covid-19: in the times of 'touch-me-not' environment, drones are the new best friends. The Economic Times. https://economictimes.indiatimes.com/small-biz/startups/features/covid-19-in-the-times-of-touch-me-not-environment-drones-are-the-new-best-friends/articleshow/74924233.cms?from=mdr. Accessed 24 Apr 2020
49. Drones take flight to carry Covid-19 tests to labs in Africa | WIRED. https://www.wired.com/story/drones-flight-carry-covid-tests-labs-africa/. Accessed 24 Apr 2020

50. Van Tilburg, C.: First report of using portable unmanned aircraft systems (drones) for search and rescue. Wilderness Environ. Med. **28**(2), 116–118 (2017). https://doi.org/10.1016/j.wem.2016.12.010
51. Karaca, Y., et al.: The potential use of unmanned aircraft systems (drones) in mountain search and rescue operations. Am. J. Emerg. Med. **36**(4), 583–588 (2018). https://doi.org/10.1016/j.ajem.2017.09.025
52. Mendelow, B., Muir, P., Boshielo, B.T., Robertson, J.: Development of e-Juba, a preliminary proof of concept unmanned aerial vehicle designed to facilitate the transportation of microbiological test samples from remote rural clinics to National Health Laboratory Service laboratories. South African Med. J. **97**(11 Pt 3), 1215–1218 (2007). https://doi.org/10.7196/SAMJ.242
53. World Health Organization. Feasibility study for deploying Drones in Bhutan for delivering medical supplies. SEARO (2016)
54. Contraception drones are the future of women's health in rural Africa. HuffPost India. https://www.huffingtonpost.in/entry/birth-control-drones-africa_n_56a8a3b4e4b0947efb65fc11?ri18n=true. Accessed 20 Apr 2020
55. Knoblauch, A.M., et al.: Bi-directional drones to strengthen healthcare provision: experiences and lessons from Madagascar, Malawi and Senegal. BMJ Glob. Heal. **4**, 1541 (2019). https://doi.org/10.1136/bmjgh-2019-001541
56. Rapid response from the air: medicines successfully delivered using a parcel drone in East Africa. https://www.giz.de/en/press/70080.html. Accessed 20 Apr 2020
57. World Health Organization, 2020. Coronavirus disease 2019 (COVID-19): situation report, 70. Available at: https://apps.who.int/iris/bitstream/handle/10665/331683/nCoVsitrep30Mar2020-eng.pdf [Last Accessed: 14 Oct, 2020].
58. What is a COVID-19 hotspot? Where are the hotspots in India? https://www.eastmojo.com/coronavirus-updates/2020/04/10/what-is-a-covid-19-hotspot-where-are-the-hotspots-in-india. Accessed 24 Apr 2020
59. India coronavirus: all major cities named Covid-19 'red zone' hotspots—BBC News. https://www.bbc.com/news/world-asia-india-52306225. Accessed 24 Apr 2020
60. Full list of 170 COVID-19 hotspot districts: what does it mean if you live in one?—The Week. https://www-theweek-in.cdn.ampproject.org/v/s/www.theweek.in/news/india/2020/04/16/full-list-of-170-covid-19-hotspot-districts-what-does-it-mean-if-you-live-in-one.amp.html?usqp=mq331AQFKAGwASA%3D&amp_js_v=0.1#aoh=15874752246110. Accessed 25 Apr 2020
61. School closures caused by Coronavirus (Covid-19). https://en.unesco.org/covid19/education-response. Accessed 19 Apr 2020
62. Only online darshan in Himachal Pradesh. Shimla News—Times of India. https://timesofindia.indiatimes.com/city/shimla/only-online-darshan-in-himachal-pradesh/articleshow/74808181.cms. Accessed 19 Apr 2020

Chapter 2
Machine Learning-Based Scheme to Identify COVID-19 in Human Bodies

Harish Kumar, Anuradha, A. K. Solanki, and Sudeep Tanwar

Abstract A virus spread from China to all around the world named COVID-19 has now become a demon. The fear of death can be easily seen in citizens of around 180 countries and fear to force us indoors. This is a demon of the twenty-first century; typically, this demon does not link with any of the evil, occultism, literature, fiction, mythology, and folklore. COVID-19 is a member of the coronavirus family and caused by the SARS-CoV-2 virus. COVID-19 was first identified in December 2019 at Wuhan, China. SARS virus is responsible for respiratory illness known as COVID-19. We have limited articles on COVID-19 with machine learning (ML) and AI. We do not have any antivirus medicine and other dataset that bring in mind about prediction, detection, and stage identification of COVID-19 in human bodies. Therefore, we decided to bring a machine learning-based technique with a list of datasets that will apply to coronavirus dataset for identification. It is believed that ML and artificial intelligence can help accelerate solutions for predicting the stage of infection. Data analysis presented in this paper helps in minimizing the virus impact with all the other research.

Keywords COVID-19 · AI · SARS · SARS-CoV-2 · CXR · WHO

H. Kumar (*) · Anuradha
Department of Computer Science and Engineering, Meerut Institute of Engineering and Technology, Meerut, India
e-mail: sudeep.tanwar@nirmauni.ac.in

A. K. Solanki
Department of Computer Science and Engineering, Bundelkhand Institute of Engineering and Technology, Jhansi, India

S. Tanwar
Department of Computer Science and Engineering, Nirma University, Gujarat, India
e-mail: sudeep.tanwar@nirmauni.ac.in

© The Author(s), under exclusive license to Springer Nature Switzerland AG 2021

F. Al-Turjman et al. (eds.), *Emerging Technologies for Battling Covid-19*, Studies in Systems, Decision and Control 324,
https://doi.org/10.1007/978-3-030-60039-6_2

2.1 Introduction

Our earth is infected by a virus that attacks our respiratory system—the nose, throat, and lungs. Commonly we called it flu, but this not the same as normal "flu" viruses that cause minimal damage. So far, there have been more than 112,000 deaths until now worldwide. The behavior of the virus is very harsh and difficult to understand. In 2020 respiratory flu is the most emerging infectious disease, causing high morbidity and mortality in society and worldwide (deadly disease). This spreading virus is an RNA virus and generally found in three types based on their protein. Generally, we termed them as A type, B type, and C type [1, 2]. The WHO publicized that the scientific name of the 2019 SARS virus is COVID-19. COVID-19 belongs to a family of coronaviruses that may cause symptoms such as sore throat, pneumonia, fever, respiratory illness, and lung infection [3–5]. In the past 3 months, the coronavirus disease 2019 (COVID-19) pandemic is spreading at a swiftly. The first genetic material (genome) of COVID-19 was given by Prof. Yong-Zhen Zhang, in January 2020 [6]. On March 13, the WHO declared it as a pandemic for the whole world [3]. Most of the devolved or developing countries are also affected by COVID-19 [3, 4, 7]. Approximately 400 billion people have become prisoners in their houses. Lockdowns are the only solution till date as a preventive measure for spreading this virus [8, 9]. COVID-19 influenza is a pandemic in human society since December 2019. At the time of writing this paper, there have been 10,000,000 confirmed cases of COVID-19 and 500,000 deaths. Using a survey of 10,000 infected people (data available online), we find that risk perception is very high in COVID-19 patients. The human body has no immunity against the coronavirus because its protein structure is similar to human body protein. Influenza pandemics have resulted in damaging human antigen and damaging human tissues of the respiratory system. Coronavirus exists in four different generations.

1. Alphacoronavirus
2. Betacoronavirus
3. Gammacoronavirus
4. Deltacoronavirus

Coronavirus is a type of RNA virus, and its mutation rate is higher than DNA viruses. The genome codes (the set of all the genes of a specific species) for at least four main structural proteins: spike, membrane, envelope, and nucleocapsid proteins [10]. Besides these proteins, the coronavirus has some accessory proteins, which helps the replicative processes and makes it possible to enter into human cells [2]. Figure 2.1 shows the basic structure of COVID-19 virus presented by Dr. Rohan Bir Singh [10] (Table 2.1).

A number of communities are working on finding the solution to COVID-19. The more fertile ground to find the solution to COVID-19 is by using machine learning algorithms [3, 11, 12]. Machine learning creates spot correlations across large amounts of data describing the viruses (Table 2.2).

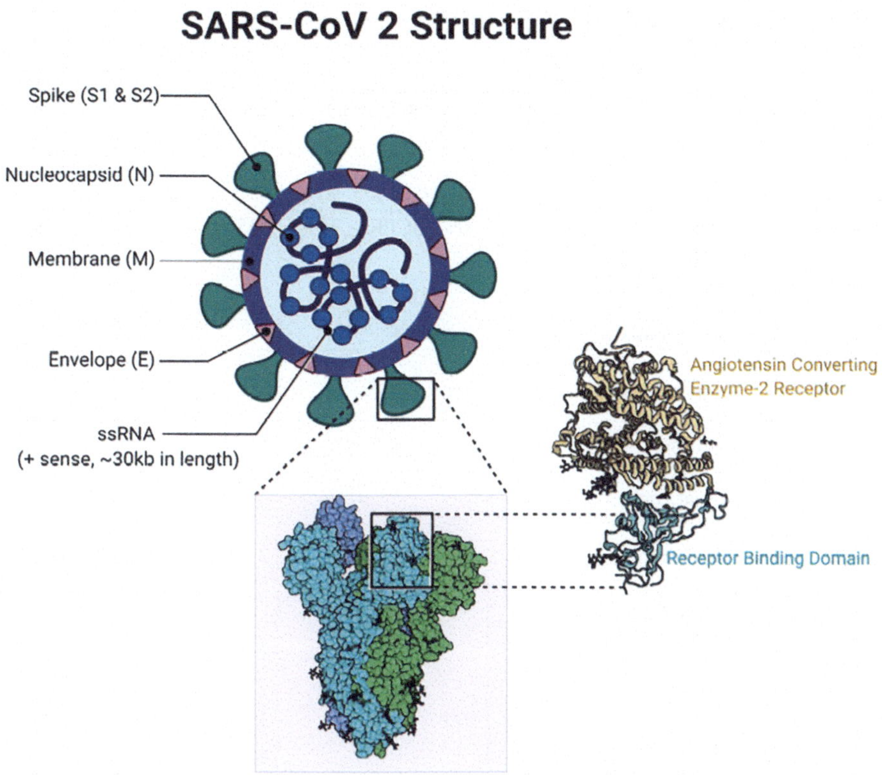

Fig. 2.1 Basic structure of coronavirus. (Proposed by Dr. Rohan Bir Singh)

Table 2.1 Basic structure of coronavirus and the function of each protein [10]

Basic structure of coronavirus	Structural protein	Function of protein
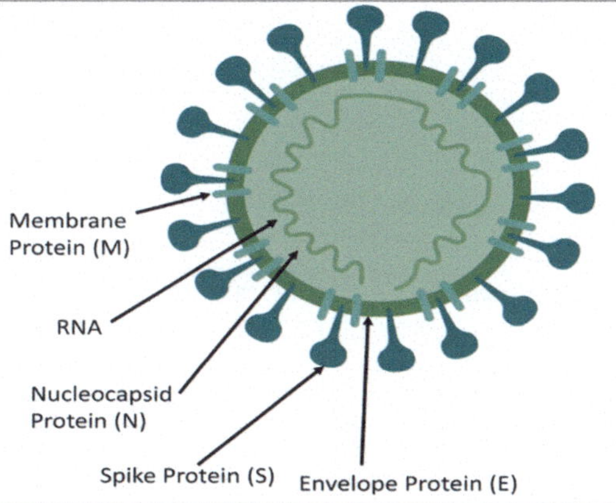	Nucleocapsid protein (N)	Bound to RNA genome to make up nucleocapsid
	Spike protein (S)	This protein is responsible for binding of host cell receptor to facilitate entry to host cell
	Envelope protein (E)	Interacts with M to form viral envelope
	Membrane protein (M)	Responsible for determining the shape of viral envelope

Table 2.2 Seven harmful influenza viruses and their impact on society

S. no	Name of virus	Symptoms	No. of country infected (approx.)	Case fatality rate (CFR)	No of persons infected	Total death	Death rate (%)
1	Marburg	Hemorrhagic fever	11	50% 24% ≤ CFR ≥ 80%	466	367	80
2	Nipah	Acute respiratory infection and fatal encephalitis	10	40% ≤ CFR ≥ 75%	513	398	77.60
3	H5N1 Bird flu	Fever (often high fever, > 38 °C) and malaise, cough, sore throat, and muscle aches	18	56%	861	455	52.8
4	Ebola	Hemorrhagic fever, rare but severe, often fatal illness in humans	9	50% 20% ≤ CFR ≥ 90%	33,557	13,562	40.4
5	H7N9	Fever, cough that produces sputum, breathing, problem and wheezing, headache, muscle pain, general malaise	11	56%	1568	619	30
6	H1N1 Swine flu	Fever, chills, cough, sore throat, runny nose, stuffy nose watery red eyes, body aches, headache	100+	1%	1,632,258	284,500	17.40
7	COVID-19	Fever, dry cough, sore throat, runny nose, and stuffy nose	176	Not yet known	8,600,000	420,000	20.47

2.1.1 Symptoms

The signs of COVID-19 are nonspecific, and the disease identification can range from no symptoms to severe pneumonia and death. As of April 13, 2020, from laboratory confirmed cases, typical signs and symptoms include the following: [3, 4, 13].

(a) Fever
(b) Cough (dry cough)
(c) Tiredness
(d) Sputum production
(e) Shortness of breath
(f) Sore throat
(g) Headache
(h) Myalgia or arthralgia
(i) Chills
(j) Nausea or vomiting
(k) Nasal congestion
(l) Diarrhea
(m) Hemoptysis
(n) Conjunctival congestion

A limited number of articles about coronavirus with artificial intelligence and machine learning are available; few have offered a truly comprehensive view. Our main aim is to design a pattern, datasets, and other aspects of analysis that will be applied to COVID-19 based on symptoms given above. In our research, decisions are according to perceived risk. Various data mining, machine learning, and AI techniques can help us to easily identify the pattern similarity in patients, which can help to accelerate solutions for predicting the stage of infection. The idea behind data mining and ML/AI techniques is to learn the hidden pattern from the available data [7, 8]. We apply various machine learning approaches to identify relationships or associations in biological data to groups with similar genetic structure, to analyze and predict infection stage. We apply machine learning techniques on sequence alignment, structure, function, and clustering structure of symptoms given in 1.1. We apply Duster algorithm which is a data filtering algorithm for refining the data. For smoothing, we use binning method. For reduction, we use parametric numerosity reduction technique and support vector machines with decision tree techniques to identify the impact of latest deadly disease damage.

2.2 Problem Definition

Fighting against COVID-19 confronts the risk of infection. Without infection, there are essentially zero risks of death. Therefore, we decide to beat COVID by prediction rules. Data mining, machine learning, and AI can contribute to the fight against COVID-19. The following are the areas where we can apply advance technology:

(a) Setting the footpath for prediction
(b) Data dashboards
(c) Before time warnings and alerts
(d) Diagnosis and prediction
(e) Treatments and cures
(f) Social control

We assume that being in a healthy state means without infection, the vector $V = (0, X, Y)$ and in an infected state with COVID-19, the vector $V = (1, X, Y)$, where X is the set of individual characteristics, Y is the set of immunity, and (0, 1) represents the infected or not infected status. COVID-19 identifications can be categorized as follows:

(a) Medical Ground: Foretell the impact of new antiviral medicines, structure of proteins, and their impact after interactions with human bodies. This study helps to identify which antiviral medicine helps the patient recover from coronavirus. According to the results of dataset, we modify the medicine to predict protein-ligand interactions [10]. Then after modification, the medicine is used to check with RNA sequence of COVID-19 and chemical composition to forecast which medicine works best.
(b) Self-Quarantine*:* To predict the infection rate in a community of patients, we apply multiple techniques that help our doctors and society to better plan resourcing and response. Till now we are having various methods for predicting the spreading rate of normal flu [14]. But all these methods are not applicable on COVID-19 due to its changing nature and availability of limited datasets.
(c) Digital Image Results: Medical images like X-ray or CT scan of coronavirus-infected people help in diagnosis. Image filtering and diagnosis help our doctors to identify the infection rate in a patient [15]. The following is the process of percentage calculation in an X-ray and CT scan method. Block diagram is a part of our identification method and is well explained in Fig 2.4.
(d) Machine Learning: The main step is to mine the data to better estimate symptoms and infection rate. The method used in mining the data helps in getting relevant information about the disease. Data received from various sites is very noisy and requires an excellent refining technique. Our main work is based on the fourth part. In an analysis, 54% had positive RT-PCR results, and 86.8% had positive chest CT scans. But in countries like India, we have limited number of laboratories and have a geographical distance between all labs. This is very typical for doctors to predict the COVID-19 patient in his geographical domain. So our aim is design a system which will help and assist society to identify a COVID-19 patient. Our approach worked on the three major tests, depending on patient requirements (Figs. 2.2, 2.3, and 2.4).

    1. OPD data collection and first-level identification (first-level quarantine).
    2. CT image or CXR report collection and identification (second-level quarantine).
    3. Main laboratory report and final prediction (third-level quarantine).

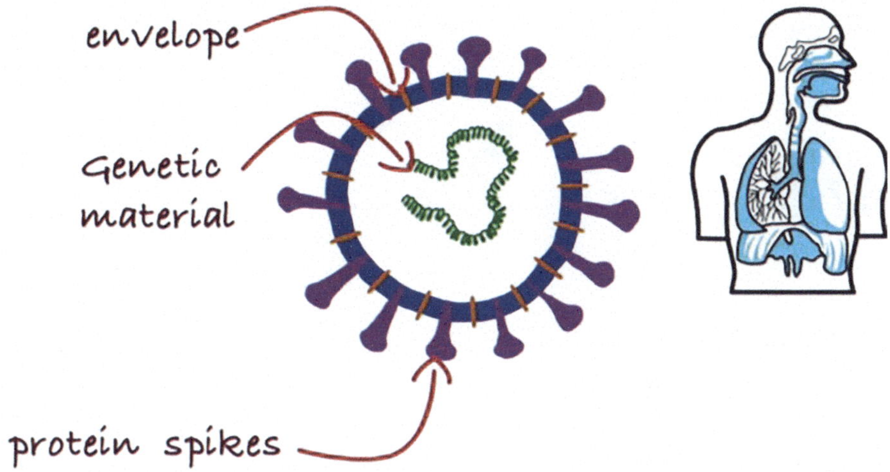

Fig. 2.2 Protein structure and the human body

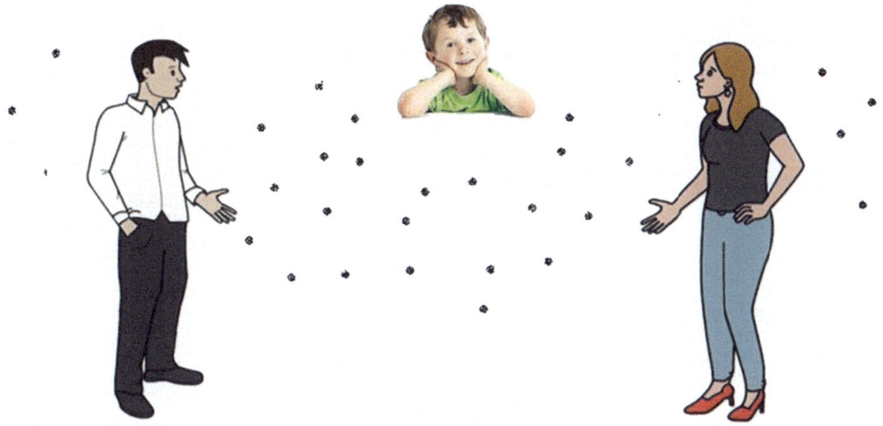

Fig. 2.3 Social distancing between a group of persons

2.3 Methodology

To control spreading of COVID-19, inspecting large numbers of cases infected with the virus for appropriate quarantine and treatment is a priority. Fast and accurate pattern recognition methods are urgently needed to fight against the disease. We decided to bring a machine learning-based technique with a list of datasets that will apply to coronavirus based on available COVID-19 dataset. Our aim is to develop a method that could extract COVID-19's features in order to provide a tentative diagnosis to our doctors. This will help in predicting the stages of infection of COVID-19

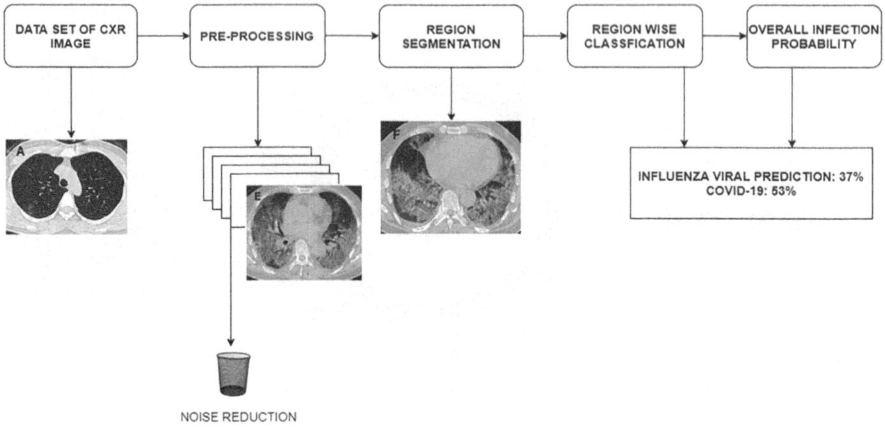

Fig. 2.4 Block diagram of CXR report classification technique and infection calculation

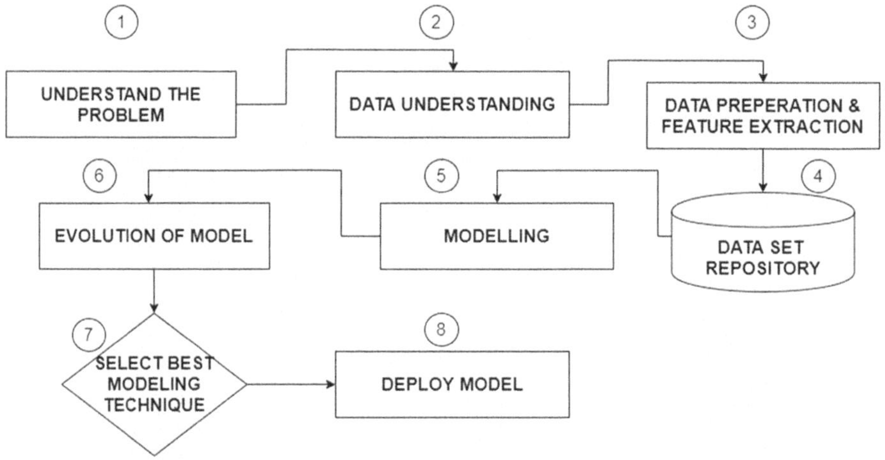

Fig. 2.5 Deployment model

patients. Our pattern matching can help to accelerate solutions for predicting the stage of infection. To achieve better results, we use recent datasets of 450 patients along with a history of previous illness. We collected approximately 350 X-ray and CT images of confirmed COVID-19 cases. Figure 2.5 represents the deployment model of the approach.

The following are the steps for data preprocessing, from steps 2 to 5.

1. Collection of data
2. Filtering of data
3. Smoothing of data
4. Reduction of data
5. Pattern analysis

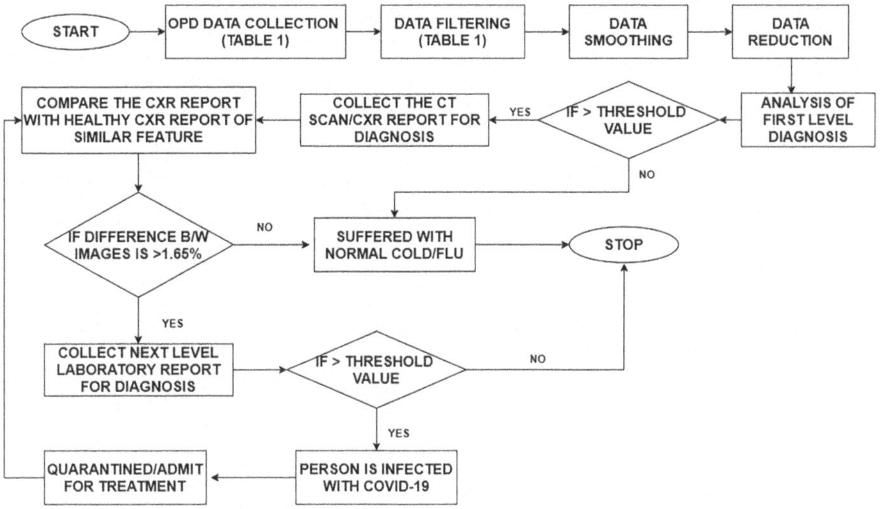

Fig. 2.6 Methodology for identification or detection of COVID-19 patients

Figure 2.6 represents the basic methodology of the detection of COVID-19. A dataset is designed for final analysis of results. Based on the results, an automated system automatically detects whether the person is infected or not and if there is any chance of recovery or not with a minimum cost and accurate results.

2.4 Dataset and Tentative Solution

Coronavirus disease 2019 (COVID-19) is a communicable disease. The virus can easily spread from one person to another. A 57-year-old Chinese woman named Wei Guixian is the patient zero of COVID-19.The disease causes respiratory illness with symptoms like cough, fever, and difficulty in breathing. A person can protect himself/herself by washing his/her hands frequently, avoiding touching the face, and avoiding close contact with infected people. On December 31, 2019, the WHO was alerted by the Chinese government of a series of corona-like cases in the city of Wuhan. The disease causes respiratory illness with symptoms like cough, fever, and difficulty in breathing. We collect all the data from various sites [3, 4, 16]. We feel that every problem seems to have a ML solution. There are various areas where ML/AI can contribute to the fight against COVID-19.

(a) OPD data collection and first-level identification: Testing is also an essential process for a suitable response to the pandemic illness [8]. Testing helps us to understand the spread processing and to take evidence-based measures to slow down the spread of the disease. OPD diagnosis allows COVID-19-infected people to know that they are infected or not. Its solution may be moved with manual

Table 2.3 First-level clinical data of COVID-19 patients

		Mild ($N = 42$)	Severe ($N = 9$)
Sex	Male	51	56
	Female	48	44
Travel history		Yes/no	Yes/no
Age	Mean (SD)	43.70 ± 11.71	52.83 ± 12.96
	Range	15–78	31–79
Cough	No	32	17
	Yes	68	83
Fever	No	16	17
	Yes	84	83
Temperature	Male	98.4	98.6
	Female	100.4	100.4
Previous case history	No	85	83
	Yes	15	17

processes; every doctor must have to fill all the following data of each patient. This is a first-stage diagnosis process or clinical features identification [17] (Table 2.3).

On the basis of above diagnosis table, doctors cannot predict if a patient is infected with COVID-19 or not, and people do not know that they suffering from COVID-19 or not. If no, one might stay at home, and others might go for quarantine stage for 14 days. This approach is applicable where a number of cases are limited and in controlled population states. But for countries like India where the population is around 135 billion, this is not possible if a disease becomes a pandemic. For finding, I strongly feel that ML/AI with data mining technique is the only solution for identification of patients (Table 2.4).

The decision tree algorithm for predictive modeling can be used to explicitly represent decisions. Its graphical representation makes the use of branching techniques to exemplify all possible outcomes. For identifying whether the person is infected with COVID-19 or not, we apply DT algorithm of machine learning technique (Figs. 2.7 and 2.8).

The supervised learning (decision tree) technique can be used for prediction [11, 12, 18, 19]. This helps in solving classification and regression issues. We complete this into two steps, as follows:

1. Classification (used to find results from a set of possible values)
2. Regression (used to find the result data where results are continuous values)

Constructing optimal binary decision trees is NP-complete. Decision trees are created through a process called splitting, and this process is also known as induction. We use recursive divide and conquer strategy. To achieve better results, we apply greedy algorithm steps, as follows.

Table 2.4 Second level clinical data of COVID-19 patient

Age	TH	Sex	Cough	Fever (°F)	Previous history
0.6	N	M	Y	97.9	N
1	N	M	Y	99.9	N
5	N	M	Y	99.9	N
10	N	M	Y	98.9	N
15	Y	F	Y	100.9	N
20	Y	F	Y	100.5	N
25	Y	M	Y	101	N
27	Y	M	Y	102	N
30	N	F	Y	100	Y
35	N	F	Y	101.7	N
40	Y	M	Y	99.9	Y
45	N	M	Y	99.9	N
50	Y	F	Y	102	N
55	Y	F	Y	101	N
60	N	F	Y	101	Y
65	N	M	Y	101	Y
7	N	M	Y	97.9	Y
75	N	M	Y	97.9	Y
80	N	F	Y	99.9	Y
85	N	F	Y	101.9	N

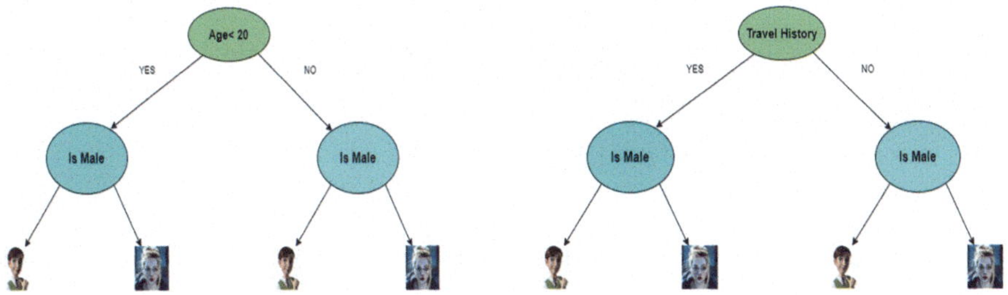

Fig. 2.7 (**a**) Tree based on age. (**b**) Tree based on travel history outside India

1. Trace the root node; we create a crack (splitting) for each attribute.
2. Calculate the cost of the split at each level.
3. Choose the split that costs the least.
4. Recur the process into the sub-trees and repeat step 1 until all leaf nodes are covered.

Information gain is the main factor that is used to construct a decision tree [12]. For calculating the splitting cost, we apply cost function and information gain function:

$$I(P,n) = \frac{P}{S}\log_2\frac{P}{S} - \frac{n}{S}\log_2\frac{n}{S} \quad (2.1)$$

where $S = P + n$.

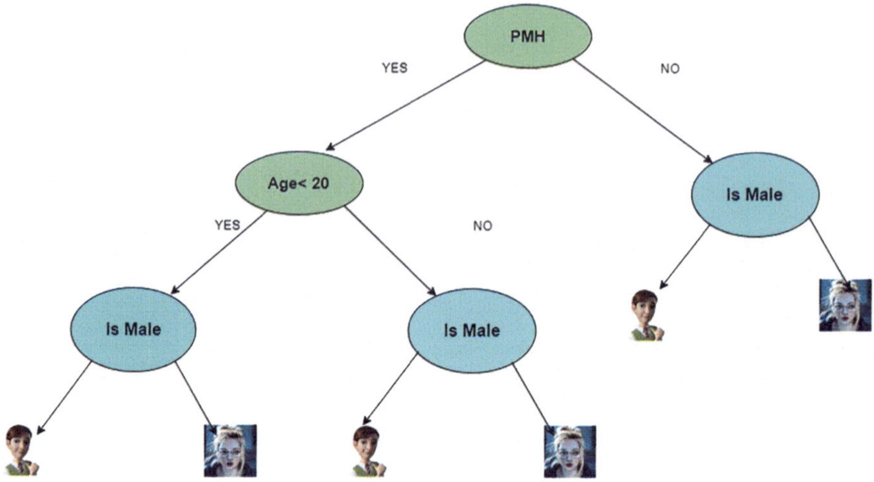

Fig. 2.8 Tree based on PMH

The two impurity measures or splitting criteria that are commonly used in decision trees are Gini impurity and entropy:

$$E(A)=\sum_{i=1}^{T}\frac{P_i+n_i}{P+n}*I(P_i+n_i) \tag{2.2}$$

$$\text{Gain}(A)=I(P,n)-E(A) \tag{2.3}$$

$$\log_2(x)=\frac{\log_{10}(x)}{\log_{10}2} \tag{2.4}$$

The above equations help us to calculate the total gain and entropy from the COVID-19 datasets and help to design and exact prediction of COVID-19 patient. According to analysis, only three possibilities are there, named COVID-19, normal cold, and flu (Table 2.5 and Fig. 2.9).

(b) CT image or CXR report collection and identification: Fig. 2.10 shows two images, one representing the healthy lungs and the other one representing infected images. We are applying a deep learning-based technique for detecting COVID-19 on CT scan and lung X-rays using MATLAB.

All the images were compared by the technique given in the flowchart and which will be well written in MATLAB (Fig. 2.11).

Codes for change in image or image comparison of healthy and infected lungs are well written in Python/MATLAB and simulate the results in WEKA, offer a list of suggestions to the doctors, and assist them in the diagnosis process, predicting results of infection (Fig. 2.12).

Table 2.5 Trained dataset with results

S.no	Disease	Sex	Age	TH	Cough	Fever (°F)	Previous history	Remark 1	Remark 2
1	COVID-19	M	0.6	N	Y	97.9	N	1	Infected
2	Influenza	M	1	N	Y	99.9	N	0	Flu
3	Influenza	M	5	N	Y	99.9	N	0	Flu
4	Influenza	M	10	N	Y	98.9	N	1	Flu
5	COVID-19	F	15	Y	Y	100.9	N	1	Infected
6	Cold	F	20	Y	Y	100.5	N	0	Normal cold
7	COVID-19	M	25	Y	Y	101	N	1	Infected
8	COVID-19	M	27	Y	Y	102	N	1	Infected
9	COVID-19	F	30	N	Y	100	Y	1	Infected
10	COVID-19	F	35	N	Y	101.7	N	1	Infected
11	Cold	M	40	Y	Y	99.9	Y	0	Normal cold
12	COVID-19	M	45	N	Y	99.9	N	1	Infected
13	Cold	F	50	Y	Y	102	N	0	Normal cold
14	COVID-19	F	55	Y	Y	101	N	1	Infected
15	COVID-19	F	60	N	Y	101	Y	1	Infected
16	Cold	M	65	N	Y	101	Y	0	Normal cold
17	Cold	M	7	N	Y	97.9	Y	0	Normal cold
18	COVID-19	M	75	N	Y	97.9	Y	1	Infected
19	Cold	F	80	N	Y	99.9	Y	0	Normal cold
20	Influenza	F	85	N	Y	101.9	N	0	Flu

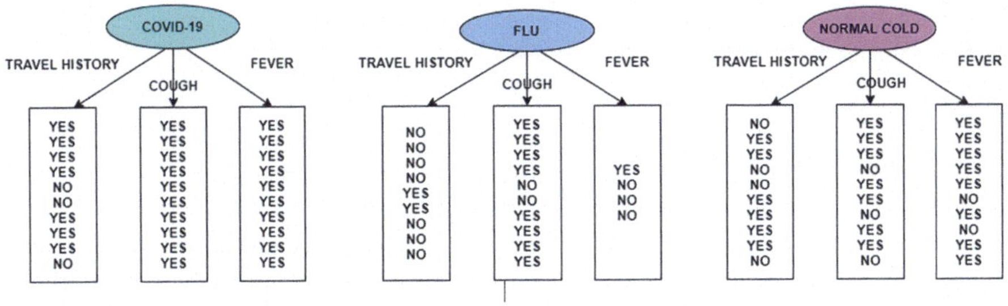

Fig. 2.9 Decision tree based on attribute selection

All the images are compared by the following code, which is well written in MATLAB. This will help us to classify the two different images and help in identifying the difference between the two images. For differentiation, we use X-ray images of a coronavirus-infected person and found that every day the infection is increasing with a growth rate of 4.75%. We are dealing with a limited dataset, and to achieve better and effective result, we use the same images for different comparison algorithm. Every CXR image of the lungs has some difficulties in the exact calculation of results, and these problems may be summarized as ABCDEF [15, 20].

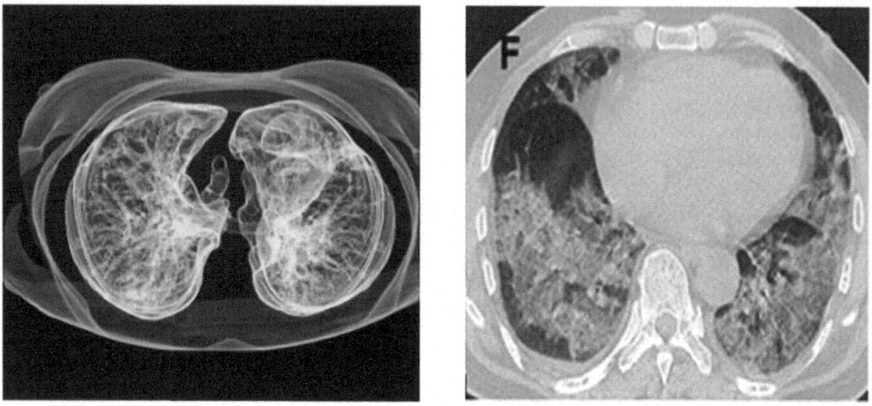

Fig. 2.10 Clinical image of healthy lungs vs infected lungs

- Airways
- Breast shadows (females)
- Bones
- Cardiac outline
- Costophrenic angles
- Diaphragm
- Edges
- Extrathoracic tissues
- Fields (lung parenchyma)
- Failure

Due to all these difficulties, we cannot rely only on CXR images [21]. We need some more accurate and authentic results including CXR images, which will help us in accurate prediction of COVID-19 stage. However, this is not the only problem in testing COVID-19. In every city, basic scanning facilities like CT scan machine and chest X-ray machine are not available especially in rural areas. To save the citizens of countries, governments are performing COVID-19 tests on people.

(c) Main laboratory report and final identification for quarantine: CXR result analysis has some limitations which were described earlier. Testing is also an essential process for a suitable response to the COVID-19 illness [8]. OPD diagnosis allows COVID-19-infected people to know that they are infected or not (first level). The changes in CT scan and lung X-ray shows the second level of diagnosis. People do not know that they suffering from COVID-19 or not. If no, one might stay at home, and others might go for quarantine stage for 14 days. For more accurate results, we require few more laboratory test results of patients infected with COVID-19 on final admission to hospital. However, this is an expensive and time-consuming process (Tables 2.6, 2.7, and 2.8).

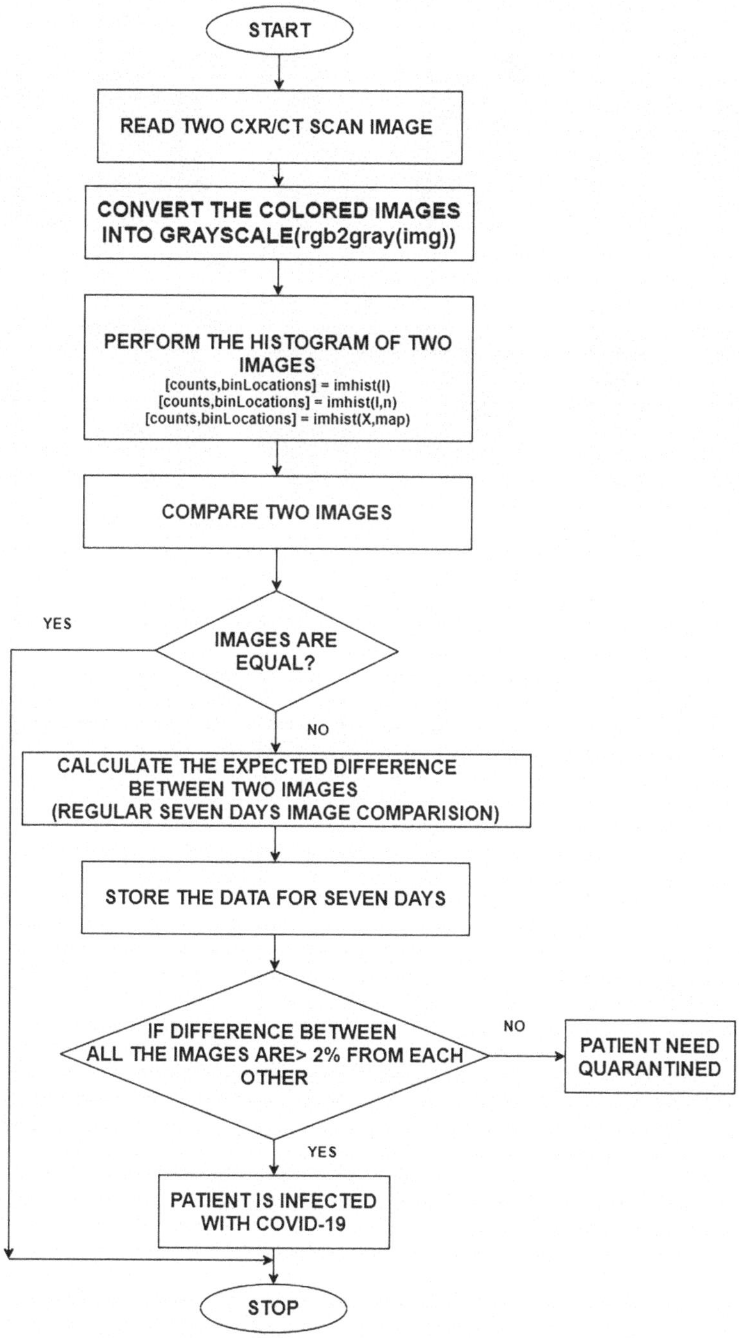

Fig. 2.11 Flowchart for comparison of two images

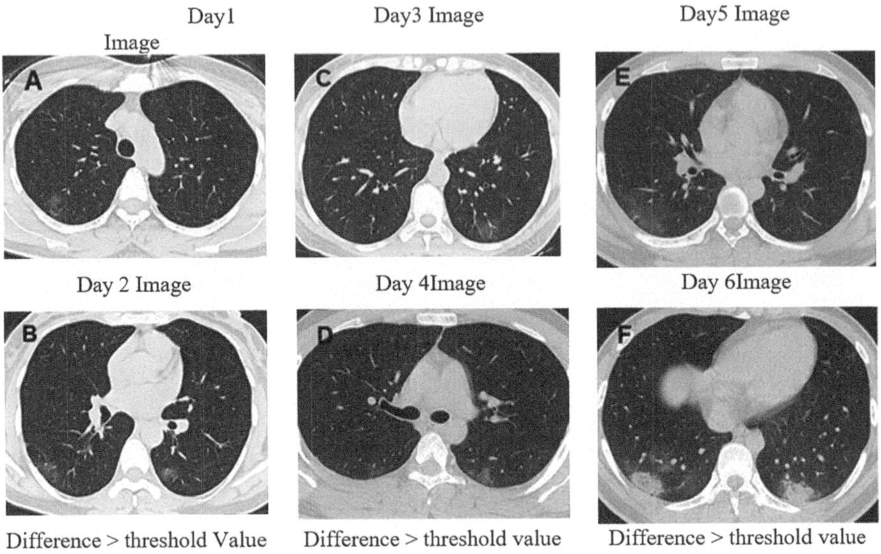

Fig. 2.12 Comparisons of day-wise CXR reports

Table 2.6 First-level clinical data

	Mild/no ICU ($N = 42$)	Severe/ICU ($N = 9$)
First-level data (from Table 2.3)		
COVID-19 RT-PCR test		
SARS-CoV-2 N1	±	±
SARS-CoV-2 N2	±	±
SARS-CoV-2 N3	±	±

2.5 Results

On the basis of above data, we design decision tree for the same. The max_depth of the COVID-19 decision tree is 3. If max_depth = 0, split the nodes. Maximum height indicates over-fitting, and the minimum value indicates under-fitting (Tables 2.9 and 2.10).

The algorithm for calculating accuracy is as follows:

Table 2.7 Second-level clinical data

Previous case history (Based on India Statistical Medical Data)			
Diabetes	No	38	8
	Yes	4	1
Hypertension	No	30	6
	Yes	12	3
Cardiovascular disease	No	35	7
	Yes	7	2
Chronic obstructive	No	38	7
	Yes	4	2
Pulmonary disease	No	34	8
	Yes	8	1
Chronic liver disease	No	41	9
	Yes	1	0
Laboratory report			
White blood cell count, * 10^9/l	(4.5–11.0)	5.85 (3.1–7.6)	11.5 (5.8–12.1)
Neutrophil count,* 10^9/l	(1.5–8.0)	4.5 (2.0–6.1)	10.7 (5.01–11.8)
Lymphocyte count	3000–9500	<4000	<3000
Hemoglobin, g/dl	Male 13.8–17.2	(13.8–15.8)	(11.2–13.0)
	Female 12.1–15.1	(12.3–14.2)	(11.1–13.1)
Platelet count,* 10^9/l		149.0 (131.0–263.0)	196.0 (165.0–263.0)
Prothrombin time, s		10.7 (9.8–12.1)	12.2 (11.2–13.4)
Activated partial thromboplastin time, s		27.7 (24.8–34.1)	26.2 (22.5–33.9)
Albumin, g/l		34.7 (30.2–36.5)	27.9 (26.3–30.9)
Total bilirubin, mmol/l		10.8 (9.4–12.3)	14.0 (11.9–32.9)
Potassium, mmol/l		4.1 (3.8–4.6)	4.6 (4.0–5.0)
Sodium, mmol/l		139.0 (137.5–140.5)	138.0 (137.0–139.0)
Creatinine, μmol/l		73.3 (57.5–84.7)	79.0 (53.1–92.7)
Creatine kinase, u/l		133.0 (61.0–189.0)	132.0 (82.0–493.0)
Lactate dehydrogenase, u/l		281.0 (233.0–357.0)	400.0 (323.0–578.0)
Hypersensitive troponin I, pg/ml		3.5 (0.7–5.4)	3.3 (3.0–163.0)

We have collected medical records relevant to COVID-19 of approximately 5000 patients (source of data is the Internet), and we try to predict it stage
*is the count (150 to 400).

```
# Train Decision Tree Classifer
Step 1: clf = clf.fit(X_train,y_train)
#Predict the response for test dataset
Step 2: y_pred = clf.predict(X_test)
```

```
# Model Accuracy
Step 3: print "ACCURACY:",met.accuracy_score(y_test, y_pred))
```

Correctly classified instances	20	100%
Incorrectly classified instances	0	0
Kappa statistic		1
Mean absolute error		0

Table 2.8 Diagnosis result of COVID-19 patients

S. no	Factor	R1	R2	R3	R4	R5
1	DCXR	1.67%	1.47%	1.42%	1.22%	1.21%
2	Cough	+	+	+	+	−
3	Fever (temperature)	+	+	±	±	±
4	Chest pain	+	+	−	−	−
5	Glucose PP	+	+			
6	Glucose fasting	+	+			
7	Qualitative PCR	+	+	+	+	−
8	SARS-CoV-2 N1	+	+	−	−	−
9	SARS-CoV-2 N2	+	+	−	−	−
10	SARS-CoV-2 N3	+	±	+	−	−
11	RNase P	±	±	±	+	−
		COVID-19 infected	COVID-19 infected	Presumptive positive	SARS-CoV-2 not detected	Invalid results

DCXR Difference between two consecutive CXR
\+ Infected above the range
− Absence
± Value increments or decrement based on recovery

Table 2.9 Detailed accuracy by class of Table 2.7

S. no	TP rate	FP rate	Precision	Recall	F-measure	MCC	ROC area	PRC area	Class
1	1.0	0.0	1.00	1.00	1.00	1.00	1.00	1.00	Infected
2	1.0	0.0	1.00	1.00	1.00	1.00	1.00	1.00	Flu
3	1.0	0.0	1.00	1.00	1.00	1.00	1.00	1.00	Normal cold
	1.0	0.0	1.00	1.00	1.00	1.00	1.00	1.00	

Table 2.10 Confusion matrix of Table 2.5

A	B	C	Classified as
10	0	0	Infected
0	4	0	Flu
0	0	6	Normal cold

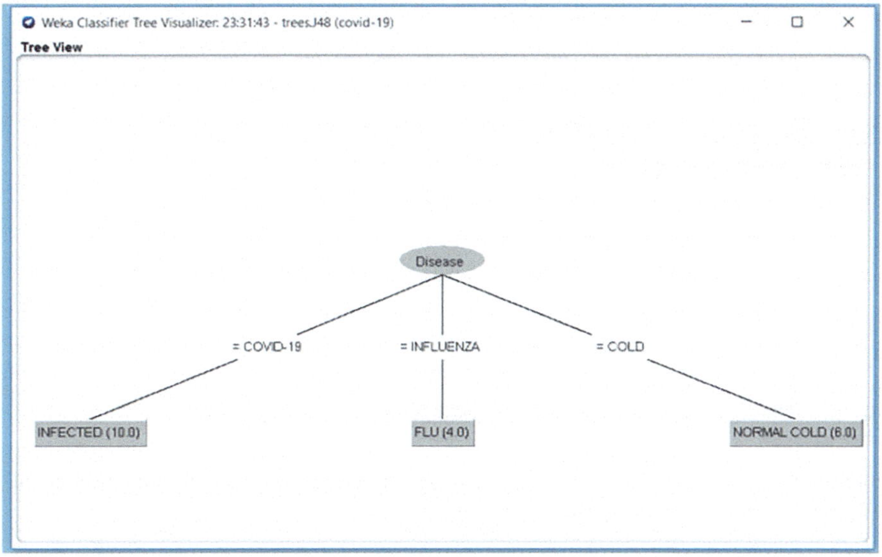

Fig. 2.13 Decision tree using WEKA

Root mean squared error		0
Relative absolute error		0%
Root relative squared error		0%
Total number of instances		20

Accuracy level is 77.53%, which is better for achieving approximation results (Figs. 2.13 and 2.14).

After 100 folds, we found the following difficulties in decision tree method:

1. COVID-19 dataset is changing every minute, and all the predictions are failing, so a small change in data causes a change in complete decision tree.
2. This method involves higher time to train the model.
3. This algorithm is quite complex and expensive, and decision trees are NP-complete (Fig. 2.15).

The estimation of COVID-19 patient can be identified by dividing the death rate by the number of infected patients [22, 23]. The mortality rate is an "estimate of the

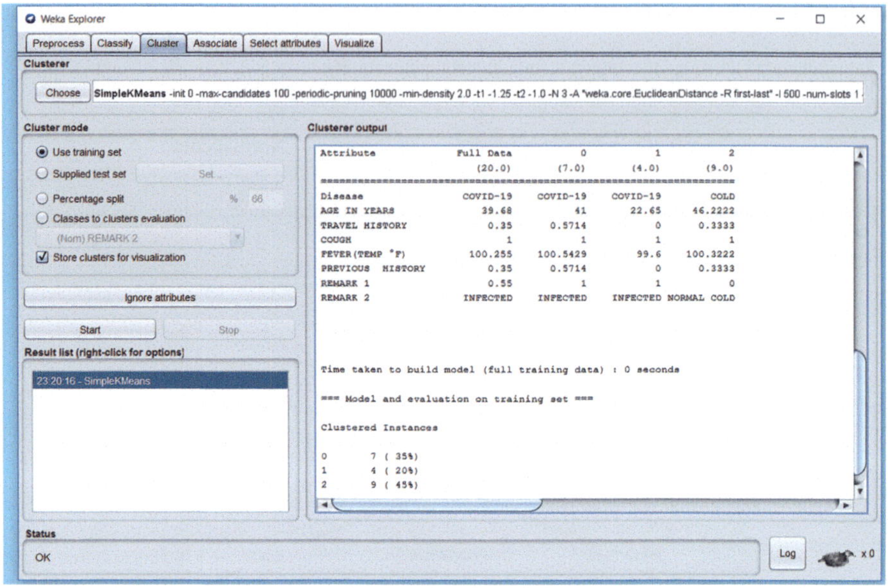

Fig. 2.14 Cluster data using the *K*-means algorithm

portion of a population that dies during a specified period"; case fatality rate is calculated by our approach by the following formula:

$$\text{CFR}(\%) = \frac{\text{No of Death from Disease}}{\text{Noof Diagnosis cases of Disease}} * 100 \tag{2.5}$$

CFR is sometimes different from original data, but crude mortality rate is also called the crude death rate and is accurate, as shown in Fig. 2.16.

Case fatality rate is sometimes called infection fatality rate [22] and calculated as:

$$\text{IFR}(\%) = \frac{\text{No of Death from Disease}}{\text{Noof Diagnosis cases of Disease}} * 100 \tag{2.6}$$

2.6 Conclusion

In this paper, we applied data mining and machine learning techniques to identify the symptoms of COVID-19. Accurate diagnosis of COVID-19 origin can be done significantly for improving influenza surveillance and treatment. Our approach is simple, accurate, and cost-effective. Our paper is based on the analysis of randomly selected data samples available on the Internet and CXR report of patients. Decision tree method helps us in diagnosing the symptoms and helps in the exact calculation of CFR and IFR rate for COVID-19.

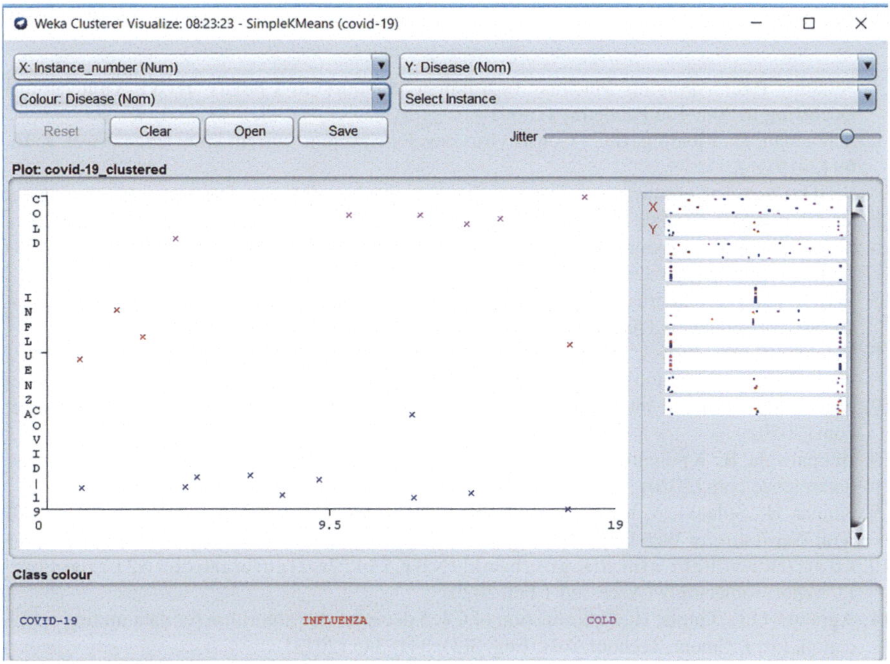

Fig. 2.15 Simple *K*-means clustering

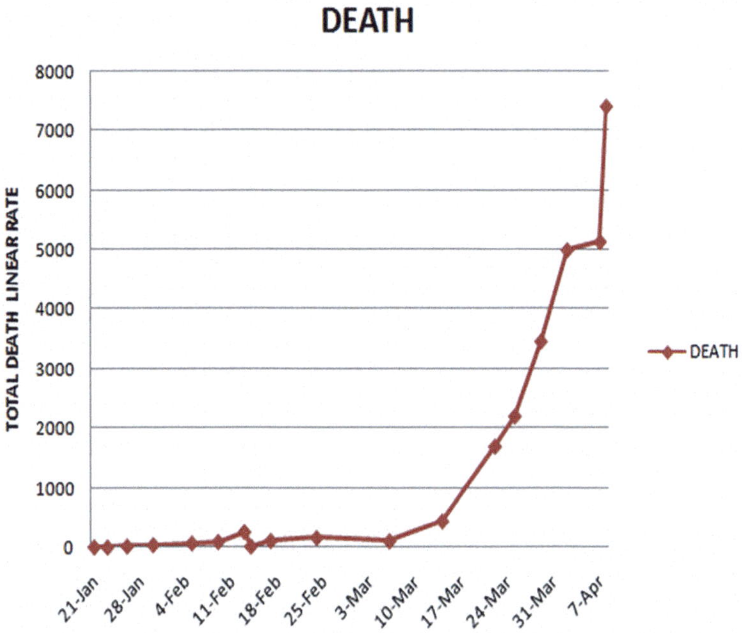

Fig. 2.16 Crude death rate globally (last modified on April 7)

References

1. Attaluri, P.K.: Applying Machine Learning Techniques to Classify H1N1 Viral Strains Occurring in 2009 Flu Pandemic (2009)
2. Schoeman, D., Fielding, B.C.: Coronavirus envelope protein: current knowledge. Virol. J. **16**, 69 (2019)
3. WHO. Novel Coronavirus—China. https://www.who.int/docs/defaultsource/coronaviruse/situation-reports/20200211-sitrep-22-ncov.pdf?sfvrsn=fb6d49b1_2. Accessed 11 Feb 2020
4. https://www.who.int/docs/default-source/coronaviruse/who-china-joint-mission-on-covid-19-final-report.pdf (Accessed 1 Feb 2020)
5. WHO. Novel coronavirus–China (2020). https://www.who.int/csr/don/12-january-2020-novel-coronavirus-china/en/ (Accessed 1 Feb 2020)
6. Virological.org. Novel 2019 coronavirus genome (2020). http://virological.org/t/novel-2019-coronavirus-genome/319 (Accessed 1 Feb 2020)
7. Naudé, W.: Artificial intelligence against COVID-19: an early review. towardsdatascience.com (2020)
8. Bhopalwala, B.: A potential machine learning approach that can help stop COVID-19. towards-datascience.com (2020)
9. Kumar, H., Solanki, A. K., & Singh, K. K. (2020). Progressive Machine Learning Approach with WebAstro for Web Usage Mining. Procedia Computer Science, 167, 1400–1410
10. https://www.ncbi.nlm.nih.gov/books/NBK554776/figure/article-52171.image.f3/?report=objectonly (Accessed 1 Feb 2020)
11. Agrawal, G.L., Gupta, H.: Optimization of C4. 5 decision tree algorithm for data mining application. Int. J. Emerg. Technol. Adv. Eng. **3**(3), 341–345 (2013)
12. Roobaert, D., Karakoulas, G., & Chawla, N. V. (2006). Information gain, correlation and support vector machines. In Feature extraction (pp. 463–470). Springer, Berlin, Heidelberg.
13. LabCorp COVID-19 RT-PCR test EUA summary. https://www.fda.gov/media/136151/download (Accessed 1 Feb 2020)
14. Haque, M., Sartelli, M., McKimm, J., & Bakar, M. A. (2018). Health care-associated infections–an overview. Infection and drug resistance, 11, 2321. https://doi.org/10.2147/IDR.S177247. Published online 2018 Nov 15. PMCID: PMC6245375
15. https://radiopaedia.org/articles/chest-x-ray-abcde-summary (Accessed 1 Feb 2020)
16. Zhu, N., Zhang, D., Wang, W., Li, X., Yang, B., Song, J., ... & Niu, P. (2020). A novel coronavirus from patients with pneumonia in China, 2019. New England Journal of Medicine. https://doi.org/10.1056/NEJMoa2001017
17. Huang, C., Wang, Y., Li, X., Ren, L., Zhao, J., Hu, Y., ... & Cheng, Z. (2020). Clinical features of patients infected with 2019 novel coronavirus in Wuhan, China. The lancet, 395(10223), 497–506. https://doi.org/10.1016/S0140-6736(20)30183-5
18. Maingi, N. N., Lukandu, I. A., & Mwau, M. Comparative Analysis of the C4. 5 and ID3 Decision Tree Algorithms for Disease Symptom Classification and Diagnosis. Int. Res. J. Adv. Eng. Sci. **4**(2), 188–194 (2019) ISSN (Online): 2455–9024
19. Shaukat, K., Masood, N., Mehreen, S., Azmeen, U.: Dengue fever prediction: a data mining problem. J. Data Mining Genomics Proteomics. **6**, 181 (2015). https://doi.org/10.4172/2153-0602.1000181
20. Mettler, F.A., Huda, W., Yoshizumi, T.T., Mahesh, M.: Effective doses in radiology and diagnostic nuclear medicine: a catalog. Radiology. **248**, 254–263 (2008)
21. Yang, R., Li, X., Liu, H., Zhen, Y., Zhang, X., Xiong, Q., ... & Zeng, W. (2020). Chest CT severity score: an imaging tool for assessing severe COVID-19. Radiology: Cardiothoracic Imaging, 2(2), e200047.
22. Spychalski, P., Błażyńska-Spychalska, A., & Kobiela, J. (2020). Estimating case fatality rates of COVID-19. The Lancet. Infectious Diseases. **20**(7), 774–775 (2020). https://doi.org/10.1016/S1473-3099(20)30246-2
23. Baud, D., Qi, X., Nielsen-Saines, K., Musso, D., Pomar, L., & Favre, G. (2020). Real estimates of mortality following COVID-19 infection. The Lancet infectious diseases. Lancet Infect. Dis. **20**(7), 773 (2020). https://doi.org/10.1016/S1473-3099(20)30195-X

Chapter 3
COVID-19 Epidemic Analysis and Prediction Using Machine Learning Algorithms

Arun Solanki and Tarana Singh

Abstract COVID-19 is a real problem, and it is spreading like a forest fire. The data of this pandemic is time-series data. The models that can handle time-series data are the ARIMA model, the Holt-Winter model, the SARIMAX model, polynomial regression, and LSTM. These models have been applied to COVID-19 data, and the results are discussed with significance. This chapter used three types of datasets. The primary dataset is the 2019 Novel Coronavirus COVID-19 (2019-nCoV) Data Repository by Johns Hopkins CSSE (https://github.com/CSSEGISandData/COVID-19). The second dataset is used from Worldometers website (https://www.worldometers.info/), and third is from Kaggle. The SARIMAX model produced 0.236 as the MAPE value, while the Holt-Winter model produced 0.249. The polynomial regression model shows that the accuracy of the model approximated for the tenth day is 85% in the prediction of the number of affected cases and the number of deaths. The LSTM model used the ADAM optimizer and calculated the root mean square error. The prediction error for training is 6.45, and the calculated overall error is 5.34.

Keywords COVID-19 · ARIMA · SARIMAX · Polynomial regression · Long short-term memory · World Health Organization

A. Solanki (✉) · T. Singh
Gautam Buddha University, Greater Noida, India
e-mail: asolanki@gbu.ac.in

© The Author(s), under exclusive license to Springer Nature Switzerland AG 2021

F. Al-Turjman et al. (eds.), *Emerging Technologies for Battling Covid-19*, Studies in Systems, Decision and Control 324,
https://doi.org/10.1007/978-3-030-60039-6_3

3.1 Introduction

The new coronavirus disease 2019 (COVID-19) pandemic started in Wuhan, China, in December 2019 and is a genuine general medical issue around the world. The infection that causes the COVID-19 pandemic is called severe acute respiratory syndrome [1, 2]. Coronaviruses (CoV) are an enormous class of infections that cause sicknesses brought about by cold, for example, the Middle East respiratory syndrome coronavirus (MERS-CoV) and severe acute respiratory syndrome coronavirus (SARS-CoV). The COVID-19 is another species of covid family which found in 2019 [3, 4]. Coronavirus is a zoonotic sickness because of sullying by human creatures. Studies show that the SARS-CoV infection contaminates civet people and the MERS-CoV infection taints dromedary people. The COVID-19 infection is accepted to be contracted by people from bats. Unhealthy respiratory diseases starting with one individual and then onto the next quickly spread the scourge [5, 6]. COVID-19 shows mild to moderate manifestations in about 82% of cases, while different cases are serious or extreme. As per data received on 30th march 2020 from WHO the number of instances of coronavirus was roughly 335,403 of which 14,611 died & 97,636 recovered and rest 223,156 were active cases [3]. While 95% of infected patients live poorly, the remaining 5% suffer from serious or severe illness. Signs of infection include respiratory symptoms, fever, cough, and dyspnoea. In more severe cases, the infection can cause pneumonia, severe acute respiratory syndrome, septic shock, multiple organ failure, and death. The infection rate in men is higher than that in women, and it is determined that no children aged 0–9 die. The respiration rate of COVID-19 pneumonia was shown to be faster compared to healthy people [3, 7, 8]. In many developed countries, the demand for intensive care units is also increasing at the same time, and the medical system is on the verge of collapse [9]. There are many patients in the intensive care unit with exacerbated COVID-19 pneumonia. The World Health Organization reports that the pandemic situation is divided into four stages. The first stage begins with a case reported about people traveling to the affected area, while the second stage is reported locally by family, friends, and other people in contact with other affected areas [10]. Currently, what is affected can be tracked. The situation worsened in the third stage, after which the cause of the infection became untraceable and was transmitted to people who had never travelled or who had no contact with the infected person. In this situation, an immediate national blockade is needed to reduce social contact between individuals and control the rate of infection. Figure 3.1 shows that the WHO detailed that COVID-19 happened in countless affirmed cases in the USA, Italy, Spain, and China. To top it all off, stage 4 gets pervasive and wild [11–13]. Figure 3.2 shows all phases of the COVID-19 epidemic. So far, some countries have entered the fourth stage. China is the primary nation to encounter the fourth phase of COVID-19 infection. However, the source of the infection is accepted to be Wuhan in China which affects the other developed nations (the USA, Italy, Spain, the UK, etc.). These nations are presently in the fourth phase of contamination and face a larger number of diseases and deaths than China [14–16]. In China, the exponential increase in

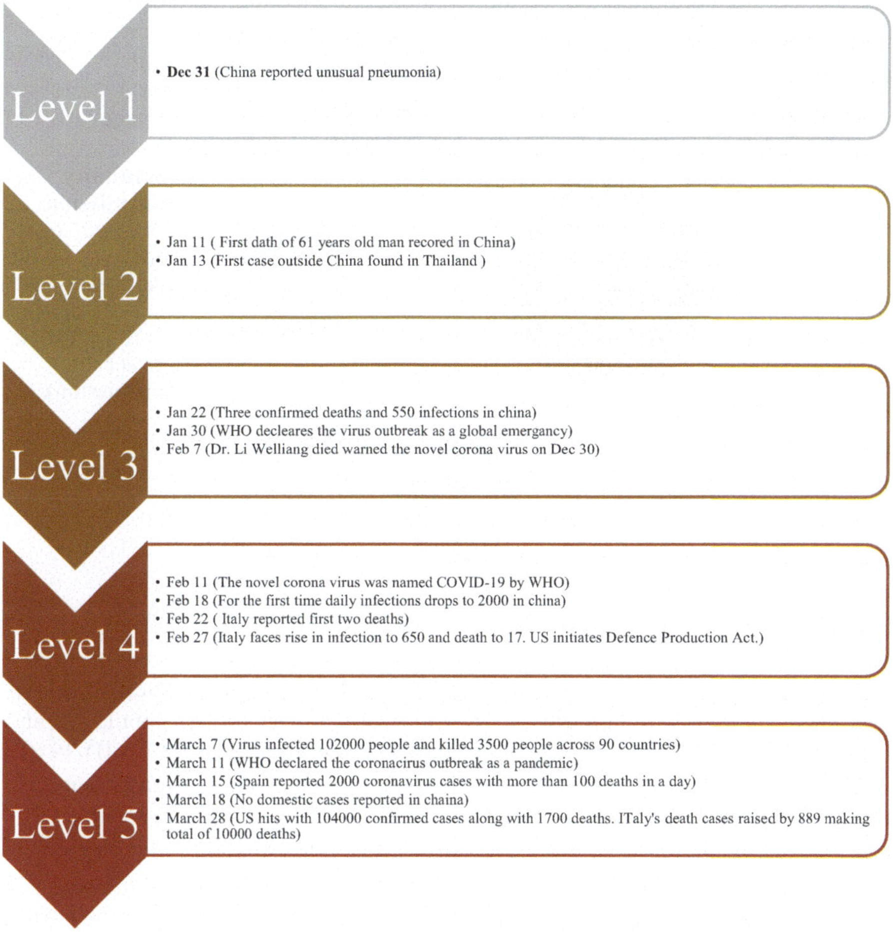
Level 1
• Dec 31 (China reported unusual pneumonia)
Level 2
• Jan 11 (First dath of 61 years old man recored in China)
• Jan 13 (First case outside China found in Thailand)
Level 3
• Jan 22 (Three confirmed deaths and 550 infections in china)
• Jan 30 (WHO decleares the virus outbreak as a global emergancy)
• Feb 7 (Dr. Li Welliang died warned the novel corona virus on Dec 30)
Level 4
• Feb 11 (The novel corona virus was named COVID-19 by WHO)
• Feb 18 (For the first time daily infections drops to 2000 in china)
• Feb 22 (Italy reported first two deaths)
• Feb 27 (Italy faces rise in infection to 650 and death to 17. US initiates Defence Production Act.)
Level 5
• March 7 (Virus infected 102000 people and killed 3500 people across 90 countries)
• March 11 (WHO declared the coronacirus outbreak as a pandemic)
• March 15 (Spain reported 2000 coronavirus cases with more than 100 deaths in a day)
• March 18 (No domestic cases reported in chaina)
• March 28 (US hits with 104000 confirmed cases along with 1700 deaths. ITaly's death cases raised by 889 making total of 10000 deaths)

Fig. 3.1 Timeline of COVID-19 across the nations in different levels

confirmed cases reached a saturation point, at which point the number of cases stopped increasing. This is due to the fact that the number of susceptible people exposed to the virus is significantly reduced [17]. It is possible to isolate infected people and reduce social contact between them, and the Chinese government has begun a period of complete blockade, thereby reducing the likelihood of further transmission.

Machine learning algorithms [18–22] play an important role in epidemiological analysis and prediction. Machine learning techniques can help mitigate epidemic patterns when large amounts of epidemiological data are present [23–25]. Therefore, you can take early steps to prevent the spread of the virus. This study used real-time information from the Johns Hopkins dashboard to observe the daily behaviour of domestic COVID-19 and predict future accessibility using machine learning and deep learning models. Since the Spanish flu epidemic in the early twentieth century,

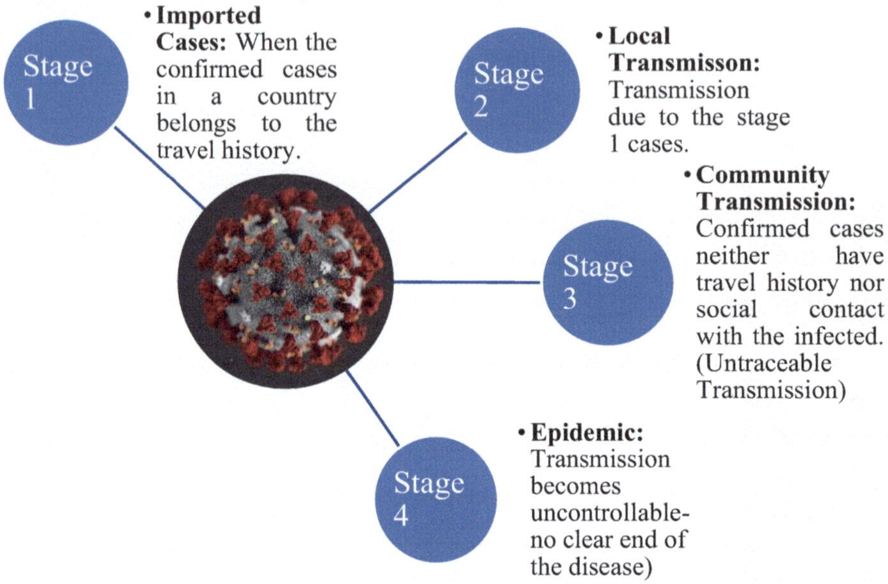

Fig. 3.2 Complete transmission stages of COVID-19

the COVID-19 pandemic is the largest pandemic, affecting approximately three million people worldwide. Pandemics have a serious impact on the population and economy of many countries. From a machine learning perspective, COVID-19 can easily be considered a random forest when mapping diseases or viruses that have recently affected human species to the decision tree. The spread of this deadly virus is unimaginable, but it is not impossible to calculate. It is therefore of great interest to be able to model this epidemiological data and provide information and better adaptation strategies to contain the effects of the virus. That is good for the people and the economy of the country [26–29]. This study uses existing data and various machine learning models to try to predict the epidemiologic spread of the virus in India [30].

The whole chapter is organized in five different sections. Section 3.1 contains the introduction. In Sect. 3.2, related work is discussed briefly. In Sect. 3.3, different models have been discussed. In Sect. 3.4, results analysis has been done. Section 3.5 discusses the final conclusion and future work.

3.2 Related Work

Over the past decade, digital technology has played a key role in key issues in the health sector, including disease prevention, and today's global health emergencies also seek technical support to resolve COVID-19. In the article, the author highlighted in trendy digital technologies, for example, the Internet of Things (IoT), big data analytics, artificial intelligence (AI), deep learning, and technology. Blockchain is being created to screen, distinguish, and forestall scourges and decide the materialness of the technique and the effect of the epidemic on the health sector [9].

In a study, Benvenuto et al. [10] proposed an autoregressive integrated moving average (ARIMA) model for foreseeing the spread of COVID-19. In light of an investigation of the predominance and frequency of COVID-19, the author anticipated different boundaries throughout the following 2 days of his article. The examination additionally indicated correlation maps of epidemic incidence and prevalence and ARIMA prediction maps. Authors [11] proposed a time-series method to dissect the occurrence model and evaluated duplicate number of the COVID-19 pestilence. Having directed factual examination, talked about scourge drifts, and featured the current epidemio-intelligent phase of the district, various arrangements can be chosen to react to COVID-19 pandemics in various areas. In the current circumstance, it is important to comprehend the early methods of contamination so as to plan and screen viable security measures. Authors proposed a significant logical model of the spread of SARS-CoV-2 utilizing different informational collections to examine COVID-19 episodes since Wuhan. In this way, they investigated the potential for outbreaks of the disease outside Wuhan [12]. Several studies have recently been conducted on the epidemiology of COVID-19 using exploratory data analysis (EDA) based on the different datasets available. These studies focus primarily on cases of diagnosis, death, and rehabilitation in Wuhan and other parts of the world to understand the plans for suspicious threats and subsequent containment activities [13]. The study by Lauer et al. raised the important question of COVID-19 latency. They investigated 181 confirmed cases, determined that the incubation period varied from 5 to 14 days, and planned better surveillance and surveillance activities accordingly [14]. In a recent study, Singer analysed data from 25 affected counties to track short-term forecasts for the COVID-19 epidemic. In this study, where there is a disease-specific infection rate, the exponential law differs according to the regular or explosive growth of the exponential law. Based on this understanding, the author analyses the effects of blockades in the world [15]. Traditionally, mathematical modelling has been used epidemiologically to model viruses and infectious diseases. The compartment model is one of these models. The most popular model is the SIR model (S stands for susceptibility, I represents infectious dose, and R represents the number of individuals who recovered or died (or immunized)). However, the authors believe that by leveraging the large amount of data currently available, machine learning can provide better predictions [24].

Based on the literature above, it is clear that exploratory data analysis can do a good job of understanding current trends in the epidemic, but there is still plenty of development and room for development. Test effective predictive models based on machine learning so that you can adopt active strategies. Make sure it meets your current needs.

3.3 Model Discussions

The study compares the predictions of multiple different models. These include the traditional statistical time-series forecasting models like ARIMA, SERIMAX, and Holt-Winter's exponential smoothing model [31–33]. Another approach is to use machine learning-based regression models. To demonstrate this approach, the study uses a regularized regression model—the ridge regression model. Deep learning is another exciting new field of research in machine learning [34–36]. Since the data in question is time series or sequential, it is not possible to model it using traditional feed-forward neural networks that do not have any concept of time [37–39]. Recurrent neural networks (RNN) are neural networks that have a feedback loop that enables them to model sequential data. Long short-term memory (LSTM) is a more developed form of a recurrent neural network that utilizes the concept of attention and has been shown to provide better results than RNNs in many applications [40–42]. An LSTM-based approach has also been used to predict the COVID 19 spread in this study [43–46].

3.3.1 Ridge Regression

The study is using a dataset prepared by the Johns Hopkins University Centre for Systems Science and Engineering (JHU CSSE) and the crowdsourced data from the Covid19india.org tracker [47, 48]. The study first discussed the nature of epidemic growth and analyses the initial exponential growth of the virus and calculates the growth ratio and growth factor of the epidemic for the case of India. The study also makes predictions for the expected number of cumulative confirmed cases using a ridge regression model and uses the growth factor and growth as features in this model [49–52].

3.3.1.1 Initial Exponential Epidemic Growth

Epidemics initially follow exponential growth due to the nature of viruses where the people infected with a virus in turn infect others. This growth is measured using a positive constant called the growth factor of the epidemic [53]. However, this exponential growth is not sustained throughout the epidemic, due to factors like intervention, a large portion of the population getting infected, etc., and starts to stabilize at a growth factor of 1 before gradually decreasing [54, 55]. This point is known as the Inflection point for a curve and can be visualized using a logistic curve. The study observes this phenomenon in the graph of the growth of the virus in China, as shown in Fig. 3.3.

Comparing this with the growth of COVID 19 in India as of April 22, shown in Fig. 3.4, it can be seen that the virus is still in the initial stages.

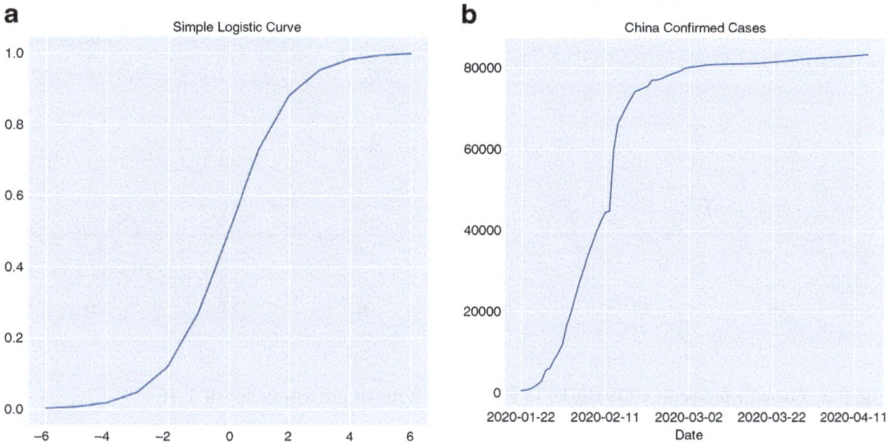

Fig. 3.3 (**a**) A simple logistic curve and (**b**) exponential growth of COVID 19 in China

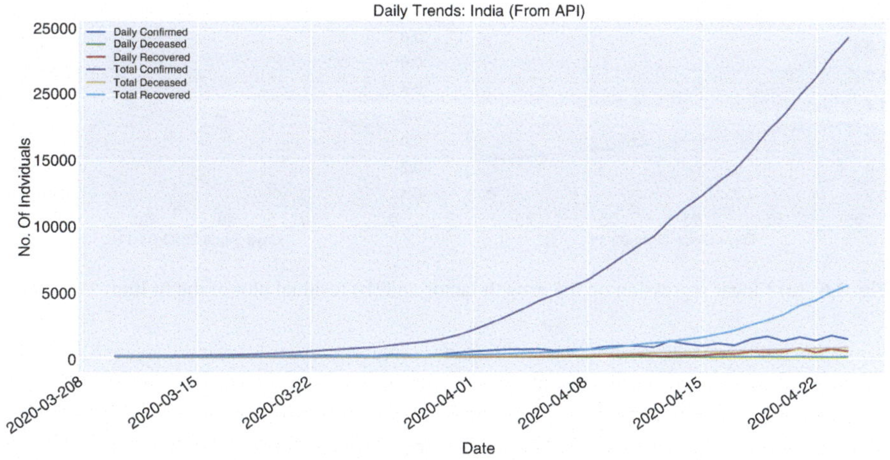

Fig. 3.4 COVID-19 statistics in India as of April 22, 2020

The question now becomes whether the growth of the virus has reached the inflection point. This can be analysed using the growth factor [56].

3.3.1.2 Growth Factor

The growth factor is a constant factor by which the total cases would be multiplied in the case of exponential growth. The growth factor on day N is the number of confirmed cases on day N minus confirmed cases on day $N - 1$ divided by the

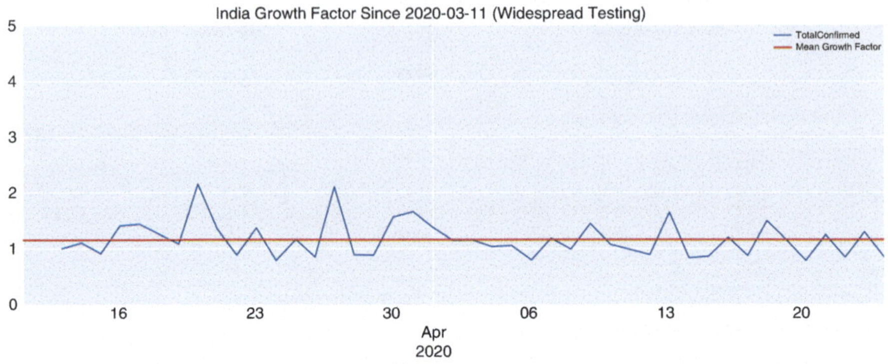

Fig. 3.5 Growth factor of COVID-19 in India with a mean growth factor of 1.16

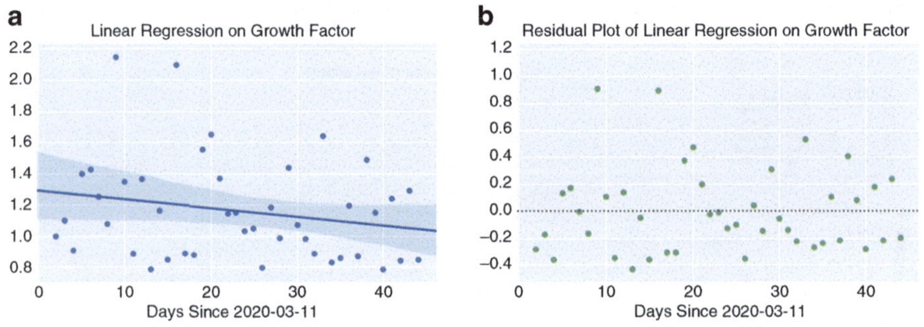

Fig. 3.6 (**a**) Linear regression on the growth factor and (**b**) residual plot of the fit line

number of confirmed cases on day $N-1$ minus confirmed cases on day $N-2$. It is a measure of whether the spread of the virus is growing or not [57]. A value of greater than 1 is associated with growth, and values of less than 1 are associated with decline. A growth factor of 1 is the inflection point, and at this point, the spread is not growing. Figure 3.5 shows the updated growth factor of the virus in India. As of April 24, the growth factor for the last 10 days is around 1.05, and it can be seen that the growth of the virus has not stabilized at the inflection point but is much lower than the mean growth factor up to this point indicating that the initial exponential growth might be over [58].

A linear regression on the growth factor points to a downward trend, but the margin of error is high as defined by a 95% confidence interval, shown in Fig. 3.6.

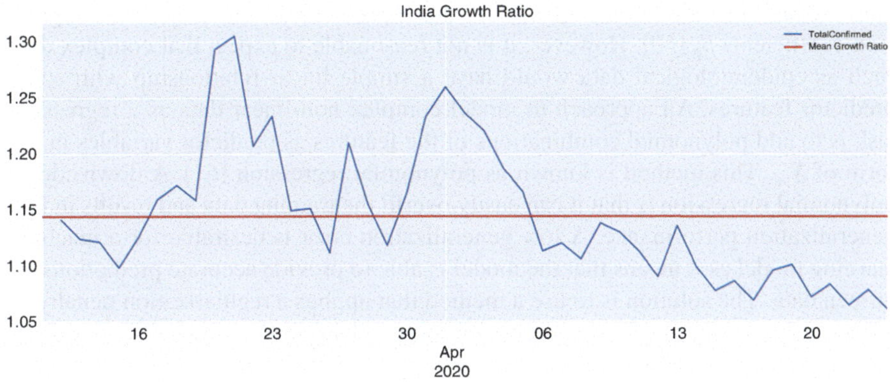

Fig. 3.7 Growth ratio of COVID-19 in India with a mean growth ratio of 1.14

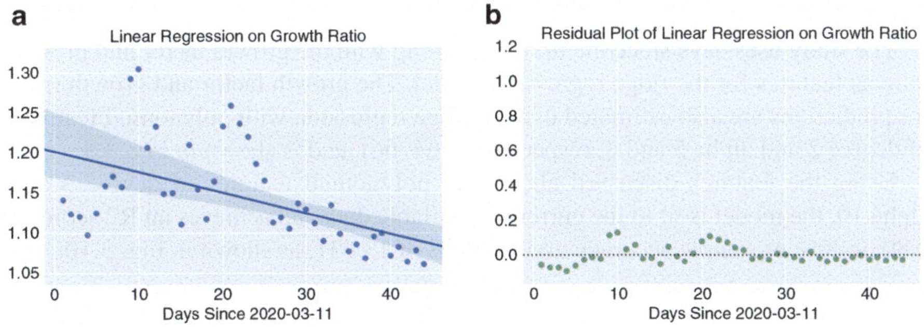

Fig. 3.8 (**a**) Linear regression on the growth ratio and (**b**) residual plot of the regression line

3.3.1.3 Growth Ratio of Virus

The growth ratio on day N is the number of confirmed cases on day N divided by the number of confirmed cases on day $N - 1$ [59]. Looking at the graph in Fig. 3.7, there is an unmistakable downward trend to the growth ratio, with a 6% growth in the number of cases occurring on April 24 compared to highs of 25–30% since the start of reliable testing. After performing a linear regression on the growth ratio, a strong downward trend can be seen in Fig. 3.8a, and in Fig. 3.8b, a linear relationship can be seen in the residual plot confirming that such an assumption is reasonable.

3.3.2 Regularized Ridge Regression

The approach discussed here attempts to model the spread of COVID-19 as a regression problem. A linear regression model in machine learning attempts to model the target or dependent variable Y, the total number of confirmed cases of COVID-19 in this case, as a linear relationship between some predictor features X_p and the regression coefficients β_p [60]. However, it is not reasonable to expect that complex data such as epidemiological data would have a simple linear relationship with some predictor features. An approach to model complex non-linear data as a regression task is to add polynomial combinations of the features as predictor variables in the form of X_{pd}. This method is known as polynomial regression [61]. A downside of polynomial regression is that it can easily overfit the training data and results in low generalization performance. A low generalization error is desirable for a machine learning model as it means that the model is able to provide accurate predictions on unseen data. The solution is to use a method that applies a regularization penalty to reduce this overfitting. Ridge regression applies half of the squared l2 norms of model parameters as a regularization term or penalty to reduce overfitting and improve generalization performance [62]. This penalty is controlled using the hyperparameter alpha and reduces in-sample training accuracy but will help the model generalize better in the absence of a large number of features and training data [63].

The study uses days since the first case, along with the growth factor and growth ratio as features for the ridge regression model. The growth factor and growth ratio for predictions are also estimated using a ridge regression with polynomial features of degree 2 and alpha 5 and 2, respectively [64–66], and is shown in Fig. 3.9.

Using the features discussed above and polynomial features of degree 3 and alpha 10, the model is fit to the currently available data and achieves an R2 score of 0.80 or 80% in-sample accuracy and an MSE of 13,631, as shown in Fig. 3.10.

3.3.3 LSTM Model

LSTM is an RNN architecture which contains memory, i.e. it remembers the state of the model at different stages. It is most suited for time-series prediction when the time gap length is unknown [54]. Thus, LSTM can be proved to be the well-suited

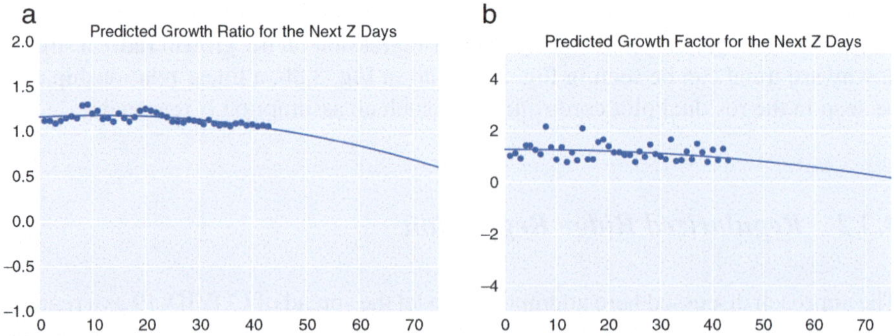

Fig. 3.9 Predicted (**a**) growth ratio and (**b**) growth factor for use with ridge regression to predict COVID-19 cases

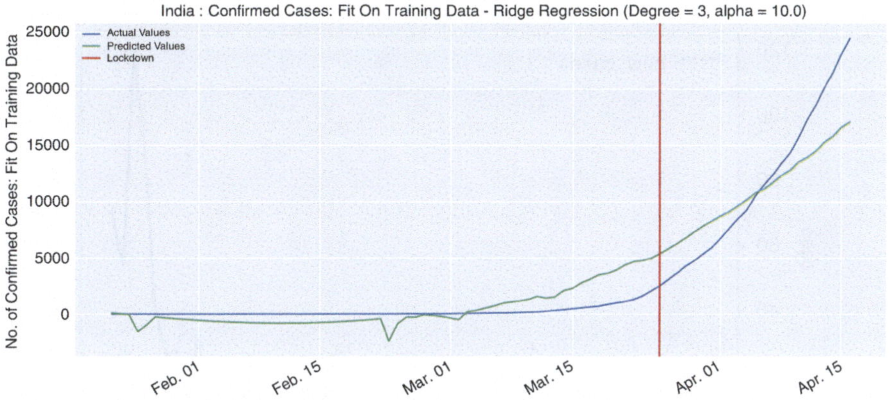

Fig. 3.10 Ridge regression model fit on the training data

date	new_cases	new_deaths	total_cases	total_deaths
2019-12-31	0	0	0	0
2020-01-01	0	0	0	0
2020-01-02	0	0	0	0
2020-01-03	0	0	0	0
2020-01-04	0	0	0	0

Fig. 3.11 Dataset depicting various parameters of COVID-19 spread in India

model for the COVID-19 spread in the world. This section investigates and estimates the number of new cases in India as compared to all over the world. The dataset is taken from Kaggle which contains four columns which are new_cases, new_deaths, total_cases, and total_deaths. The dataset contains the country-wise data describing the above columns for each country on an everyday basis. The data is available from December 31, 2019, to March 25, 2020. The dataset for India is depicted in Fig. 3.11.

The number of actual cases based on new cases can be represented by a graph shown in Fig. 3.12. The number of new cases depends upon the number of active cases, as this pandemic is communicable and spreads from an infected person. Thus, the greater the number of active cases, the greater the number of new cases. The growth rate of actual cases, therefore, becomes exponential.

- Training the model: The model is built to train the dataset in order to predict the number of new cases which can be infected by COVID-19 based on the data provided. The LSTM model is a recurrent neural network whose architecture is shown in Fig. 3.13.

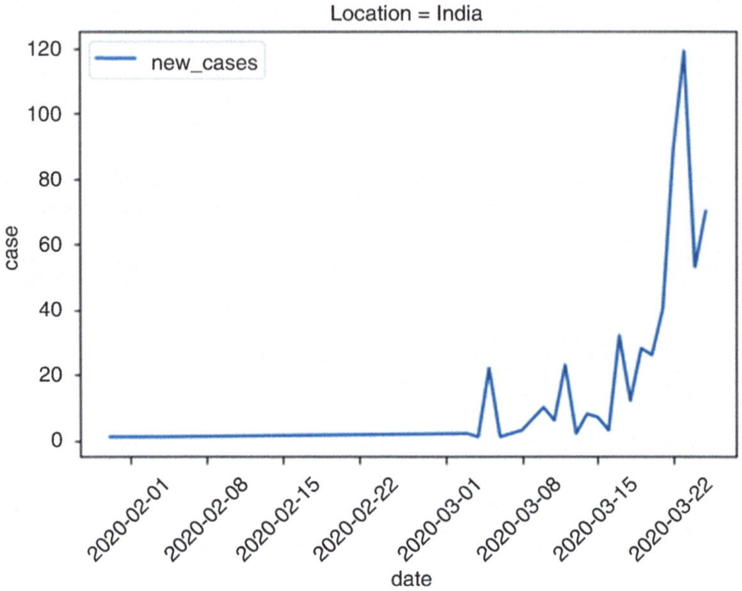

Fig. 3.12 New cases based on actual cases in India

```
Model: "sequential_1"
_________________________________________________________________
Layer (type)                 Output Shape              Param #
=================================================================
lstm_1 (LSTM)                (1, 1, 4)                 96
_________________________________________________________________
lstm_2 (LSTM)                (1, 1)                    24
_________________________________________________________________
dense_1 (Dense)              (1, 1)                    2
=================================================================
Total params: 122
Trainable params: 122
Non-trainable params: 0
_________________________________________________________________
```

Fig. 3.13 Model architecture

The model is trained on the dataset for 2000 iterations in each epoch. A total of 16 epochs were run for complete training. The training loss came out to be 0.0081. The loss during the training is shown in Fig. 3.14.

3.3.4 SARIMA Model

The SARIMA model stands for seasonal autoregressive integrated moving average or seasonal ARIMA and belongs to the family of the ARIMA model. It is an extension of the ARIMA model which deals with the univariate time-series data

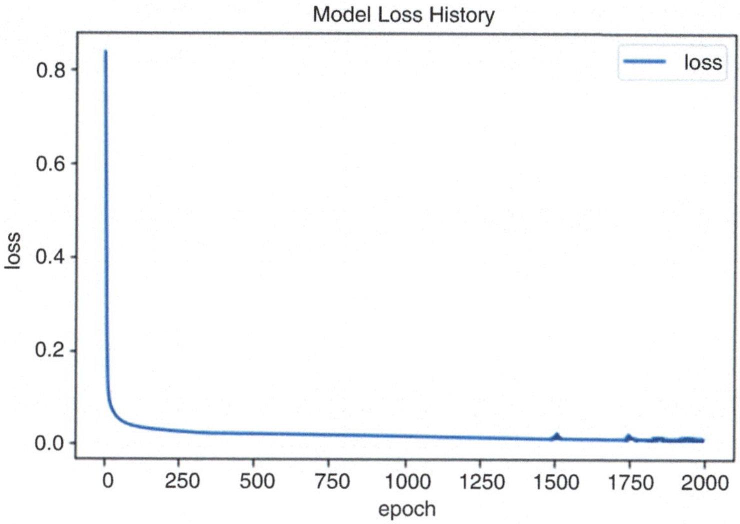

Fig. 3.14 Training loss history

	Deaths	Confirmed_cases	Recovered_cases
1/22/20	0.0	0.0	0.0
1/23/20	0.0	0.0	0.0
1/24/20	0.0	0.0	0.0
1/25/20	0.0	0.0	0.0
1/26/20	0.0	0.0	0.0
1/27/20	0.0	0.0	0.0
1/28/20	0.0	0.0	0.0
1/29/20	0.0	0.0	0.0
1/30/20	0.0	1.0	0.0
1/31/20	0.0	1.0	0.0

Fig. 3.15 Dataset for COVID-19 spread in India

containing the seasonality component. It adds three new hyperparameters to specify the autoregression (AR), differencing (I), and moving average (MA) for the seasonal component of the series, as well as an additional parameter for the period of the seasonality. The SARIMAX model is nothing but a SARIMA model having an exogenous variable represented by *X*. This work is an attempt to calculate the rate of spread of this virus and thus to predict the deaths, recoveries, and confirmed cases, so that it may help us to prepare better and survive. The dataset used in this research work is the 2019 Novel Coronavirus COVID-19 (2019-nCoV) Data

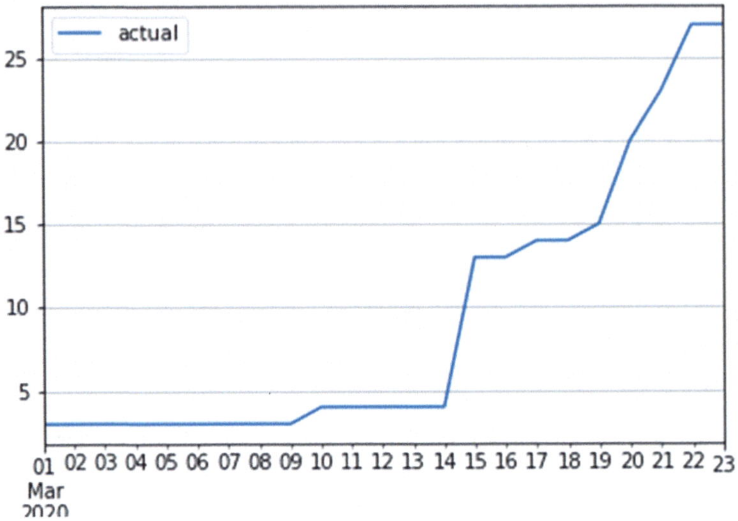

Fig. 3.16 Trend line for recovered cases

Repository by Johns Hopkins CSSE (https://github.com/CSSEGISandData/COVID-19). As the dataset used had trend and seasonality in it, the models that have been used here are the SARIMAX model and the Holt-Winter model. Figure 3.15 displays the values for deaths, confirmed cases, and recovered cases for India.

This is no news that COVID-19 has turned into a pandemic because it is communicable and can spread by the medium of contact.

It means that the number of new cases or future cases is in one way or another related to the present cases. This is a prime reason why the past data can be tuned into a machine learning model and then use it to predict new cases. There is an upward trend in the dataset which can be observed from graphical representation of the data. One such representation has been displayed in Fig. 3.16.

- Model Training: The model is trained on a time period ranging from January 22, 2020, to March 23, 2020. A summary of the training is displayed in Fig. 3.17 in order to understand the various parameters of training.

The stationarity of the time series was checked with the help of augmented Dickey-Fuller test, and the p-value for different datasets (deaths, recovered, and confirmed) lied in the range of 0.00–0.07.

Statespace Model Results

Dep. Variable:	Recovered	No. Observations:	62
Model:	SARIMAX(0, 1, 0)x(1, 1, 1, 12)	Log Likelihood	-95.992
Date:	Sun, 10 May 2020	AIC	197.984
Time:	16:33:53	BIC	203.659
Sample:	01-22-2020	HQIC	200.137
	- 03-23-2020		
Covariance Type:	opg		

	coef	std err	z	P>|z|	[0.025	0.975]
ar.S.L12	0.0469	28.257	0.002	0.999	-55.336	55.430
ma.S.L12	-0.1626	28.304	-0.006	0.995	-55.637	55.312
sigma2	2.9353	0.205	14.314	0.000	2.533	3.337

Ljung-Box (Q):	29.54	Jarque-Bera (JB):	461.04
Prob(Q):	0.89	Prob(JB):	0.00
Heteroskedasticity (H):	14.20	Skew:	3.33
Prob(H) (two-sided):	0.00	Kurtosis:	16.47

Fig. 3.17 Model fit summary for recovered cases

3.4 Result and Discussion

3.4.1 Scenario 1: Ridge Regression—Regularized Regression Model

Using the model to predict the total confirmed cases, we see a maximum or plateau of 140,000 confirmed cases before the total number of active cases starts to slow down around the middle of September. This is shown in Fig. 3.18. The predictions also indicate that the inflection point of the virus will be reached around July. The results appear to follow similar curves when compared to China and Italy. Upon observation the middle portion of the graph corresponding to slowing growth and the crossover to the inflection point seems prolonged. This can be due to a lack of features in the training data and the high predictive power of the days since the first case feature. It is a shortcoming of the model and is basis for future work.

3.4.2 Scenario 2: LSTM Model

This data is trained by using the LSTM model. The error is calculated using root mean square error, and the optimizer used is ADAM. The prediction error for training came out to be 6.45, and the overall calculated error is calculated to be 5.34. The number of new cases of people infected with coronavirus is predicted by the LSTM model, which gave the results as shown in Fig. 3.19.

The comparative study of the predicted cases as compared to the actual cases in India is shown in Fig. 3.20. This is done to estimate the accuracy of the model.

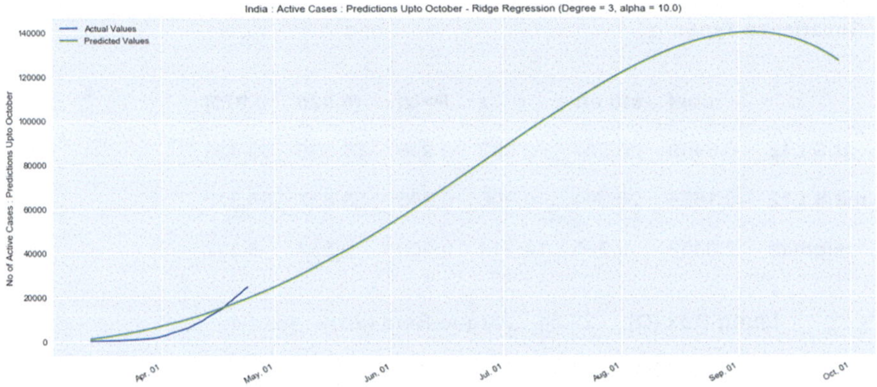

Fig. 3.18 Predictions for coronavirus cases in India using ridge regression

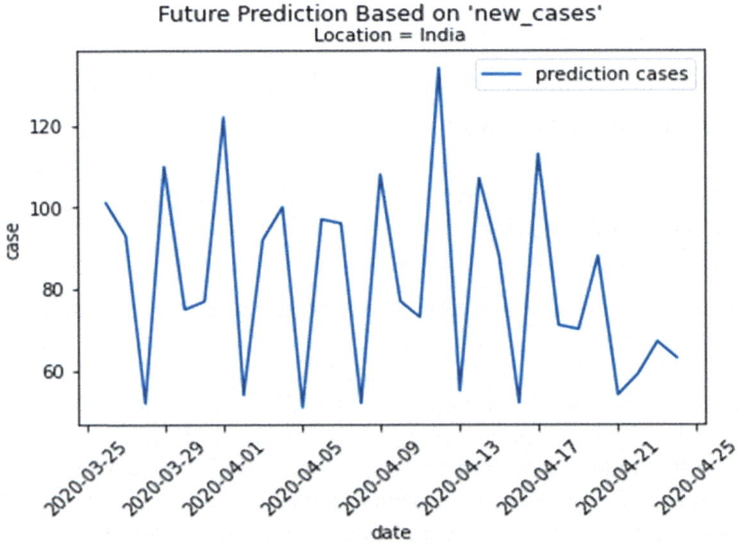

Fig. 3.19 Future prediction of the number of new cases

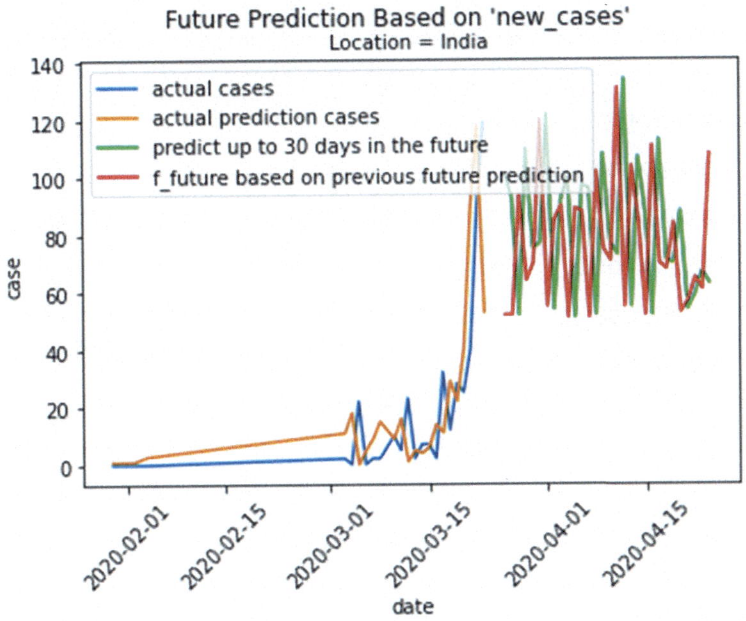

Fig. 3.20 Future prediction of new cases

3.4.3 Scenario 3: SARIMA Model

The model has then been used in order to make predictions for deaths and confirmed and recovered cases for the time period of April 1, 2020, to April 23, 2020. These predictions have been depicted in Fig. 3.21. Mean absolute percentage error (MAPE) has been used to measure the accuracy of predictions made by the model. MAPE is inversely proportional to the accuracy of a model, i.e. the higher the value of MAPE, the lower is the model accuracy and vice versa (Fig. 3.22).

3.5 Conclusion

The conclusion is divided according to the model discussed in the chapter, i.e. regression, LSTM, and SARIMA models.

	Deaths	Confirmed_cases	Recovered_cases
2020-04-01	10	10	41
2020-04-02	9	9	43
2020-04-03	11	11	47
2020-04-04	11	11	47
2020-04-05	11	11	47
2020-04-06	12	12	47
2020-04-07	12	12	47
2020-04-08	12	12	55
2020-04-09	12	12	55
2020-04-10	13	13	56
2020-04-11	13	13	56
2020-04-12	14	14	57
2020-04-13	15	15	61
2020-04-14	14	14	64
2020-04-15	16	16	67

Fig. 3.21 The predicted values for confirmed cases, deaths and recovered cases

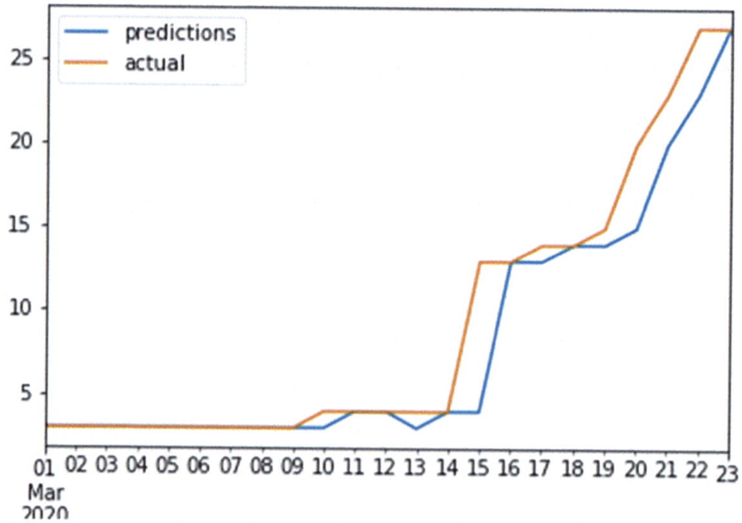

Fig. 3.22 Predicted vs actual value for recovered cases

3.5.1 Regression

The study has analysed the growth of COVID-19 in India and performed ridge regression to predict the growth of cases in the country. The model is fit to the currently available data with an R2 score of 0.80 or 80% in-sample accuracy. The analysis of the results shows that the growth of the virus has still not stabilized, and the expected total cases are 140,000 by the middle of September. The total active cases are expected to decrease after this point. The lack of features to fit the model on is a limitation of the study and an opportunity for future work.

3.5.2 LSTM

The study has analysed the growth of COVID-19 in India and used the LSTM model to predict the number of new cases in the country. The analysis of the results shows that the growth of the virus has still not stabilized, and the expected total cases will be 2000 new cases every day by the end of July. The extension of relaxation in lockdown will greatly affect the spread of this pandemic.

3.5.3 SARIMA

The predictions made by model have the MAPE value ranging between 0.38 and 0.08 for different cases. The COVID-19 virus is spreading like a forest fire, and if sufficient measures are not taken, it could get out of hand. The various parameters of the SARIMA(X) model, like the seasonal order, etc., can be tweaked to decrease the MAPE value and make more accurate predictions.

References

1. Stoecklin, S.B., Rolland, P., Silue, Y., Mailles, A., Campese, C., Simondon, A., Mechain, M., et al.: First cases of coronavirus disease 2019 (COVID-19) in France: surveillance, investigations and control measures, January 2020. Euro Surveill. **25**(6), 2000094 (2020)
2. Github repository. 2019 Novel Coronavirus COVID-19 (2019-nCoV) Data Repository by Johns Hopkins CSSE. https://github.com/CSSEGISandData/COVID-19. Accessed 31 Mar 2020
3. WHO coronaviruses (COVID-19). https://www.who.int/emergencies/diseases/novel-coronavirus-2019. Accessed 30 Mar 2020
4. Prasad, S., Potdar, V., Cherian, S., Abraham, P., Basu, A.: Transmission electron microscopy imaging of SARS-CoV-2. Indian J. Med. Res. **151**, 241–243 (2020)
5. Leppard, G.G.: Evaluation of electron microscope techniques for the description of aquatic colloids. In: Environmental Particles, pp. 231–289. CRC Press, Boca Raton (2019)

6. Jia, L., Li, K., Jiang, Y., Guo, X.: Prediction and analysis of coronavirus disease 2019. arXiv preprint arXiv:2003.05447 (2020)
7. Kalipe, G., Gautham, V., Behera, R.K.: Predicting malarial outbreak using machine learning and deep learning approach: a review and analysis. In: 2018 International Conference on Information Technology (ICIT), pp. 33–38. IEEE (2018)
8. Singh, R., Singh, R., Bhatia, A.: Sentiment analysis using machine learning technique to predict outbreaks and epidemics. Int. J. Adv. Sci. Res. **3**(2), 19–24 (2018)
9. Ting, D.S.W., Carin, L., Dzau, V., Wong, T.Y.: Digital technology and COVID-19. Nat. Med. **26**(4), 459–461 (2020)
10. Benvenuto, D., Giovanetti, M., Vassallo, L., Angeletti, S., Ciccozzi, M.: Application of the ARIMA model on the COVID-2019 epidemic dataset. Data in brief (2020): 105340. It is made available under a CC-BY-NC-ND 4.0 International license . (which was not certified by peer review) is the author/funder, who has granted medRxiv a license to display the preprint in perpetuity. medRxiv preprint. https://doi.org/10.1101/2020.04.08.20057679. This version posted April 11, 2020. The copyright holder for this preprint 10 Narinder Singh Punn et al
11. Deb, S., Majumdar, M.: A time series method to analyze incidence pattern and estimate reproduction number of COVID-19. arXiv preprint arXiv:2003.10655 (2020)
12. Kucharski, A.J., Russell, T.W., Diamond, C., Yang, L., Edmunds, J., Funk, S., Eggo, R.M., et al.: Early dynamics of transmission and control of COVID-19: a mathematical modelling study. Lancet Infect. Dis. **20**(5), 553–558 (2020)
13. Dey, S.K., Rahman, M.M., Siddiqi, U.R., Howlader, A.: Analyzing the epidemiological outbreak of COVID-19: a visual exploratory data analysis (EDA) approach. J. Med. Virol. **92**(6), 632–638 (2020)
14. Lauer, S.A., Grantz, K.H., Bi, Q., Jones, F.K., Zheng, Q., Meredith, H.R., Azman, A.S., Reich, N.G., Lessler, J.: The incubation period of coronavirus disease 2019 (COVID-19) from publicly reported confirmed cases: estimation and application. Ann. Intern. Med. **172**, 577 (2020)
15. Singer, H.M.: Short-term predictions of country-specific Covid-19 infection rates based on power law scaling exponents. arXiv preprint arXiv:2003.11997 (2020)
16. Awad, M., Khanna, R.: Support vector regression. In: Efficient Learning Machines, pp. 67–80. Apress, Berkeley, CA (2015)
17. De Castro, Y., Gamboa, F., Henrion, D., Hess, R., Lasserre, J.-B.: Approximate optimal designs for multivariate polynomial regression. Ann. Stat. **47**(1), 127–155 (2019)
18. Pandey, S., Solanki, A.: Music instrument recognition using deep convolutional neural networks. Int. J. Inf. Technol. **13**(3), 129–149 (2019)
19. Rajput, R., Solanki, A.: Real-time analysis of tweets using machine learning and semantic analysis. In: International Conference on Communication and Computing Systems (ICCCS2016), Taylor and Francis, at Dronacharya College of Engineering, Gurgaon, 9–11 Sept, vol. 138(25), pp. 687–692 (2016)
20. Ahuja, R., Solanki, A.: Movie recommender system using K-means clustering and K-nearest neighbor. In: Accepted for Publication in Confluence-2019: 9th International Conference on Cloud Computing, Data Science & Engineering, Amity University, Noida, vol. 1231(21), pp. 25–38 (2019)
21. Tayal, A., Kose, U., Solanki, A., Nayyar, A., Saucedo, J.A.M.: Efficiency analysis for stochastic dynamic facility layout problem using meta-heuristic, data envelopment analysis and machine learning. Comput. Intell. **36**(1), 172–202 (2019)
22. Tayal, A., Solanki, A., Singh, S.P.: Integrated frame work for identifying sustainable manufacturing layouts based on big data, machine learning, meta-heuristic and data envelopment analysis. Sustain. Cities Soc. **62**, 102383. https://doi.org/10.1016/j.scs.2020.102383
23. Greff, K., Srivastava, R.K., Koutnik, J., Steunebrink, B.R., Schmidhuber, J.: LSTM: a search space odyssey. IEEE Trans. Neural Netw. Learn. Syst. **28**(10), 2222–2232 (2016)
24. Chen, Y.-C., et al.: A time-dependent SIR model for COVID-19 with undetectable infected persons. arXiv:2003.00122 (2020)
25. Chowell, G., Sattenspiel, L., Bansal, S., Viboud, C.: Mathematical models to characterize early epidemic growth: a review. Phys. Life Rev. **18**, 66–97 (2016)

26. Ma, J.: Estimating epidemic exponential growth rate and basic reproduction number. Infect. Dis. Modell. **5**, 129–141 (2020)
27. Brauer, F.: Age of infection models and the final size relation. Math. Biosci. Eng. **5**, 681–690 (2008)
28. Davoudi, B., Pourbohloul, B., Miller, J.C., Meza, R., Meyers, L.A., Earn, D.J.D.: Early real-time estimation of infectious disease reproduction number. arXiv 0905 0728 (2009)
29. Diekmann, O., Heesterbeek, J.A.P.: Mathematical Epidemiology of Infectious Diseases. Wiley, Chichester (2000)
30. Yan, P., Feng, Z.: Variability order of the latent and the infectious periods in a deterministic SEIR epidemic model and evaluation of control effectiveness. Math. Biosci. **224**(1), 43–52 (2010)
31. Chowell, G., Brauer, F.: The basic reproduction number of infectious diseases: computation and estimation using compartmental epidemic models. In: Chowell, G., Hyman, J.M., Bettencourt, L.M.A., Castillo-Chavez, C. (eds.) Mathematical and Statistical Estimation Approaches in Epidemiology. Springer, Dordrecht (2009)
32. Chowell, G., Ammon, C.E., Hengartner, N.W., Hyman, J.M.: Transmission dynamics of the great influenza pandemic of 1918 in Geneva, Switzerland: Assessing the effects of hypothetical interventions. J. Theor. Biol. **241**, 193–204 (2006)
33. Nishiura, H., Chowell, G.: The effective reproduction number as a prelude to statistical estimation of time-dependent epidemic trends. In: Chowell, G., Hyman, J.M., Bettencourt, L.M.A., Castillo-Chavez, C. (eds.) Mathematical and Statistical Estimation Approaches in Epidemiology. Springer, Dordrecht (2009)
34. De Jong, M.C., Diekmann, O., Heesterbeek, J.A.: The computation of R0 for discrete-time epidemic models with dynamic heterogeneity. Math. Bioci. **119**, 97–114 (1994)
35. Chowell, G., Nishiura, H.: Quantifying the transmission potential of pandemic influenza. Phys Life Rev. **5**, 50–77 (2008)
36. Anderson, R.M., May, R.M.: Infectious Diseases of Humans: Dynamics and Control. Oxford University Press, Oxford (1991)
37. Davidian, M., Giltinan, D.M.: Nonlinear models for repeated measurement data. In: Monographs on Statistics and Applied Probability 62. Chapman and Hall, New York (1995)
38. Ying, S., et al.: Spread and control of COVID-19 in China and their associations with population movement, public health emergency measures, and medical resources, p. 24 (2020)
39. Bai, Y., et al.: Presumed asymptomatic carrier transmission of COVID-19. J.A.M.A. **323**(14), 1406–1407 (2020)
40. Greff, K., Srivastava, R.K., Koutník, J., Steunebrink, B.R., Schmidhuber, J.: LSTM: a search space odyssey. IEEE Trans. Neural Netw. Learn. Syst. **28**(10), 2222–2232 (2017)
41. Chen, B., et al.: Data visualization analysis and simulation prediction for COVID-19. arXiv:2002.07096 (2020)
42. Lin, I.: Real-Time Data API for COVID-19 Epidemic (2020). **22**(12), 1013–1033 (2020). Accessed 3 Feb 2020
43. Hong, X.: Predicting Alzheimer's Disease Using LSTM. **35**(18), 2034–2048 (2019)
44. Gers, F.A.: Learning to forget: continual prediction with LSTM. In: Proc. 9th Int. Conf. Artif. Neural Netw. (ICANN), pp. 850–855 (1999)
45. Chen, X., Yu, J., Wu, Z.: Temporally identity-aware SSD with attentional LSTM. IEEE Trans. Cybern. **18**(11), 2228–2245 (2019)
46. Wang, L.: MCPL-Based FT-LSTM: medical representation learning-based clinical prediction model for time series events. **22**(10), 1825–1840 (2019). Accessed 12 March 2019
47. Li, F., Tran, L., Thung, K.H., Ji, S., Shen, D., Li, J.: A robust deep model for improved classification of AD/MCI patients. IEEE J. Biomed. Health Inform. **19**(5), 1610–1616 (2015)
48. Hou, B.: LSTM-Based Auto-Encoder Model for ECG Arrhythmias Classification References for Potential Neutralizing Antibodies Discovered for Novel Corona Virus Using Machine Learning
49. Computational predictions of protein structures associated with COVID-19/research/opensource/computational-predictions-of-protein-structures-associated-with-COVID-19. Accessed 9 Mar 2020

50. Seber, G.A.F., Lee, A.J.: Linear Regression Analysis Ser, Wiley Series in Probability and Statistics. Wiley (2003)
51. Lall, U., Moon, Y.I., Kwon, H.H., Bosworth, K.: Locally weighted polynomial regression: parameter choice and application to forecasts of the Great Salt Lake. Water Resour. Res. **42**, W05422 (2006). https://doi.org/10.1029/2004WR003782
52. Cleveland, W.S., Devlin, S.J.: Locally weighted regression: an approach to regression analysis by local fitting. J. Am. Stat. Assoc. **83**(403), 596–610 (1988)
53. Jakobsson, E., Farimani, A.B., Tajkhorshid, E., Aluru, N.: Combining physics-based and evolution-based methods to design antibodies against an evolving virus. Biophys. J. **118**(3), 482a (2020). https://doi.org/10.1016/j.bpj.2019.11.2669
54. Hochreiter, S., Schmidhuber, J.: Long short-term memory. Neural Comput. **9**(8), 1735–1780 (1997)
55. Zheng, M., Song, L.: Novel antibody epitopes dominate the antigenicity of spike glycoprotein in SARS-CoV-2 compared to SARS-CoV. Cell. Mol. Immunol. **17**(5), 536–538 (2020)
56. JCI Insight. Predicting the broadly neutralizing antibody susceptibility of the HIV reservoir https://insight.jci.org/articles/view/130153. Accessed 13 Mar 2020
57. Yoon, H., Macke, J., West, A.P., Foley, B., Bjorkman, P.J., Korber, B., Yusim, K.: CATNAP: a tool to compile, analyze and tally neutralizing antibody panels. Nucleic Acids Res. **43**(W1), W213–W219 (2015). https://doi.org/10.1093/nar/gkv404
58. Ekiert, D.C., Bhabha, G., Elsliger, M.-A., Friesen, R.H.E., Jongeneelen, M., Throsby, M., Goudsmit, J., Wilson, I.A.: Antibody recognition of a highly conserved influenza virus epitope. Science. **324**(5924), 246–251 (2009). https://doi.org/10.1126/science.1171491
59. Schmid, N., Eichenberger, A.P., Choutko, A., Riniker, S., Winger, M., Mark, A.E., van Gunsteren, W.F.: Definition and testing of the GROMOS force-field versions 54A7 and 54B7. Eur. Biophys. J. **40**(7), 843 (2011). https://doi.org/10.1007/s00249-011-0700-9
60. Darden, T., York, D.M., Pedersen, L.G.: Particle mesh Ewald: an N·log(N) method for Ewald sums in large systems. J. Chem. Phys. **98**(12), 10089–10092 (1993). https://doi.org/10.1063/1.464397
61. Bakibayev, T., Kulzhanova, A.: Common movement prediction using polynomial regression. In: 2018 IEEE 12th International Conference on Application of Information and Communication Technologies (AICT), Almaty, Kazakhstan, pp. 1–4 (2018). https://doi.org/10.1109/ICAICT.2018.8747047
62. Omelchenko, A.V., Fedorov, O.V.: Polynomial regression coefficients estimation in finite differences space. In: 2015 25th International Conference Radioelektronika (RADIOELEKTRONIKA), Pardubice, pp. 257–260 (2015). https://doi.org/10.1109/RADIOELEK.2015.7129024
63. Chen, X.: Recursive local polynomial regression estimation and its applications. In: Proceedings of the 31st Chinese Control Conference, Hefei, pp. 2043–2048 (2012)
64. Su, W., Yang, H., Liu, Z.: System identification based on orthogonal polynomial regression analysis method. In: Proceedings of the 29th Chinese Control Conference, Beijing, pp. 1441–1446 (2010)
65. Rallis, M., Vazirgiannis, M.: Rank prediction in graphs with locally weighted polynomial regression and EM of polynomial mixture Models. In: 2011 International Conference on Advances in Social Networks Analysis and Mining, Kaohsiung, pp. 515–519 (2011). https://doi.org/10.1109/ASONAM.2011.44
66. Krzyzak, A., Pawlak, M.: Almost everywhere convergence of a recursive regression function estimate and classification (Corresp.). IEEE Trans. Inform. Theory. **30**(1), 91–93 (1984). https://doi.org/10.1109/TIT.1984.1056833

Chapter 4
Big Data and Modern-Day Technologies in COVID-19 Pandemic: Opportunities, Challenges, and Future Avenues

Mohd Abdul Ahad, Sara Paiva, Gautami Tripathi, Zeeshan Ali Haq, Md. Tabrez Nafis, and Noushaba Feroz

Abstract The COVID-19 pandemic has emerged as one of the most crucial health emergencies in the last decade where almost all entities of a nation's ecosystem like inhabitants, businesses, governments, economies, and environment are impacted. The large volumes of epidemiological, clinical, personal, and environmental data generated during any pandemic can provide useful insights about the underlying causes, symptoms, relations, and correlations, which if analyzed can assist in mitigating the impact to a great extent. The cheap and easy connectivity and communication provided by the social media platforms (SMP) have established them as one of the most preferred mediums of communications among the masses. The data generated by these platforms can be analyzed in context of the ongoing COVID-19 crisis to provide critical information and insights related to the ground level realities like spread and severity of infection, the state of implementation of control measures, the mental state of individuals, and their needs. The tweets and comments of the users can provide information about the current situation and intensity of the problems in the affected regions. With the help of techniques like sentiment analysis and web mining, we can identify the emergent requirements and needs (like food, shelter, medicine, medical emergencies, security, etc.) of the population in the COVID-19-affected areas. With this chapter we aim to identify several use cases where the big medical data from the patients, epidemiological data, social media data, and environment-related data can be used to identify patterns, causes, and other growing factors of the COVID-19 pandemic with a goal to mitigate the damages and contain further spread of the disease. The chapter also discusses the impact of a preferred mitigation measure of nationwide lockdown on the number of new

M. A. Ahad (✉) · G. Tripathi · Z. A. Haq · M. T. Nafis · N. Feroz
Department of Computer Science and Engineering, Jamia Hamdard, New Delhi, India
e-mail: aahad@jamiahamdard.ac.in

S. Paiva
Instituto Politécnico de Viana do Castelo, Viana do Castelo, Portugal

© The Author(s), under exclusive license to Springer Nature Switzerland AG 2021

F. Al-Turjman et al. (eds.), *Emerging Technologies for Battling Covid-19*, Studies in Systems, Decision and Control 324,
https://doi.org/10.1007/978-3-030-60039-6_4

novel coronavirus-positive patients as well as the impact on the environment by analyzing the available data. Since the tourism industry is now of the worst hit businesses, we also discussed the impact of COVID-19 on tourism industry. Furthermore, we identify the challenges associated with handling the massive amount of data generated during such pandemics. Finally, the future avenues of using big data for effectively devising predictive mechanisms and techniques to contain such pandemics in the initial stages are discussed. The chapter also discusses the importance of edge/fog technologies and IoT to identify possible use cases and where immediate point of contact actions is needed to mitigate the situations. Since edge computing facilitates calculations near the origin of data, it is imperative to understand the potential use cases in times of COVID-19-like pandemics.

Keywords COVID-19 · Big data · SMP · Epidemiological data · IoT · Nanotechnology

4.1 Introduction

The recent COVID-19 pandemic has created a situation of panic across the globe. The hysteria surrounding the novel coronavirus is already having devastating effects on the individual well-being and the nations as a whole. First reported in Wuhan City in China, the overall impact of the COVID-19 pandemic is so far reaching that it was declared as "public health emergency of international concern" by the "World Health Organization (WHO)." The exponential rise in the coronavirus-positive cases is creating an environment of fear and emergency where the nations across the globe are taking extreme control measures like lockdown. Considering the impact of COVID-19 pandemic, it is estimated that the after-effects may last for several years to come. The majority of the developed and developing nations (including the USA, Europe, and Asia) around the world are witnessing the devastation caused by this pandemic. However, this is not the first time that we have been hit by a novel kind of virus. In the past there were also several such cases of virus epidemics like plague, N1H1, Ebola, etc. Today, technologies have advanced to a level where if used efficiently they can lend promising support to fight such adverse situations. The modern-day technologies like big data, IoT, data analytics, sensors, etc., have enormous potential to develop solutions at various levels (individual, national, and global). Data analytics is one such technology that can provide useful insights into the various aspects of an infectious disease. The data generated from the personal records of the patients can be analyzed to identify the following as shown in Fig. 4.1:

- Which sex and age group is most affected by the epidemics?
- What are the common symptoms of the patients?
- What is the degree of potential threat to the population in general?

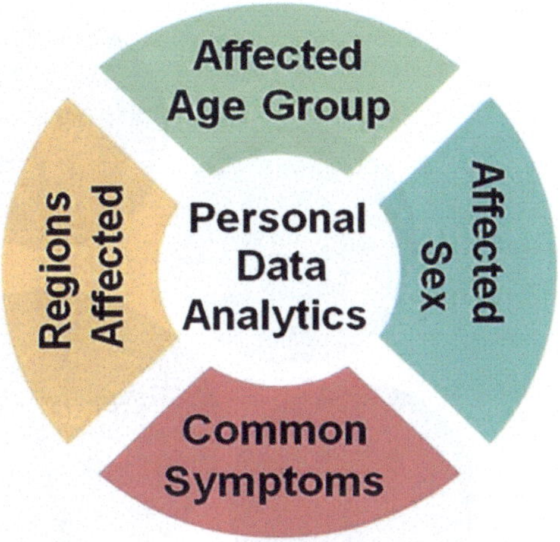

Fig. 4.1 Outcomes from analysis of demographic data

Similarly, the clinical data analysis can provide the causes and remedy of the epidemics. With effective analysis of clinical datasets, we are able to identify the following:

- What type of virus is affecting the population?
- Virological assessments.
- Receptor-binding and receptor recognition analysis.
- Which family of virus does it belong to?
- Which parts of the body are being affected by the virus?
- Does patient medical history (BP, sugar, hypertension, cardiac, etc.) affect the effect of virus on the person?
- Diagnostic mechanisms (testing kits and other means).
- Possible therapeutic solutions for the virus.
- Propose precautionary measures and containment plan.

In order to extract accurate insights about the pandemic, it is imperative to ensure that the data and information must be authentic, valid, verifiable, immutable, and traceable. Such information can be useful in tracking the outbreak, identifying the epicenter of the pandemics, track the carrier of the disease, and other contacts.

4.1.1 What Makes Big Data So Unique

"Big data" has been considered as one of the most widely used terms used in the computing domain in recent years. There is no quantifiable definition of big data in terms of its size. It is a relative term whose definition differs with different organizations. In general, we can define big data as any massive amount of data which is beyond the managing capacities of the legacy tools, devices, and systems [1, 2]. As

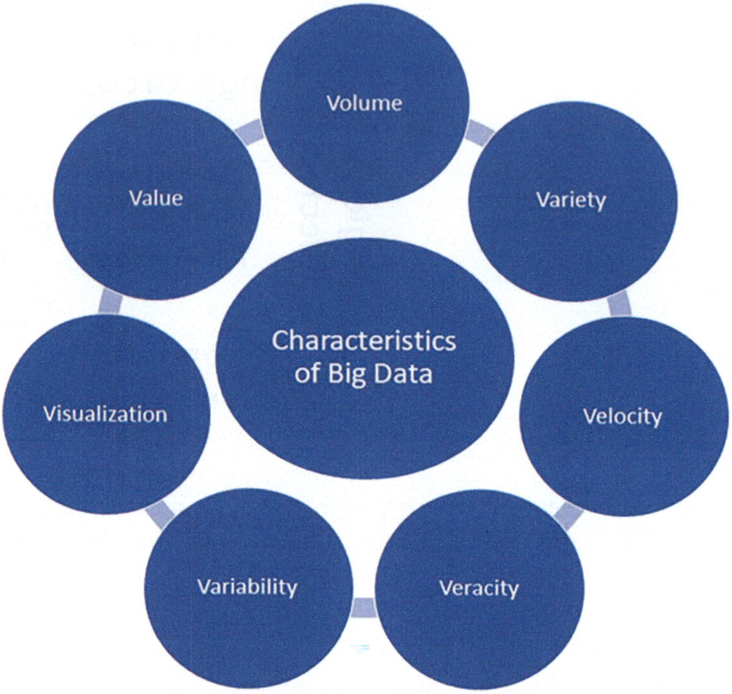

Fig. 4.2 Characteristics of big data

shown in Fig. 4.2, there are several inherent characteristics of big data which make it unique in several ways. These characteristics include [1–3]:

Volume: It includes the gigantic amount of data generated with time along with the archival data.

Velocity: It defines the rate of generation of new data. With the new age technological advancements, the data is getting generated at an exponential rate.

Variety: This constitutes the heterogeneity of the data at our disposal. Big data may include text, numbers, image, audios, videos, logs, etc.

Veracity: It defines the correctness and trustworthiness of the data. It is one of the most important characteristics of big data.

Variability: It defines the changing nature and type of the data. The data which is relevant at one point of time may become irrelevant in other time or situation.

Visualization: It is the ability to depict or portray the data using visual charts, bar graphs, and other diagrams.

Value: This is the most important quality of big data and the most complex one too. The ultimate goal of playing with big data resides in extracting meaningful value from the data.

Each of these characteristics makes the management of big data an intricate task. Big data includes data which may or may not be structured. Therefore, special storage devices and procedures are adopted for storing such types of datasets. There are several solutions prevalent for managing big data which includes Hadoop, Quantcast, Cassandra, HDInsight, Andrews File System, etc. Each of these solutions has their own set of advantages, disadvantages, and use cases. Some are preferred for archival datasets, while others are used for managing real-time datasets [3].

4.1.2 Sources of Big Data in a Pandemic

Big data may be generated from several sources including social media data, news, blogs, seismic activities, weather forecasting, sensors, videos, audios, images, etc. Broadly, the sources of big data can be characterized in six parts, as shown in Fig. 4.3 [4–6].

- **Medical**: The big data generated through medical cases, tests and scan reports, prescriptions, medical history, symptoms, etc.
- **Transactional**: The data generated through online and offline transactions.
- **Logs**: This constitutes the log of the activities performed during any work or transaction.

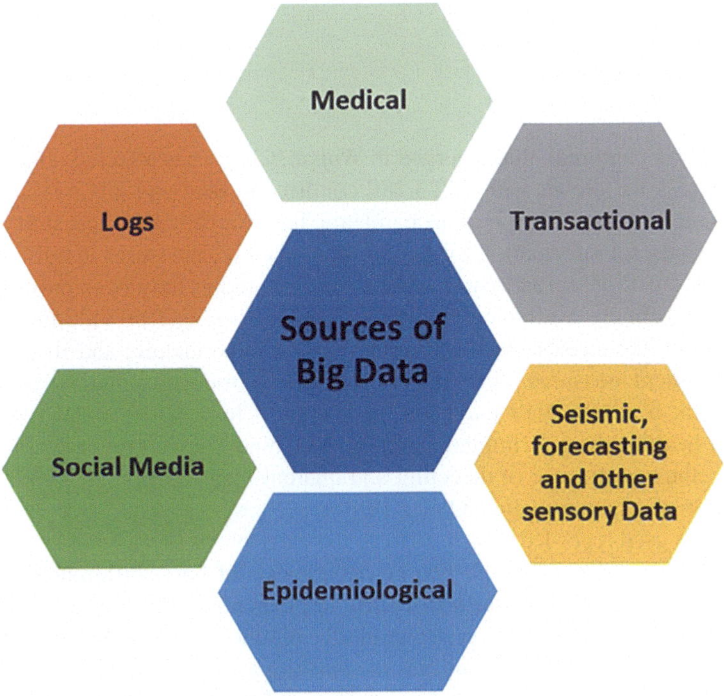

Fig. 4.3 Sources of big data in a pandemic

- **Social Media**: This is the primary source of big data with more than 500 million tweets per day, 300 h of video uploaded on YouTube per minute, etc., and 29 million messages are sent via WhatsApp per minute.
- **Epidemiological**: This includes the non-experimental observations, including "population exposure levels" and "health effect values" observed from the samples.

4.1.3 Chapter Organization

The complete chapter is divided into seven sections. Section 4.2 discusses some of the recent researches and related works in the area of COVID-19 and big data management. Section 4.3 highlights how big data can be utilized for managing pandemics. Section 4.4 discusses the challenges in the implementation of big data solutions for combating pandemics. Section 4.5 presents the impact of social distancing and nationwide lockdowns on COVID-19 pandemics in India, the UK, Italy, France, and Spain. The impact of lockdown on tourism industry is also discussed. The role of IoT and nanotechnology in managing Covid-19 is highlighted in Sect. 4.6. Section 4.7 presents the conclusion and further scope for the integration of modern-day technologies for providing solutions in time of pandemics.

4.2 Related Works

The COVID-19 outbreak that emerged in Wuhan, China, has affected almost all the nations across the globe, with 7,823,289 confirmed cased and 431,541 confirmed deaths as on June 15, 2020 [7]. This pandemic has compelled the research community to mine useful information to support the preventive measures in mitigating the impact of COVID-19 spread. Many researches and studies have been published that analyze the publicly available data about the pandemic and provide many useful insights about the causes, potential threats from the pandemic, and its preventive and containment measures. The authors in [8] have introduced a model that portrays the outbreak of COVID-19 pandemic in Wuhan, China. This model reflects the impact of health strategies implemented by the Chinese government to control this epidemic, the significance of detecting and quarantining unrecorded cases, and the contribution of asymptomatic COVID-19-positive cases to virus transmission. The authors have used recorded case data from the early phase of this pandemic to estimate the final number of cases. The layout consists of basic differential equation scheme. The model demonstrates that early implementation of precautionary measures leads to dramatic reduction in cumulative number of cases. An analysis of the COVID-19 is given in [9] that outlines the existing awareness related to the worldwide COVID-19 epidemic. The paper presents a chronological sequence of events from the origin of the virus in Wuhan City to being labeled as a "global pandemic" by the World Health Organization (WHO). The paper highlights the measures taken by countries around the world to combat this virus with an emphasis on UK cases and response. An elaboration of COVID-19 virus characteristics such as physiology, detection, treatment, prevention, prediction, and containment measures has been presented. Furthermore, the authors have discussed the impact of this outbreak on global economy and the imperative need for effective governance following COVID-19 epidemic. The authors in [10] have built a statistical model to predict COVID-19 cases in Wuhan City of China. The model derives the number of unreported cases from the data of reported symptomatic cases in Wuhan, and the forecasts obtained highlight the significance of public health policies to contain this outbreak. The authors have addressed the implications of reported and unreported cases and public safety interventions on the growth of this epidemic in Wuhan. From the model, it is observed that interventions such as lockdown and quarantine, when implemented at early stages, dramatically decrease the final scale of the outbreak. In [11], the authors have explored the COVID-19 epidemic from an urban viewpoint and focus on smart city network potential for improving standardization protocols to enhance the exchange of information in case of epidemics, contributing to greater awareness and control globally. The authors have emphasized the need of communication standardization by means of globally accepted standardized protocols and for smart city technologies to be democratized to foster equality and clarity among stakeholders, thereby allowing further collaboration in the wake of an outbreak. The author in [12] has discussed various applications in which artificial intelligence (AI) could help contain the global pandemic of COVID-19. These applications include forecasting the location of another epidemic, molecules engineered by AI algorithms to inhibit the replication of novel coronavirus, forecasting the impact of changing seasons on COVID-19 epidemic, stabilizing current economy, and rapid detection of COVID-19 from lung CT scans, among others. In [13], the author has advocated the integration of big data and advanced models for upgrading surveillance infrastructure and global cooperation for epidemic preparation. The author has discussed the benefits of big data in tackling an epidemic such as outbreak prediction and policymaking. Moreover, the paper discusses though real-time big data can enhance monitoring and control techniques in a quick-growing outbreak, the resulting challenges and privacy concerns need to be addressed. The paper recommends that versatile, dispersed teams should cover the systematic and functional dimensions of the outbreak response, in the implementation of big data schemes. In [14], the authors detail public safety approaches to contain the outbreak of COVID-19 on cruise vessels. The authors discuss that cruise passengers are highly vulnerable to outbreaks with accelerated disease transmission, requiring vigorous attempts to curb spread. Two cruise ships have been mentioned in particular, “Diamond Princess” and “Grand Princess”, both acting as COVID-19 clusters, with numerous reported cases. It is also observed that due to the closed setting of cruise ships, the COVID-19 cases increased gradually after the passengers and crew were quarantined on the vessels. The authors have highlighted that vigorous attempts were made to curb COVID-19 spread on the vessel and prevent community transmission. The authors in [15] have presented a comparison of

COVID-19 clinical traits with other types of pneumonia. For their study, the authors have selected 19 COVID-19-positive cases and 15 non-COVID-19 pneumonia cases from Hubei province of China. The authors have observed that for COVID-19 patients, the mean incubation period is 8 days, while for non-COVID-19 patients, the period is 5 days. Although both the conditions display similar symptoms, liver damage is more prevalent in COVID-19 patients, and the tests are strikingly atypical. The authors recommend CT scan for testing suspected COVID-19 cases, with "α-HBDH" and "LDH" as indicators for analysis. In [16], the authors have presented a chronology of efforts by various institutions of the USA to discover and track all individuals who had come in close proximity with reported COVID-19 patients. The paper presents elaborate statistics related to COVID-19 monitoring in the USA in the months of January and February, to facilitate swift identification, diagnosis, and treatment as well as minimize further spread. The paper stresses on disease management and prevention measures, in tandem with contact tracing initiatives, to minimize the transmission of the disease in a community. The authors in [17] have selected 1099 confirmed COVID-19 cases from 552 hospitals in China to study the clinical features of novel coronavirus. It is observed that the patients are mostly male with an average age of 47 years. Moreover, except for a small percentage, most of the patients had never come in contact with wild animals. The authors have observed that cough and fever are common, while diarrhea is rare in patients. The average duration from exposure to onset is 4 days. The results have confirmed the three-stage sequence of the epidemic, asymptomatic transmission and family cluster outbreaks. The authors in [18] have discussed the available knowledge related to other coronaviruses (SARS and MERS) in an effort to understand the effects of coronavirus virus disease 2019 (COVID-19) on pregnancy. The authors have noted that scarce information regarding COVID-19 is available and attempt to create awareness about the treatment of pregnant women with confirmed COVID-19. The authors observe that there is no data available to demonstrate higher vulnerability of pregnant women to COVID-19 or increased severity of symptoms in them.

According to Fitzpatrick et al. [19], artificial intelligence (AI) provides tremendous potential in preventing and managing infections (IPC). "Big data" determines AIs to find the correlations that may point to medically related conditions or to identify potential risk factors. AIs can also occasionally ignore small clusters of data that may be clinically relevant and unable to utilize deep knowledge of core processes. Rather than concentrating on the AI tools themselves, the emphasis should be on the IPC problem that needs to be tackled through the development of priorities, plans, and processes to support this that could involve AI. In [20] the authors discussed how Chinese government agencies explored social media to engage citizens during the COVID-19 crisis. To achieve this, they systematically examined the impact of dialogic loops, media prosperity, and type of content on citizen engagement through government social media based on "media wealth theory (MRT)" and "dialogic communication theory (DCT)." The authors in [21] suggested that large-scale data collection may help curb the COVID-19 pandemic, but it should not ignore public trust and privacy. To maintain accountable standards of data collection and data processing at a global scale, finest practices should be recognized.

According to [22], a mathematical modeling is a critical method for forecasting and estimating the severity and length of epidemics, determining the effectiveness of public health initiatives, and informing public health policy. Their study showed the challenges modelers face in predicting outbreaks of this nature and providing a partial justification for the wide variability in earlier model predictions of the COVID-19 epidemic. Their study suggested that due to the larger number of model parameters to be estimated, more complex models may not inevitably be more confident in making predictions, given the same dataset of incorrigible cases.

Through their research, the authors in [23] offer a new perspective for the inspection of epidemiological and behavioral data by proposing networks for migrants. They showed that they did not analyze traffic data (e.g., number of train or flight frequencies) but instead studied the causes of traffic relocation on social networks. This is more scientific, and it is possible to prepare simple tools to provide a method for forecasting disease transmission and calculating risk even in complex circumstances. It is hoped that as long as the approximations are clear and accurate, a continually changing understanding of the complexities of the real world can be obtained, and the approach will continue to assist in the detection and control of diseases. The authors in [24] provided extensive clinical, demographic, radiological, epidemiologic, and laboratory characteristics, and technical hitches, cure, and results of non-severe and severe COVID-19 hospitalized patients in Wuhan. They suggested that half of the patients in their study were identified as serious cases, which may vary from previous study results. In their study, the proportion of patients who were 65 years of age or older was higher than in the study conducted by Nanshan Zhong (38.8% vs. 15.1%, respectively).

Sarkodie et al. (2020) in [25] showed that their analysis was focused on phenomenological models. They demonstrated that the influence of confirmed cases on COVID-19 attributable deaths is perfectly linear, while a nonlinear direction is followed by the impact of confirmed cases on recovery cases. They used a mix of estimation approach to increase model sensitivity and robustness.

4.3 Managing Pandemics with Big Data

In the time of Ebola crisis, UNICEF used big data-based apps and solutions like EduTrac and U-Report to enhance the collective efforts against the crisis [26, 27]. Data was one of the most valuable assets that helped UNICEF to plan the emergency response in areas of high alerts. This was backed by the data analysis that provided valuable insights into the exact needs and conditions of the affected regions. Moreover, the data collected during the whole process was also used to develop educational resources for spreading awareness about the epidemic along with its probable causes and symptoms. Real-time data and tools can assist in emergency response systems and help the authorities to efficiently and precisely monitor, manage, and contain the spread of diseases and can play a vital role in eventually saving human lives.

A data-based global surveillance system can assist in disease tracking and mapping, for example, MagicBox v0.5 which is a data mapping tool that can provide valuable services in emergency situations.

The different types of data which can be analyzed in cases of epidemics and pandemics include [26, 27]. Table 4.1 provides the specific role of big data in each stage of the pandemic.

Table 4.1 Phases of pandemics and role of big data

Phases of pandemic	Responses	Role of big data	Type of data analytics
Phase 1: Emergence	Anticipation Early detection of disease	Data from various sources can be analyzed to predict the possibility of any infection or emergence of a new/existing disease Data analysis techniques can be applied on the historical data for investigating the possible causes and sources of the spread and can assist in investigating the future possibilities	Predictive and cognitive
Phase 2: Local transmission	Mapping of spread and containment	Data from geospatial apps and location tracking devices can be used to map the spread of infectious diseases	Diagnostic and prescriptive
Phase 3: Community transmission	Mapping of spread and containment	Social networking websites, web news, and individual GPS data of the affected patients can be analyzed to • Keep track of the movements of the affected patients • Isolate and quarantine the suspected cases • Identify the opinions and sentiments of the affected populations • Identify urgent needs and requirements of the affected populations • Plan the future course of actions in terms of infrastructure and logistics	Diagnostic and prescriptive
Phase 4: Global spread/ amplification	Control and mitigation	• Analyze the clinical data of the patients along with the epidemiological data • Identify relations and correlations and mapping them with historical datasets of similar such incidents • Identify the therapeutic solutions	Diagnostic and prescriptive
Phase 5: Reduced transmission	Elimination	The data from regular monitoring of patients and mapping of the spread can provide information related to the rate of spread of disease Decline in the number of new cases and containment of spread points toward the reduced transmission of diseases and start of elimination phase	Prescriptive and predictive

1. **Genetic data collection and monitoring**: The genetic data collected over time can be analyzed to study the mutations of microbes and predicting outbreaks. It can also identify classes of viruses and their correlations.
2. **Mobility data analysis**: The mobility data of the infected person and other individuals from the epidemic hit areas can be used for mapping the spread of disease and predicting the potential areas where outbreak may occur. The mobility data also helps in tracking of the infected carriers and studying the pattern of spread and backtracking the source.
3. **Social media data analysis**: The data collected from various social media platforms can help to understand the sentiments of the affected population and give insights into the immediate needs of the masses and the points to address since with any epidemics, providing only the healthcare facilities cannot work. There must be a provision to identify the relating needs of the affected population like food, security, and other essential services. All this can be analyzed with the help of social media data, and preventive measures can be planned accordingly.
4. **Mapping of affected geographical areas**: The data collected from the hospitals and medical facilities at various locations can be analyzed and later mapped to identify the affected areas and populations. The data from the travel history of the individuals from the affected areas can provide valuable insights into the potential spread of the disease.
5. **Simulating epidemic spread on global scale**: Big data collected from population census, demographics, short-range mobility data like commuting patterns between subpopulations of an area, and long-range mobility data like air travel, frequency, and connectivity of different geographical locations, etc., can be analyzed to simulate the spread of an outbreak on a global scale.
6. **Preparedness**: Medical records of patients, symptoms, data from past pandemics and epidemics, and the corresponding preventive measures can be analyzed to take precautions to prevent future outbreaks and develop solutions and contingency plans for emergency situations.

4.3.1 Big Data for Containment of Pandemics

The most critical stage of any epidemics or pandemics is the community transfer stage. It is really important to restrict the spread and outbreak of the disease as much as possible before the start of such stage. Once this stage arrives in the lifetime of any epidemics, it becomes very difficult to identify the original source of disease since the spread gets exploded exponentially. Big data can provide unprecedented results in the tracking of affected patients and avoiding the community spread [26, 28–31]. Since ensuring and maintaining the veracity of big data is the most critical step in order to extract accurate value from the datasets, there must be standardized mechanisms and protocols for handling the authenticity of the source and contents of the data. The architecture presented in Fig. 4.4 explains the typical process of containing community transfer in case of any pandemics or epidemics. At the time

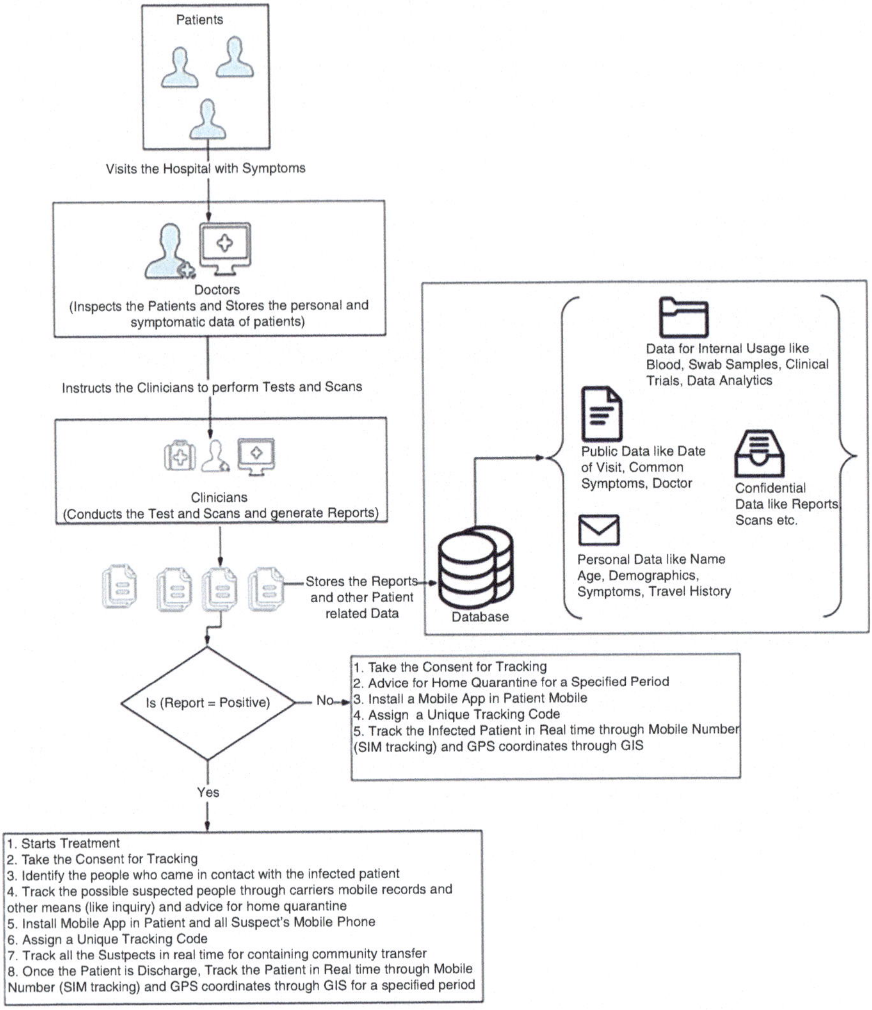

Fig. 4.4 Architecture for restricting community transfer during pandemics

of disease discovery and confirmation, consent must be taken from the infected person to access the contacts in order to track the people who came in contact with the infected person. This consent can be made a mandatory step to curb the chances of spread and community transfer. Apart from the infected patients, the doctor and other medical staff involved in treating the patients may also be tracked as they are the most vulnerable classes who are in constant contact with the infected patients. Such care providers must be periodically tested even if they show no signs of any symptoms related to the deadly pandemics. This periodic testing will ensure early detection, isolation, and treatment of the care providers as well. A GPS-based physical tracker may be provided to all the infected patients who must be instructed to carry that tracker always on and close to them so that they can be tracked. It must be ensured at all time that the data being collected from the patients conforms the standard data collection, sharing, and storage norms like prescribed in GDPR by the European Union. Further, since the community transfer cannot be solely restricted by the authorities and governments, the communities themselves are the major players who can stop the spread of such transfer of disease, and thus the consent is their responsibility to obey government directions and precautionary measures.

We can use two-way tracking of the infected person. First tracking can be done easily in coordination with the mobile service providers. Since the mobile companies always keep track of the SIM location, the infected person can be tracked using the mobile phone SIM location. Secondly a GPS-based tracking application can be installed on the infected person mobile so that they can be tracked using the application in real time through GPS/GPRS coordinates. This tracking serves two purposes. Since the tracking is done with the help of GIS system, it can be used to provide location-based services to the infected individuals. The infected person can be tracked, and necessary medical help may be provided in case of the any emergency since the patient is being continuously monitored. The healthcare officials and the government agencies can use this tracking data to identify whether the person is on the move or not and thus can restrict the movement and prevent community spread. Figure 4.5 shows the use of big data analytics in an event of pandemics like COVID-19.

4.4 Challenges with Big Data Analytics

This section provides the various challenges associated with analyzing the big data generated from multiple sources in events of any pandemics [26, 27, 32–35].

- **Infodemics**: The widespread use of social media had led to the emergence of "infodemics" that describes the spread of information which may include rumors, unreliable information, gossips, and guesses related to the concerned issues, conspiracy theories, etc. This rapid spread is facilitated by the popularity of the social media platforms and discussion forums. This false information circulated at a global scale may create panic among the masses resulting in a situation of chaos and mismanagement. Such data when reaches the data repositories may adversely affect the analysis process by manipulating the outcomes. In such situations the data needs to be checked at the source to avoid any kind of misuse and spread of misinformation.
- **Correlation and Causation**: One of the major concerns with big data analytics is the lack of causation. Data analytics majorly focuses on finding the correlations between data and establishing statistical patterns rather than figuring out the question what causes what and how. The tech giant Google felt prey to one such situation where they claimed to have successfully tracked the spread of influenza without any medical checkups [36]. This claim was made purely on the

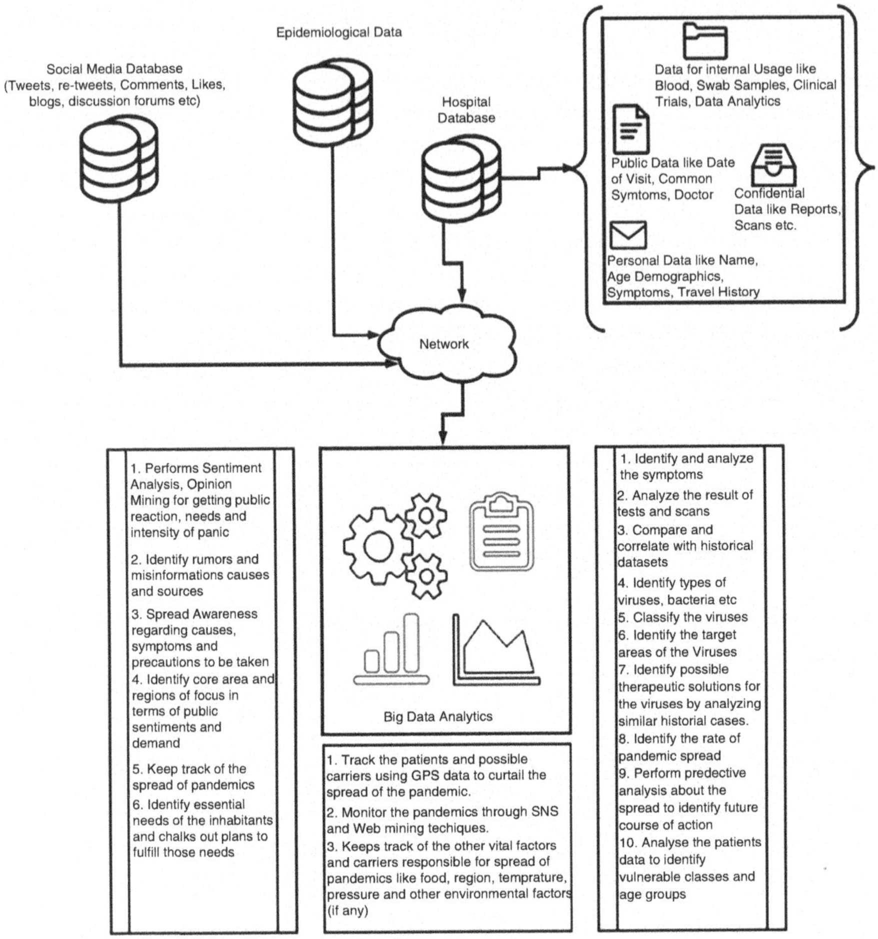

Fig. 4.5 Big data analytics at work in COVID-19

basis of data analysis on the Google search data. The most significant aspect of the claim was that Google was faster than the Centers for Disease Control and Prevention (CDC) in tracking the spread with only a day's delay as compared to weeks taken by CDC. The Google Flu Trends were later found to be overstated by almost a factor of two, thus concluding that theory-free correlation can be highly fragile and inaccurate [37].

- **Multiple Comparison Problem**: The size and choice of data highly affects the final outcomes. In [38] the authors presented a similar study discussing how the claims made by any scientific study cannot be considered completely accurate. This conclusion was derived based on the fact that the results of any study are dependent on various factors including the size of data, related researches and studies, relationships, number of tested relationships and correlations, etc. While predicting the outcomes using big data analysis especially in critical situations like epidemics, similar issues may arise jeopardizing the final outcomes.

- **Heterogeneity**: The heterogeneity of the data poses the most critical challenge in managing big data. Several types of data exist which may be structured, semi-structured, or unstructured. Tackling all such data in a similar manner cannot be an optimal solution since each of these data types requires different processing and management techniques [32–34, 39].
- **Multiple Formats and Schema**: The varied formats and schemas of big data also pose inherent complexities for its management. It is difficult to standardize the data so as to bring it to a common format for further processing. Several big data handling tools like Hadoop, Cassandra, and HDInsight process the data in their own respective formats. For example, Hadoop does not differentiate between the types of files and process them in the same manner irrespective of their type. This can cause severe performance issue for certain types of files which are much smaller in size as compared to Hadoop block size [3, 32, 40, 41].

4.5 Impact of Nationwide Lockdown

This section investigates the impact of social distancing and nationwide lockdowns on COVID-19 pandemics in India, the UK, Italy, France, and Spain. In order to analyze the effect of social distancing and lockdown, we have used the COVID-19 dataset from "Johns Hopkins University Center for Systems Science and Engineering (JHU CCSE)." This work also uses the publicly available data and reports about the COVID-19 spread from various government sources and analyzes the patterns in the spread of infection under various circumstances. Apart from the pandemic data, we have also analyzed the effect of social distancing and lockdowns on the environment. Specifically, we have compared the air quality index pre- and post-enforcement of lockdown in India. The results of the study and analysis indicate that social distancing and nationwide lockdown are indeed highly effective in mitigating the spread of the coronavirus with only 11.67% new cases after 1 week of lockdown for India, 12.60% for Italy, 24.32% for Spain, 23.96% for France, and 13.41% for the UK which is much less as compared to the number of new cases coming up before the lockdowns were announced.

For the empirical evaluations, we have considered India, Italy, Spain, France, and the UK in order to measure the effect of lockdowns and social distancing in COVID-19 in these countries. We analyzed the COVID-19 patient information dataset available from "JHU CCSE," uploaded on "Kaggle" and "Github" [42–44]. This dataset contains time-series data about the number of patients found positive, number of deceased patients, and number of patients recovered from COVID-19 infection. We have analyzed the number of coronavirus-positive cases on five different intervals each before the date of lockdown and after the date of lockdown (inclusive) as shown in Table 4.2 and Figs. 4.6 and 4.7.

Table 4.2 Number of coronavirus-positive cases before and after lockdown

Country	Date of lockdown	Before 10 days	Before 8 days	Before 6 days	Before 4 days	Before 1 day	On the day of lockdown	After 2 days	After 4 days	After 6 days	After 1 week
India	March 24, 2020	102	119	156	244	499	536	727	987	1251	1397
Italy	March 10, 2020	1128	2036	3089	4636	9172	10,149	12,462	21,157	27,980	31,506
Spain	March 14, 2020	222	400	673	1695	5232	6391	9942	13,910	20,410	25,374
France	March 16, 2020	653	1126	1784	2281	4499	6633	9043	12,612	16,018	19,856
UK	March 23, 2020	798	1140	1950	2689	5683	6650	9529	14,543	19,522	22,141

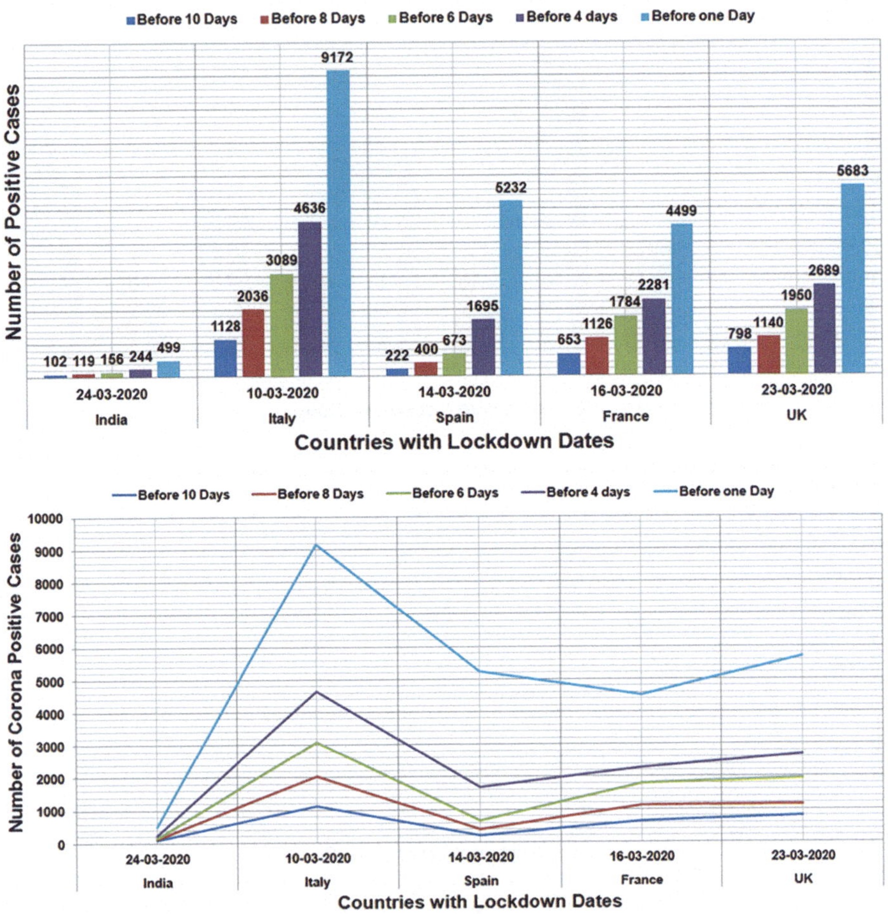

Fig. 4.6 Number of coronavirus-positive cases before lockdown

The result of this analysis can be found in Table 4.3 where we have calculated the percentage increase of the number of coronavirus-positive cases before and after the date of lockdowns.

As it can be observed from Table 4.3, the percentage increase in the number of new coronavirus-positive cases is consistently decreasing with only 11.67% new cases after 1 week of lockdown for India, 12.60% for Italy, 24.32% for Spain, 23.96% for France, and 13.41% for the UK.

Finally, in order to measure the effect of lockdown on environment in India, we have analyzed the air quality index (AQI) of the past 3 years (2017–2019) with the current year (2020) at the five different intervals before and after the date of lockdown [45, 46]. The analysis is shown in Fig. 4.5. The chart clearly depicts the AQI for specific dates before and after lockdown from 2017 to 2020. It can be inferred from Fig. 4.8 that there is a significant improvement in the AQI after the lockdown,

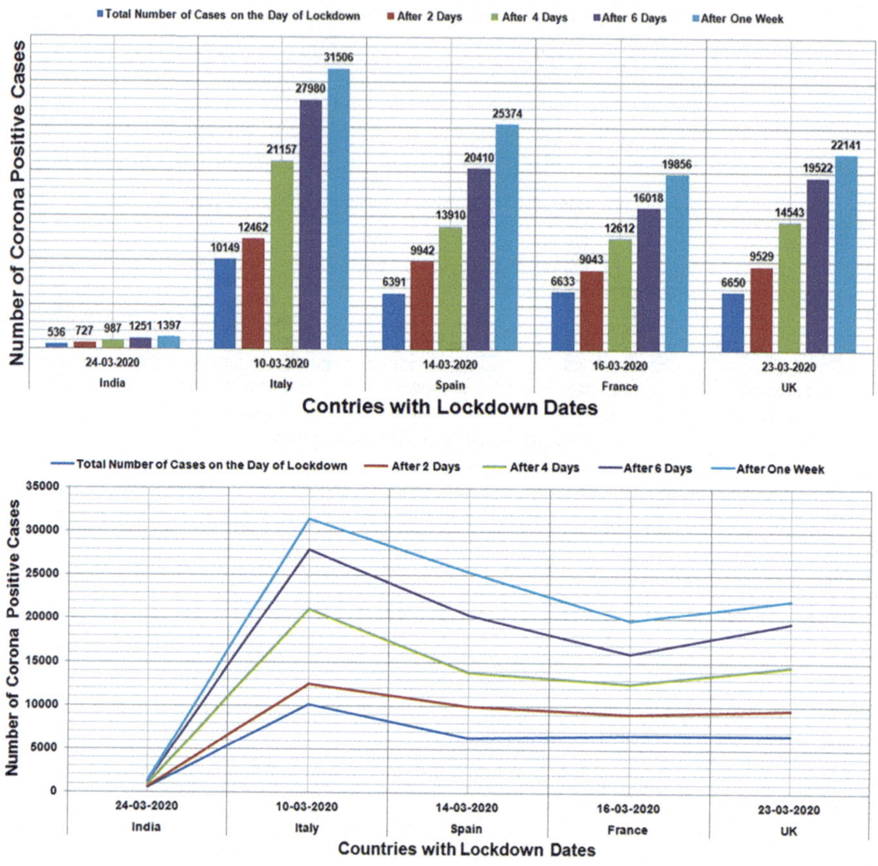

Fig. 4.7 Number of coronavirus-positive cases after lockdown

Table 4.3 Percentage increase in the number of cases before and after lockdown

Country	Percentage increase in the number of new cases								
	Date of lockdown	Before 8 days	Before 6 days	Before 4 days	Before 1 day	After 2 days	After 4 days	After 6 days	After 1 week
India	March 24, 2020	16.67	31.09	56.41	104.51	35.63	35.76	26.75	11.67
Italy	March 10, 2020	80.50	51.72	50.08	97.84	22.79	69.77	32.25	12.60
Spain	March 14, 2020	80.18	68.25	151.86	208.67	55.56	39.91	46.73	24.32
France	March 16, 2020	72.43	58.44	27.86	97.24	36.33	39.47	27.01	23.96
UK	March 23, 2020	42.86	71.05	37.90	111.34	43.29	52.62	34.24	13.42

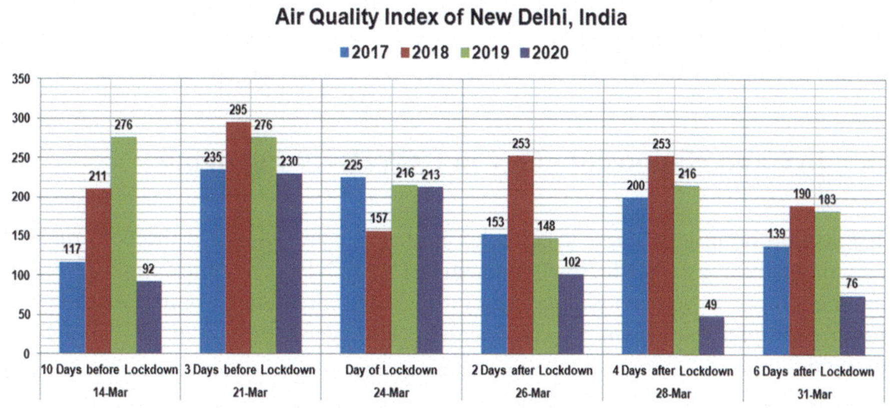

Fig. 4.8 Air quality index (2017–2020) at New Delhi, India

which was announced on March 24, 2020. On a similar pattern, other countries around the world have shown improvements in the AQI as a result of nationwide lockdowns [46].

4.5.1 Impact of COVID-19 on Tourism

The outbreak of coronavirus virus disease 2019 (COVID-19) has plummeted global travel with flights grounded, ships docked, trains cancelled, and borders closed. The entire tourism sector including transportation means, hotels, travel operators, tourist destinations, restaurants, etc., has been affected severely. The pandemic has caused substantial damage to the global travel industry, risking 50 million jobs worldwide and estimated to shrink the travel industry up to 25%. Nearly 10% of global GDP is contributed by the tourism sector, and the current travel restrictions are expected to result in a loss of approximately 30–50 billion US dollars worldwide, according to UNWTO [47]. As reported by the "International Air Transport Association" (IATA), air travel revenues will decline by 5%, amounting to $29.3 billion globally in 2020 [48]. The aviation authorities in China, where the virus originated in late December, have reported a loss of 21 billion yuan [49]. A report by US Travel Association warns of a staggering loss of 910 billion dollars to the US economy in 2020 due to the travel restrictions [50]. Though the COVID-19 pandemic poses an imminent threat to economies throughout the world, some countries are facing more severe implications than others. This can be illustrated by the instance of Saudi Arabia that could lose nearly 12 billion dollars due to Hajj and Umrah cancellation [51]. It is estimated that the tourism industry would require 10 months to 3 years to recover completely from the losses incurred. Subsequently, international bodies such as the "United Nations World Travel Organization" (UNWTO) and "World Travel and Tourism Council" (WTTC) have emphasized the need of global cooperation and discussion, financial and political assistance, as well as easing travel regulations, once the pandemic is contained [52].

4.6 IoT and Nanotechnology in COVID-19 Pandemic

This section highlights the role of technological advancements in the field of IoT and nanotechnology for effectively managing COVID-19 pandemics. Since IoT and nanotechnology have been widely used in several application domains and are providing exemplary solutions, it is imperative to discuss their role in COVID-19 pandemics.

4.6.1 IoT in COVID-19

The advent of the Internet of Things (IoT) and smart technologies has brought about significant changes in the way many businesses operate and in the potential that opens up, facilitating people's lives in different ways that we did not imagine a few years ago. In times of crisis, like the one that now happens with the appearance of COVID-19 in December 2019, we have seen a suspension of some activities and the appearance of new opportunities. In the case of IoT and smart technologies, the times we live make clear the opportunity to create new solutions that make use of the combination of emerging technologies, to combat the current crisis, but mainly to act upon future pandemic crises such as the one we are experiencing today.

Detecting the spread of the virus at an early stage is of great importance to avoid spreading contamination. The use of sensor networks that can help in the detection phase is considered a very viable option by specialists, mainly in countries like China or Japan, which lead the adoption of IoT technologies. A network of surveillance sensors was once implemented by China, so the creation of an infrastructure of virus detection sensors becomes a possibility to act from an early stage in the detection of new pandemics that may exist, avoiding loss of human lives and the great impact they have on the economy and on the lives of all citizens [53].

On the other hand, aspects related to the mobility of citizens are a fundamental and crucial aspect for decision-making by the government and other responsible entities. Knowing where people are, how much time they spend outside home, and in which places is something that can bring valuable information to understand transmission chains, especially those people who are recommended to be in isolation. This monitoring can also help to regulate and better adjust the quarantine periods imposed on citizens. One of the critical factors for this location of people to be possible has to do with privacy issues, and only with legal changes at this level may it be possible to move forward with integrated and official solutions that can be used across the board by decision-making bodies. The use of monitoring solutions is already in use in countries like Taiwan (to ensure compliance with quarantine rules), South Korea (infected monitoring and proximity alert with someone infected), or Israel (monitoring infected through your mobile phone) [54].

Drones have been widely used in several countries for various purposes, asserting themselves as an intelligent solution for a variety of applications. In some countries they are being used to guarantee social distance, for example, in China and India [55]. Drones are also being used to broadcast information relevant to the community, as in the case of Spain where a drone with a loudspeaker was used to announce measures of a state of emergency [56]. Other countries used the same method to announce measures to be taken into account to ensure social distance [57]. Mass measurement of temperature by the population has also been done using a drone with an infrared camera. In some cases, it can measure the temperature of several people simultaneously [58]. Remote monitoring of symptoms (such as respiratory diseases) is being developed in Australia by monitoring temperature and heart rate [59]. The disinfection of spaces [60] and the delivery of essential medical goods [61–63] are also other features that have been attributed to drones in these times of epidemic.

The health domain is where the greatest applications of IoT and smart technologies exist at this time of crisis. The interconnection of medical devices with devices on patients (such as smartphones or wearables) and even the medical infrastructure of information systems has brought the possibility of cross-checking data and verification and decision-making almost in real time [64]. During this pandemic crisis, there is a multiplication of remote consultations, which may open new paths for telemedicine and for remote monitoring of patients (especially for those who continue to need it and cannot be exposed due to possible viruses). The Internet of Medical Things (IoMT), or healthcare IoT, which refers to the set of medical devices, software as well as the health services offered, has known significant advances also due the ease with which today the various devices can interconnect among themselves through various protocols such as Bluetooth or NFC [65]. Regarding IoT and IoMT, some of the technologies, devices, and services currently in use in this pandemic phase include smart thermometers, robots, autonomous vehicles, drones, telemedicine, and RFID readers [66, 67].

RFID robots have been used to distribute medicines to medical teams, as has been done at Geisinger Medical Center in Danville, Pennsylvania, USA. Likewise, the collection and processing of medical waste can be done by a robot, allowing safer treatment and avoiding unnecessary contagions on the part of medical assistants. Augmented reality (AR), in conjunction with an IoT network, can be used in patient care and early diagnosis that have to be done by doctors with experience. But the number may be limited in some circumstances, preventing doctors from being available in all necessary places. AR technologies can allow nurses or other professionals to be at the forefront assisted by doctors through computer systems that allow remote diagnosis and assistance [67].

4.6.2 Nanotechnology in COVID-19

The nanotechnology-based solutions and medical aid equipment for the patients and frontline care providers including doctors, nurses, other hospital staff along with security personnel, law makers, etc., have the potential to provide promising solutions at all levels in this fight against COVID-19, including prevention, diagnostics, and treatments [68–75]. The reusable nano-materials for face masks, nano-medicine for COVID-19 patients, and nano-based test kits are few applications of nanotechnology in COVID-19 pandemic. Many products are already available in the market, and many are being developed by scientists. Figure 4.9 presents the application areas of nanotechnology for fighting COVID-19 [68–75, 80].

In a recent development, scientists have claimed to have developed preventive products for COVID-19 using nanotechnology. A Japanese company "Nanotera Group" has developed an antimicrobial spray that coats almost all surfaces except the human skin and kills any pathogens [69]. The company claims that once sprayed, the coating works for 5 years. This spray provides promising solutions to fight pathogens, but it comes with a cost. The spray costs $3000 per hundred square meters [69, 70]. Nanofibers developed using the electro-spinning production technique are used to manufacture N95 respirators, which claims to block almost 95% of airborne particles that are more than 2.5 μm [71]. A research team from Korea

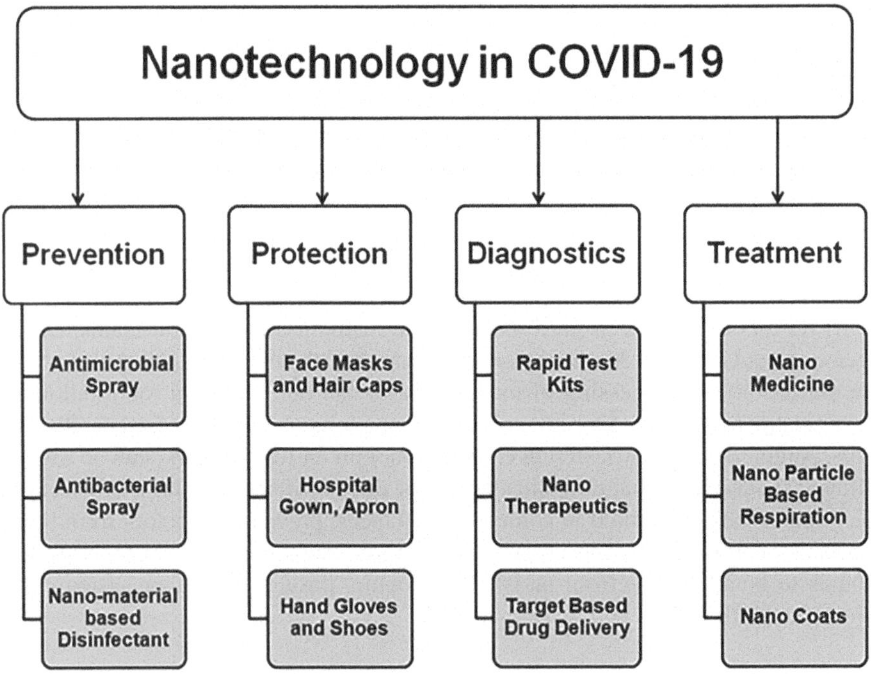

Fig. 4.9 Application domains of nanotechnology in COVID-19

Advanced Institute of Science and Technology claims to have used the insulation block electro-spinning process to manufacture nanofiber masks that are reusable even after 20 hand washes [72]. In Norway, a research team from NTNU and St. Olav's Hospital is developing a silica coated iron oxide nanoparticle for testing of COVID-19 [73]. With all such unprecedented features and applications of nanotechnology, there exist several challenges in the mass adoption of nanotechnology-based solutions.

1. Cost and underlying infrastructure: There is a considerable amount of cost involved in the adoption of nanotechnology-based solutions. Further it involves precision-based infrastructure facilities which are hard to set up.
2. Skilled personnel to use the technology: Nanotechnology is a highly specialized domain, and thus there is a scarcity of trained professionals.
3. Awareness among masses: As a growing field of research, nanotechnology has expanded its domain and range to a large section of areas including agriculture, healthcare, transportation, building constructions, etc. However, there is still a lack of awareness among the general public about its potential.
4. Availability in marketplace: Nanotechnology-based products are very rarely available in the market. Since there are only few takers, the production is also limited or made to order.

Nanotechnology has a huge potential to help in COVID-19 pandemic. It is already being used for prevention and diagnostics of COVID-19. Further research is still going on, and very soon a breakthrough can happen with the invention of nanomedicine to cure COVID-19.

4.7 Conclusion and Future Scope

COVID-19 has been declared as a medical emergency of international concern by the WHO. Till date this outbreak has claimed thousands of lives all across the globe. The novel coronavirus is a unique class of virus which attacks the lungs of the patients. Since its emergence in Wuhan City of China along with its exponential outbreak in several other nations including Italy, the UK, the USA, France, Germany, India, etc., several measures are taken by the authorities to contain the damage and stop the further spread of the novel coronavirus pandemics.

This paper discusses the role of big data analytics techniques in curbing the affects and impact of pandemics [76–79]. The results of analysis on the publicly available data about COVID-19 show that the preventive measures like social distancing can help in the containment of the spread of the disease to a great extent. The impact of lockdown is also studied and presented. It is observed that the decrease in the human activities due to the lockdown at several locations worldwide had a positive impact on the environmental aspects like improvement of the air quality. The results of the study show that data analytics can provide significant insights related to the emergence, spread, and impact of pandemics and can also help in predicting outbreaks and prescribing solutions based on diagnostics and symptoms. Therefore, if used efficiently, data analytics can be a potential tool in the fight against pandemics.

The nations worldwide are also spreading awareness about personal hygiene and sanitation as a preventive measure against COVID-19. The other preferred measures adopted worldwide are social distancing and lockdown. Apart from these, other mitigation measures that can reduce the impact of such pandemics may include [33, 76–79]:

- Changing the attitude of people.
- Understanding and conveying the nature and intensity of the threat to the vulnerable masses.
- Stringent rules, regulations, and laws.
- Policy to check all international travel with basic tests and health procedure which can be done at the time of visa processing.
- Helping the underprivileged groups in case of quarantine and relocations.
- Global corpus funds for such unexpected epidemics and pandemics.
- Grass-root level counseling of the inhabitants.
- Standardized environment, health, hygiene, and disaster management education must be made mandatory for all at UG and PG level of education.

Furthermore, it is imperative to track and contain the outbreak of epidemics and pandemics like COVID-19 in order to stop community transfer. The authenticity and validity of the epidemiological data are highly crucial for planning the mitigation measures. For effective and authentic tracking of the disease carriers and possible doubtful cases along with the epicenter of the pandemics, blockchain technology can be used. Blockchain is a distributed ledger technology which is immutable and transparent and thus makes it the most appropriate candidate for tracking the COVID-19 transmitters and epicenters. Blockchain consortiums like MiPasa and several other companies like "Acoer," "Telos," and "Algorand" have already rolled out applications to track and share the data of the patients in a transparent, secured, and privacy preserved manner. In future other modern-day enabling technologies like edge computing, blockchain, deep learning, etc., can be explored to devise novel, effective, and efficient mechanisms for tracking and containing the pandemics and epidemics.

References

1. Chen, M., Mao, S., Liu, Y.: Big data: a survey. Mobile Netw. Appl. **19**(2), 171–209 (2014)
2. McAfee, A., Brynjolfsson, E., Davenport, T.H., Patil, D.J., Barton, D.: Big data: the management revolution. Harv. Bus. Rev. **90**(10), 60–68 (2012)
3. Ahad, M.A., Biswas, R.: Comparing and analyzing the characteristics of Hadoop, Cassandra and Quantcast file systems for handling big data. Indian J. Sci. Technol. **10**(8), 1–6 (2017)
4. Kitchin, R., McArdle, G.: What makes big data, big data? Exploring the ontological characteristics of 26 datasets. Big Data Soc. **3**(1), 2053951716631130 (2016)

5. Alonso, S.G., de la Torre Diez, I., Rodrigues, J.J., Hamrioui, S., Lopez-Coronado, M.: A systematic review of techniques and sources of big data in the healthcare sector. J. Med. Syst. **41**(11), 183 (2017)
6. Sources of big data: where does it come from? https://www.cloudmoyo.com/blog/data-architecture/what-is-big-data-and-where-it-comes-from/
7. https://www.who.int/emergencies/diseases/novel-coronavirus-2019
8. Liu, Z., Magal, P., Seydi, O., Webb, G.: Predicting the cumulative number of cases for the COVID-19 epidemic in China from early data. arXiv preprint arXiv:2002.12298 (2020)
9. Sohrabi, C., Alsafi, Z., O'Neill, N., Khan, M., Kerwan, A., Al-Jabir, A., et al.: World Health Organization declares global emergency: a review of the 2019 novel coronavirus (COVID-19). Int. J. Surg. **76**, 71–76 (2020)
10. Liu, Z., Magal, P., Seydi, O., Webb, G.: Understanding unreported cases in the COVID-19 epidemic outbreak in Wuhan, China, and the importance of major public health interventions. Biology. **9**(3), 50 (2020)
11. Allam, Z., Jones, D.S.: On the coronavirus (COVID-19) outbreak and the smart city network: universal data sharing standards coupled with artificial intelligence (AI) to benefit urban health monitoring and management. Healthcare. **8**(1), 46 (2020) Multidisciplinary Digital Publishing Institute
12. McCall, B.: COVID-19 and artificial intelligence: protecting health-care workers and curbing the spread. Lancet Digit. Health. **2**(4), e149–e208 (2020)
13. Buckee, C.: Improving epidemic surveillance and response: big data is dead, long live big data. Lancet Digit. Health. **2**(5), e218–e220 (2020)
14. Moriarty, L.F.: Public health responses to COVID-19 outbreaks on cruise ships—worldwide, February–March 2020. MMWR Morb. Mortal. Wkly. Rep. **69**(12), 347–352 (2020)
15. Zhao, D., Yao, F., Wang, L., Zheng, L., Gao, Y., Ye, J., et al.: A comparative study on the clinical features of COVID-19 pneumonia to other pneumonias. Clin. Infect. Dis. (2020)
16. Burke, R.M.: Active monitoring of persons exposed to patients with confirmed COVID-19—United States, January–February 2020. MMWR Morb. Mortal. Wkly. Rep. **69**(9), 245–246 (2020)
17. Guan, W.J., Ni, Z.Y., Hu, Y., Liang, W.H., Ou, C.Q., He, J.X., et al.: Clinical characteristics of coronavirus disease 2019 in China. N. Engl. J. Med. **382**, 1708–1720 (2020)
18. Rasmussen, S.A., Smulian, J.C., Lednicky, J.A., Wen, T.S., Jamieson, D.J.: Coronavirus disease 2019 (COVID-19) and pregnancy: what obstetricians need to know. Am. J. Obstet. Gynecol. **222**(5), 415–426 (2020)
19. Fitzpatrick, F., Doherty, A., Lacey, G.: Using artificial intelligence in infection prevention. Curr. Treat. Options Infect. Dis., 1–10 (2020)
20. Chen, Q., Min, C., Zhang, W., Wang, G., Ma, X., Evans, R.: Unpacking the black box: how to promote citizen engagement through government social media during the COVID-19 crisis. Comput. Hum. Behav. **110**, 106380 (2020)
21. Lenca, M., Vayena, E.: On the responsible use of digital data to tackle the COVID-19 pandemic. Nat. Med. **26**(4), 463–464 (2020)
22. Roda, W.C., Varughese, M.B., Han, D., Li, M.Y.: Why is it difficult to accurately predict the COVID-19 epidemic? Infect. Dis. Modell. **5**, 271–281 (2020)
23. Fan, C., Cai, T., Gai, Z., Wu, Y.: The relationship between the migrant population's migration network and the risk of COVID-19 transmission in China—empirical analysis and prediction in prefecture-level cities. Int. J. Environ. Res. Public Health. **17**(8), 2630 (2020)
24. Li, X., Xu, S., Yu, M., Wang, K., Tao, Y., Zhou, Y., et al.: Risk factors for severity and mortality in adult COVID-19 inpatients in Wuhan. J. Allergy Clin. Immunol. **146**(1), 110–118 (2020)
25. Sarkodie, S.A., Owusu, P.A.: Investigating the cases of novel coronavirus disease(COVID-19) in China using dynamic statistical techniques. Heliyon. **6**(4), e03747 (2020)
26. From chaos to coherence: managing pandemics with data, can data analytics prevent future pandemics? https://expectexceptional.economist.com/managing-pandemics-with-data.html. Accessed 16 Mar 2020

27. Managing pandemics, key facts about the deadly disease. World Health Organization (2018). https://www.who.int/emergencies/diseases/managing-epidemics-interactive.pdf. Accessed 20 Mar 2020
28. Singh, R., Singh, R., Bhatia, A.: Sentiment analysis using machine learning technique to predict outbreaks and epidemics. Int. J. Adv. Sci. Res. **3**(2), 19–24 (2018)
29. Peng, L., Yang, W., Zhang, D., Zhuge, C., Hong, L.: Epidemic analysis of COVID-19 in China by dynamical modeling. arXiv preprint arXiv:2002.06563 (2020)
30. Wang, C.J., Ng, C.Y., Brook, R.H.: Response to COVID-19 in Taiwan: big data analytics, new technology, and proactive testing. J.A.M.A. **323**(14), 1341–1342 (2020). https://doi.org/10.1001/jama.2020.315
31. https://spectrum.ieee.org/the-human-os/biomedical/devices/big-data-helps-taiwan-fight-coronavirus
32. Madaan, N., Ahad, M.A., Sastry, S.M.: Data integration in IoT ecosystem: information linkage as a privacy threat. Comput. Law Secur. Rev. **34**(1), 125–133 (2018)
33. Ahad, M.A., Tripathi, G., Agarwal, P.: Learning analytics for IoE based educational model using deep learning techniques: architecture, challenges and applications. Smart Learn. Environ. **5**(1), 1–16 (2018)
34. Ahad, M.A., Biswas, R.: Dynamic merging based small file storage (DM-SFS) architecture for efficiently storing small size files in Hadoop. Procedia Comput. Sci. **132**, 1626–1635 (2018)
35. Ahad, M.A., Paiva, S., Tripathi, G., Feroz, N.: Enabling technologies and sustainable smart cities. Sustain. Cities Soc. **61**, 102301 (2020)
36. Gostin, L.O., Lucey, D., Phelan, A.: The Ebola epidemic: a global health emergency. J.A.M.A. **312**(11), 1095–1096 (2014)
37. Harford, T.: Big data: a big mistake? Significance. **11**(5), 14–19 (2014)
38. Ioannidis, J.P.: Why most published research findings are false. PLoS Med. **2**(8), e124 (2005)
39. Paiva, S., Ahad, M.A., Zafar, S., Tripathi, G., Khalique, A., Hussain, I.: Privacy and security challenges in smart and sustainable mobility. SN Appl. Sci. **2**, 1175 (2020)
40. Ahad, M.A., Biswas, R.: PPS-ADS: a framework for privacy-preserved and secured distributed system architecture for handling big data. Int. J. Adv. Sci. Eng. Inf. Technol. **8**(4), 1333–1342 (2018)
41. Ahad, M.A., Biswas, R.: Request-based, secured and energy-efficient (RBSEE) architecture for handling IoT big data. J. Inf. Sci. **45**(2), 227–238 (2019)
42. COVID-19 Datasets. https://github.com/CSSEGISandData/COVID-19/tree/master/csse_COVID_19_data/csse_COVID_19_daily_reports
43. COVID-19 Complete Dataset (Updated every 24hrs), number of confirmed, death and recovered cases every day across the globe. https://www.kaggle.com/imdevskp/corona-virus-report
44. Johns Hopkins University Center for Systems Science and Engineering (JHU CCSE). https://data.humdata.org/dataset/novel-coronavirus-2019-ncov-cases
45. National Air Quality Index, Central Pollution Control Board, Ministry of Environment, Forests and Climate Change. https://app.cpcbccr.com/AQI_India/
46. https://epha.org/air-pollution-clears-in-cities-globally-maps/
47. This is how coronavirus could affect the travel and tourism industry. World Economic Forum (2020). https://www.weforum.org/agenda/2020/03/world-travel-coronavirus-covid19-jobs-pandemic-tourism-aviation/
48. Corona virus affecting the tourism industry worldwide. Travel Daily News (2020). https://www.traveldailynews.com/post/corona-virus-affecting-the-tourism-industry-worldwide
49. Virus 'could cost millions of tourism jobs'. BBC News (2020). https://www.bbc.com/news/business-51852505
50. Thiessen, T.: U.S. travel industry warns of $910 B coronavirus losses: seven times 9/11, Forbes. https://www.forbes.com/sites/tamarathiessen/2020/04/01/us-travel-industry-warns-of-910b-coronavirus-losses/#15e6b3746c9d

51. WhatwouldcancelingHajjmeanforSaudiArabia'seconomy?MSNnews(2020).https://www.msn.com/en-ae/news/coronavirus/what-would-canceling-hajj-mean-for-saudi-arabias-economy/ar-BB127Drj?li=BBqrPye
52. Tourism and Covid-19, United Nations World Travel Organization (2020). https://www.unwto.org/tourism-covid-19
53. DQIndia online. Can Coronavirus like Outbreaks be Controlled with IoT? DQIndia (2020). https://www.dqindia.com/can-coronavirus-like-outbreaks-controlled-iot/
54. Mackenzie, M.: COVID-19: IoT has a limited role in dealing with the current crisis, but could help with future pandemics (2020). https://www.analysysmason.com/Research/Content/Comments/covid19-iot-role-rdme0-rma17/. Accessed 18 May 2020
55. Marr, B.: Robots and drones are now used to fight COVID-19 (2020). https://www.forbes.com/sites/bernardmarr/2020/03/18/how-robots-and-drones-are-helping-to-fight-coronavirus/#2a8bfbca2a12. Accessed Mar 2020
56. Gascuena, D.: Drones to stop the covid-19 epidemic (2020). https://www.bbva.com/en/drones-to-stop-the-covid-19-epidemic/. Accessed Apr 2020
57. Sharma, M.: How drones are being used to combat COVID-19 (2020). https://www.geospatial-world.net/blogs/how-drones-are-being-used-to-combat-covid-19/. Accesses Apr 2020
58. Singh, P.: Thermal scan: drones check people for fever in Delhi: Delhi news—Times of India (2020). https://timesofindia.indiatimes.com/city/delhi/thermal-scan-drones-check-people-for-fever/articleshow/75088774.cms. Accessed Apr 2020
59. UniSA working on 'pandemic drone' to detect coronavirus (2020). https://www.unisa.edu.au/Media-Centre/Releases/2020/unisa-working-on-pandemic-drone-to-detect-coronavirus/. Accessed Mar 2020
60. Pan, C.: Spain's military uses DJI agricultural drones to spray disinfectant in fight against Covid-19 (2020). https://www.scmp.com/tech/gear/article/3077945/spains-military-uses-dji-agricultural-drones-spray-disinfectant-fight. Accessed Apr 2020
61. NUI Galway makes Aviation History by Completing the World's First Diabetes Drone Mission from Mainland to Aran Islands (2020). https://www.nuigalway.ie/about-us/news-and-events/news-archive/2019/september/nui-galway-makes-aviation-history-by-completing-the-worlds-first-diabetes-drone-mission-from-mainland-to-aran-islands.html. Accessed Sep 2019
62. Ackerman, E. Zipline wants to bring medical drone delivery to U.S. to fight COVID-19 (2020). https://spectrum.ieee.org/automaton/robotics/drones/zipline-medical-drone-delivery-covid19. Accessed Apr 2020
63. Yang, J.: 3 ways China is using drones to fight coronavirus. https://www.weforum.org/agenda/2020/03/three-ways-china-is-using-drones-to-fight-coronavirus/. Accessed 7 Apr 2020
64. Son, J., Kim, Y., Zhou, S.: Recommending clinical interventions to patients via Iot-enabled health information system considering trust-dependent patient adherence (2020). SSRN: https://ssrn.com/abstract=3528921. Accessed 30 Jan 2020
65. Rouse, M.: What is IoMT (Internet of Medical Things) or healthcare IoT?—definition from WhatIs.com (2015). https://internetofthingsagenda.techtarget.com/definition/IoMT-Internet-of-Medical-Things. Accessed Aug 2015
66. Chamola, V., Hassija, V., Gupta, V., Guizani, M.: A comprehensive review of the COVID-19 pandemic and the role of IoT, drones, AI, Blockchain and 5G in managing its impact. IEEE Acces, p. 1 (2020). https://doi.org/10.1109/ACCESS.2020.2992341
67. Song, Y., Jiang, J., Wang, X., Yang, D., Bai, C.: Prospect and application of Internet of Things technology for prevention of SARIs (Severe Acute Respiratory Infections). Clin. eHealth. **3**, 1–4 (2020). https://doi.org/10.1016/j.ceh.2020.02.001
68. Hu, T.Y., Frieman, M., Wolfram, J.: Insights from nanomedicine into chloroquine efficacy against COVID-19. Nat. Nanotechnol. **15**, 247–249 (2020). https://doi.org/10.1038/s41565-020-0674-9
69. https://nano-magazine.com/news/2020/3/11/scientists-create-most-effective-anti-coronavirus-spray
70. https://statnano.com/nanotechnology-in-battle-against-coronavirus

71. https://statnano.com/news/67490/Nanotechnology-enabled-N95-Masks-Can-Halt-the-Spread-of-Coronavirus
72. https://statnano.com/news/67527/Nanofiber-based-Face-Mask-Preserves-Its-Filtering-Function-and-Sturdiness-After-20-Washes
73. https://statnano.com/news/67573/Norway-Turns-Silica-coated-Iron-Oxide-Nanoparticles-into-150-000-COVID-19-Tests-Per-Week
74. Chan, W.C.W.: Nano research for COVID-19. ACS Nano. acsnano.0c02540 (2020). https://doi.org/10.1021/acsnano.0c02540., https://www.ncbi.nlm.nih.gov/pmc/articles/PMC7123821/pdf/nn0c02540.pdf
75. Kouzegaran, V.J.: COVID-19 and nanotechnology (2020). https://nanografi.com/blog/covid19-and-nanotechnology/. Accessed Apr 2020
76. Datta, R., Yadav, A.K., Singh, A., Datta, K., Bansal, A.: The infodemics of COVID-19 amongst healthcare professionals in India. Med. J. Armed Forces India. **76**(3), 276–283 (2020)
77. Kouzy, R., Abi Jaoude, J., Kraitem, A., El Alam, M.B., Karam, B., Adib, E., et al.: Coronavirus goes viral: quantifying the COVID-19 misinformation epidemic on twitter. Cureus. **12**(3), e7255 (2020)
78. https://www.thelancet.com/journals/lancet/article/PIIS0140-6736(20)30461-X/fulltext#coronavirus-linkback-header
79. https://rss.onlinelibrary.wiley.com/doi/full/10.1111/j.1740-9713.2014.00778.x
80. Udugama, B., Kadhiresan, P., Kozlowski, H.N., Malekjahani, A., Osborne, M., Li, V.Y., et al.: Diagnosing COVID-19: the disease and tools for detection. ACS Nano (2020)

Chapter 5
Applications of Artificial Intelligence and Internet of Things for Detection and Future Directions to Fight Against COVID-19

Akshat Agrawal , Rajesh Arora , Ranjana Arora , and Prateek Agrawal

Abstract Recently, coronavirus disease 2019 (COVID-19) has become a prevalent threat for the human life all over the world. The propagation of this virus is very fast, and due to its contagious nature, it is infecting millions of people globally. Scientists and researchers are continuously working to find out the ways, i.e., medicine/vaccine for its cure. In the current scenario, spreading awareness regarding detection and prevention of this pandemic can save numerous lives in whole community. In this context, applications of artificial intelligence (AI) and Internet of Things (IoT) techniques could be a boon to mankind, as they can help in prevention, detection, forecasting, mortality risk of patients and remote operation of curing devices like ventilators, drone sanitization/surveillance, resource management, etc. In the present study, all possible applications of AI technology, viz., collection of infected blood samples, detection of virus, forecasting, etc., have been undertaken. Furthermore, the relevance of IoT in terms of monitoring and controlling electrical and mechanical devices for the cure of COVID-19, communication of interconnecting devices, and supervision of curing appliances has been reviewed here. The use of various AI and machine learning (ML) algorithms in view of detecting the most threatening symptoms and features of this dangerous virus has been demonstrated in the present work. This will significantly enhance the lifesaving probability of human beings and can help in exploring the new methods of prevention and detection of COVID-19.

A. Agrawal · R. Arora (✉) · R. Arora
Amity University Haryana, Gurugram, India
e-mail: rarora64@ggn.amity.edu

P. Agrawal
University of Klagenfurt, Klagenfurt, Austria

Lovely Professional University, Phagwara, Punjab, India

© The Author(s), under exclusive license to Springer Nature Switzerland AG 2021

F. Al-Turjman et al. (eds.), *Emerging Technologies for Battling Covid-19*, Studies in Systems, Decision and Control 324,
https://doi.org/10.1007/978-3-030-60039-6_5

Keywords Artificial Intelligence · COVID-19 · Internet of Things · Machine learning

5.1 Introduction

The COVID-19 pandemic has emerged as a very substantial catastrophe globally, since the time of the Second World War. It has exceedingly affected all the countries of our planet, and its health consequences are quite disturbing and alarming. Till date, nearly 400,000 people have died due to this virus, and unfortunately this data is ordained to rise exponentially in the near future. Besides, the situation has directed to unparalleled social penalties and turmoil. The stupendous fact is projected that more than four billion people (a half of the entire mankind) are today pretentiously facing radical constraints in their activities and social associations [1]. A massive global financial disaster unlike the former eras might tremor the world in the years to come. This prevalent pandemic has majorly affected our customs, trading protocols, communal and financial conventions, devices, working philosophies, and political administrations in a diverse manner globally. It is very astonishing that globally our governing bodies, social administration, and health organizations were improvised to accomplish such circumstances, but now the time has come to handle and improve the situation with all possible apparatuses and tools in order to make this world a safer and healthier place for our upcoming generations.

There is a persistent and abrupt requirement for the community of science and technology, to join hand in hand for delivering innovative and improved procedures, policies, models, and forecasting practices in view to comprehend and diminish the outcomes of this and forthcoming epidemics. These efforts are required in both the nearby and coming future to apprise operative and impartial protocols and procedures to handle such situations. The whole world is looking for new techniques and technologies in this worldwide health crisis, for monitoring and controlling COVID-19 (coronavirus) spread much effectively. Artificial intelligence and machine learning are the answer to such problems which can easily monitor and predict the spreading of such viruses, can categorize the prone patients, and can be highly beneficial to control this contamination in real time. It is also helpful in predicting the mortality rate by effectively investigating the previously obtained data of the sufferers. These tools are effective for fighting against this virus through population airing, medical aids, reports, and ideas regarding its contagious spread [2–7].

The proposed technologies can forecast and predict the pattern of the spreading of the disease with the help of data available, social platforms, and media, rate of the infections and is contagious spreading risk globally. Furthermore, it could also find the number of active cases and deaths that occurred in any area since the time of inception of this virus. These techniques can be helpful in recognizing the most susceptible sections, individuals, and nations to adopt all the safety measures consequently [8–10].

In the present work, a critical review on the applications of artificial intelligence and Internet of Things for detection and future directions to fight against COVID-19 has been presented in view of identifying the high-risk areas and individuals and to adopt the safety measures consequently. The work is highly beneficial for monitoring and controlling the spread of this life-threatening virus and can significantly improve the situation by making the world a safer and a healthier place for the upcoming generations.

5.1.1 *Motivation of the Study*

The study has considered the following critical points to present a thorough and a comprehensive review to overcome the COVID-19 pandemic.

1. To analyze the artificial intelligence and machine learning tools for their effectiveness in monitoring of COVID-19 spread.
2. To investigate the effect of IoT on estimation, prediction, monitoring, and controlling of the COVID-19 spread.
3. To explore various forecasting tools to monitor the spread of virus in different regions of the nations.
4. To check the possible effectiveness on the application of artificial intelligence, machine learning, and IoT on the lifesaving devices like ventilators, drone sanitization/surveillance, resource management, etc.
5. To spread awareness in the society for fighting against the virus and save the lives globally.

5.2 Machine Learning and Artificial Intelligence Techniques Used for Forecasting of Spread of COVID-19

The artificial intelligence and machine learning technologies have the great utility to improvise the scheduling, handling, and testified consequences of the COVID-19 sufferer, using the tools based on facts and evidence collected in the near past cases.

These can make up a smart and effective platform for the prediction, monitoring, and cure of the spread of the disease. A neural network technique could be developed in order to get the prominent characteristics of the virus and can be highly beneficial in the treatment of the infected lot. It can also give the updates and current number of cases active in a particular area and their probable solutions for the prevention of its spread.

The huge range of data for active COVID-19 cases can be amalgamated and investigated by latest machine learning and AI algorithms in view of providing a much better understanding of the spread of the virus. It can further help in improving the diagnosis speed and precision and development of novel therapies and

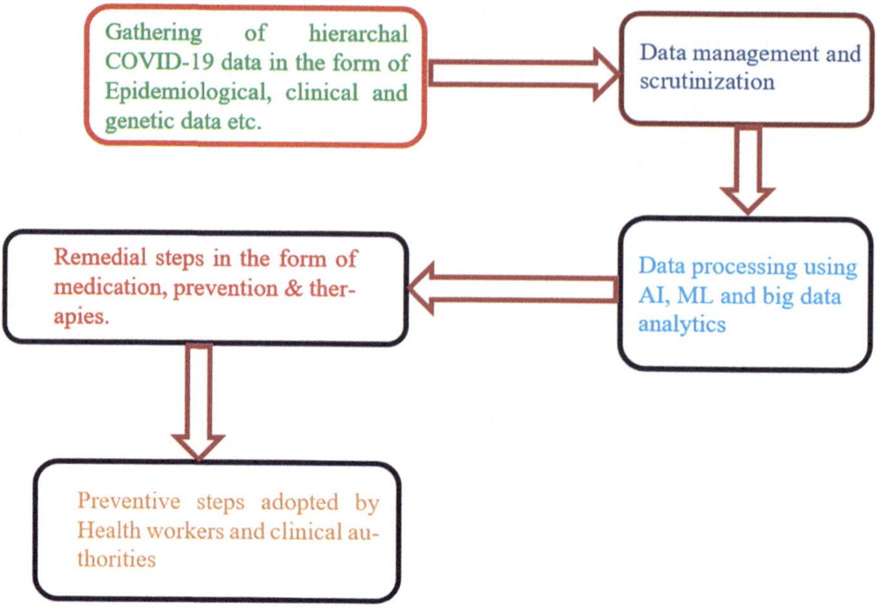

Fig. 5.1 Applications of AI/machine learning in fighting against COVID-19

psychological treatments to genetically cure the disease at faster rate. Stupendously, in a short span of time since the spread of this pandemic, these advanced AI and machine learning technologies have been employed in hieratical arrangement of COVID-19 genomes [11–15]. Figure 5.1 shows the procedural steps followed by AI and machine learning tools for helping out the health workers in order to identify COVID-19 symptoms and active infections.

5.3 IoT Applications for Surveillance of Various Virus Detection Devices

Internet of Things is playing a vital role in online monitoring, area tracking, SMS alerting, and gear up scheduling for favorable detection, monitoring, scheduling, and treatment provided for COVID-19 patients. Figure 5.2 shows the linkages of schedule management, off route maintenance, instruction management, and database decision-making of COVID-19 with respect to the prescheduled guidelines and real-time updates on standardized protocols of the disease spread. Recently, a number of researchers [16–30] have applied advanced optimization techniques, viz., genetic algorithm, NSGA-II, PSO, etc., to carry out optimum values of various design variables for different systems. In the present work, applications of these AI and ML techniques are reviewed for surveillance of various virus detection devices.

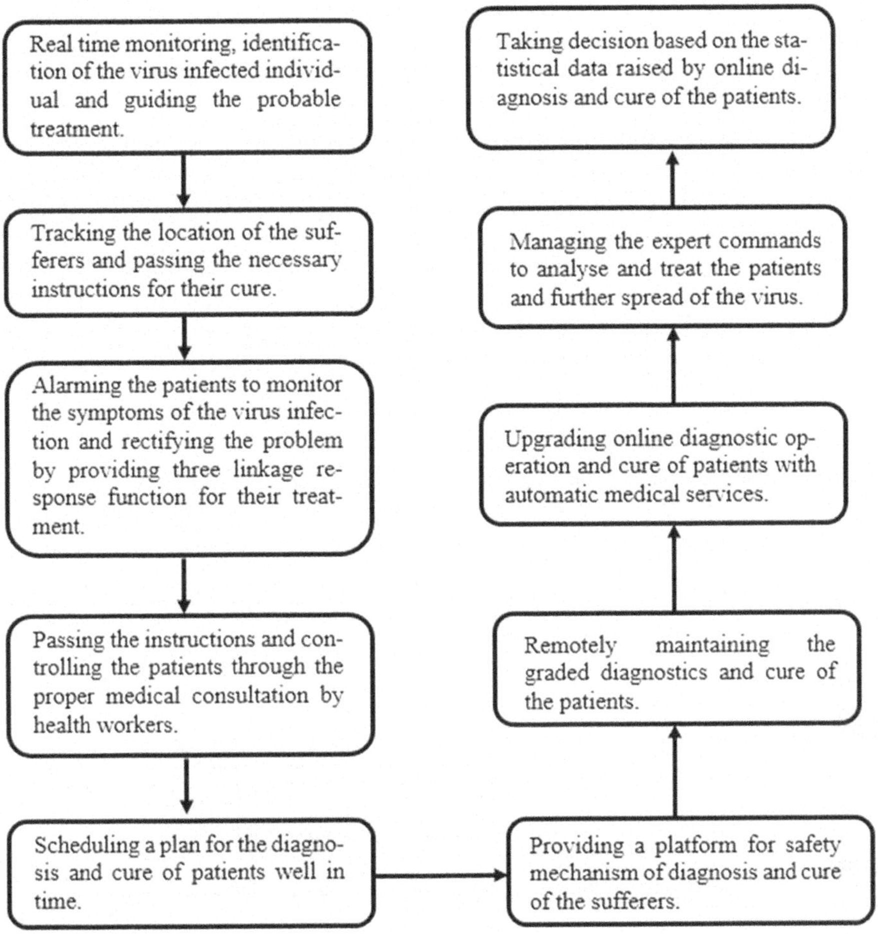

Fig. 5.2 Major functions of IoT diagnosis and curing system for COVID-19

Further, ten major functions of IoT diagnosis and curing system for COVID-19 are shown in Fig. 5.2:

5.4 Analysis of Available Data

The data pertaining to COVID-19 active cases is demonstrated through various platforms like media channels, research community, and government agencies/ websites which are increasing day by day due to the deadly spread of this dangerous virus. The presentation of the data is very important as it can significantly help in obtaining the pattern of its spread and ultimately the knowledge to prevent it. In this study, the data has been categorized in three different forms, viz., countries having active patients less than 10,000, active patients between 10,000 and 100,000, and countries with above 100,000 patients globally.

Figure 5.3 demonstrates the data pertaining to various countries having less than 10,000 active COVID-19 cases. This data is helpful for other countries to adopt their model to control the spread of COVID-19 at their place. The data of active patients is recorded from January 25, 2020, to May 30, 2020, in view of thoroughly monitoring the spread of COVID-19 in the whole world. It has been observed that there is a steep rise in the number of active patients from mid-March in almost all the countries shown in the time line. It is further observed that feeble rise in the activity of virus is found in the countries having average temperature more than

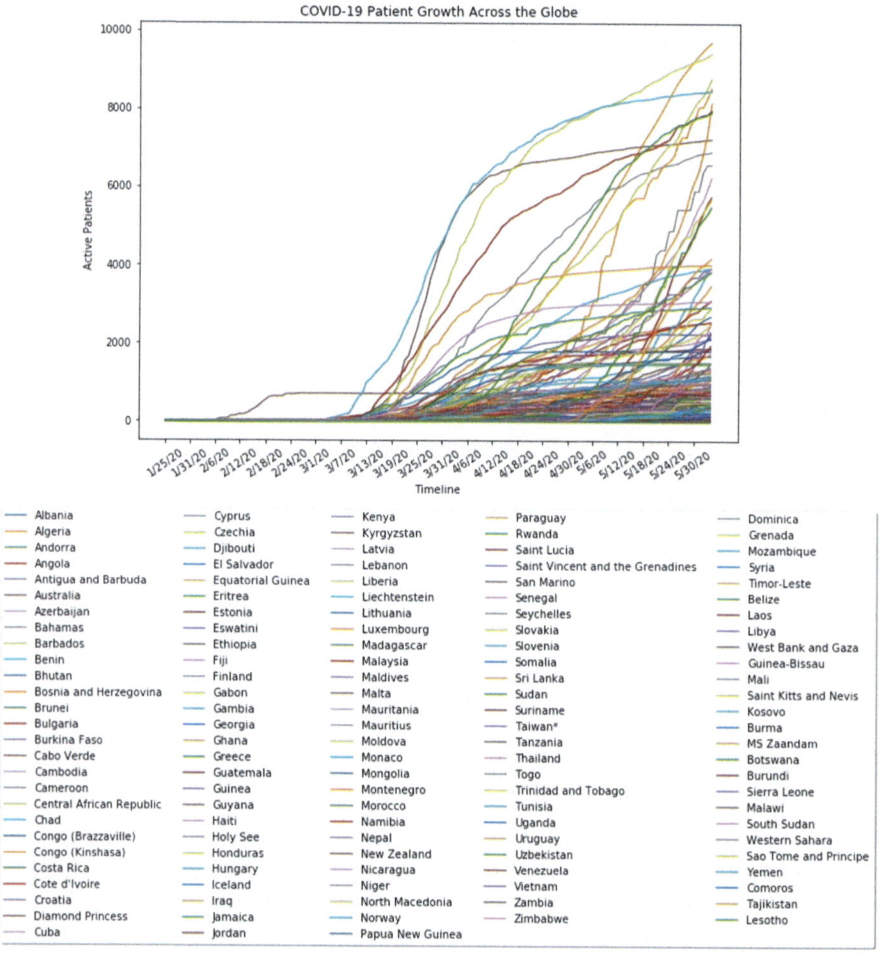

Fig. 5.3 Countries having active patients less than 10,000

50 °C. Depending upon the number of cases, these countries may be kept in the green zone in the safety scale.

Figure 5.4 demonstrates the data pertaining to various countries having less than 100,000 and more than 10,000 active COVID-19 cases. The data of active patients is recorded from January 25, 2020, to May 30, 2020, in view of thoroughly monitoring the spread of COVID-19 in the whole world. It has been observed that there is a steep rise in the number of active patients from mid-March in almost all the countries shown in the time line except China. A stringent rise in the number of active cases is observed in China from January 25, 2020, to February 20, 2020. After that the situation has been controlled as shown in the saturation in the number of active cases in the country. It is further observed that an alarming situation has arrived due to rise in the number of sufferers in all other countries around the world. The cases in these countries have not been stabilized and still

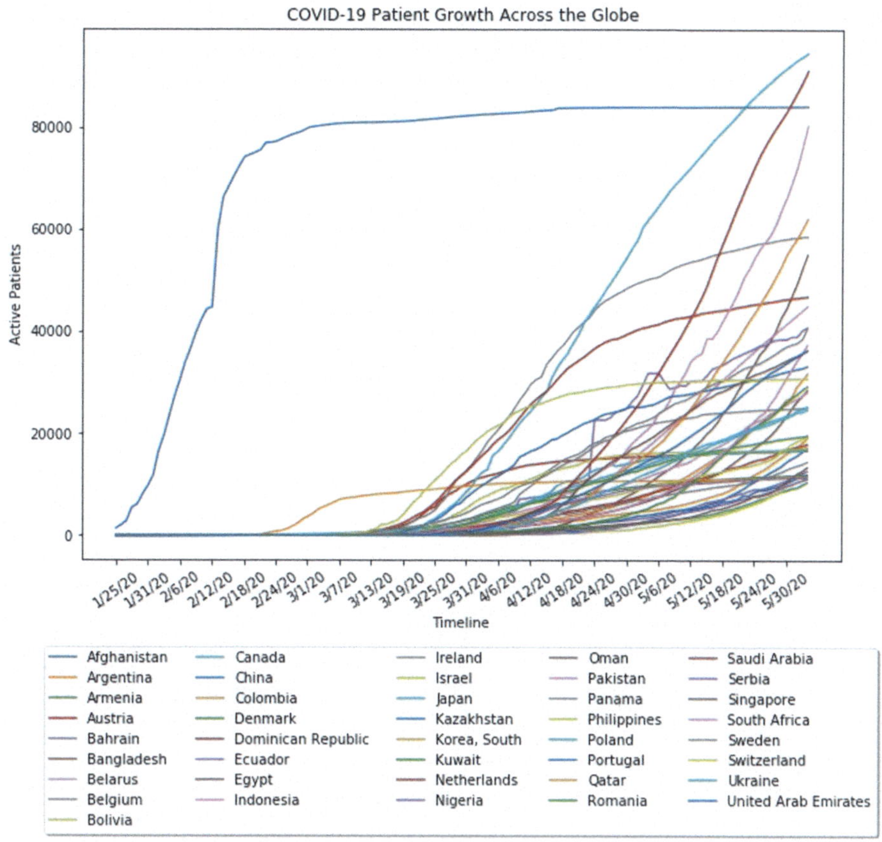

Fig. 5.4 Countries having active patients between 10,000 and 100,000

increasing day by day as shown in Fig. 5.4. These countries may be kept in the orange range.

Figure 5.5 demonstrates the data pertaining to various countries having more than 100,000 active COVID-19 cases. The data of active patients is recorded from January 25, 2020, to May 30, 2020, in view of thoroughly monitoring the spread of COVID-19 in the whole world. These are the countries which are marked in the red zone as observed from the very sharp rise in the number of active cases. It has been observed that there is a steep rise in the number of active patients from mid-March in the USA as compared to other countries shown in the time line. The situation is still not under control, and the cases are not stabilized till date. Further, the number of active cases in top ten countries around the world is shown in Fig. 5.6.

The daily rise in the number of active cases of COVID-19 in top four countries of the world is demonstrated in Figs. 5.7, 5.8, 5.9, and 5.10. The utmost rise is observed in the USA followed by Brazil, Russia, and Italy. It is found that the rise in US active cases steeply rises from mid-March and has not attained a saturation till date, as shown in Fig. 5.7. On the other hand, Brazil has shown a rise in active case from the last week of April 2020 as shown in Fig. 5.8, and still the life is in threat in this country. Likewise, Russia is showing rise in the number of active COVID-19 cases from mid-March, and the situation is not still under control in this country (refer to Fig. 5.9). Whereas in

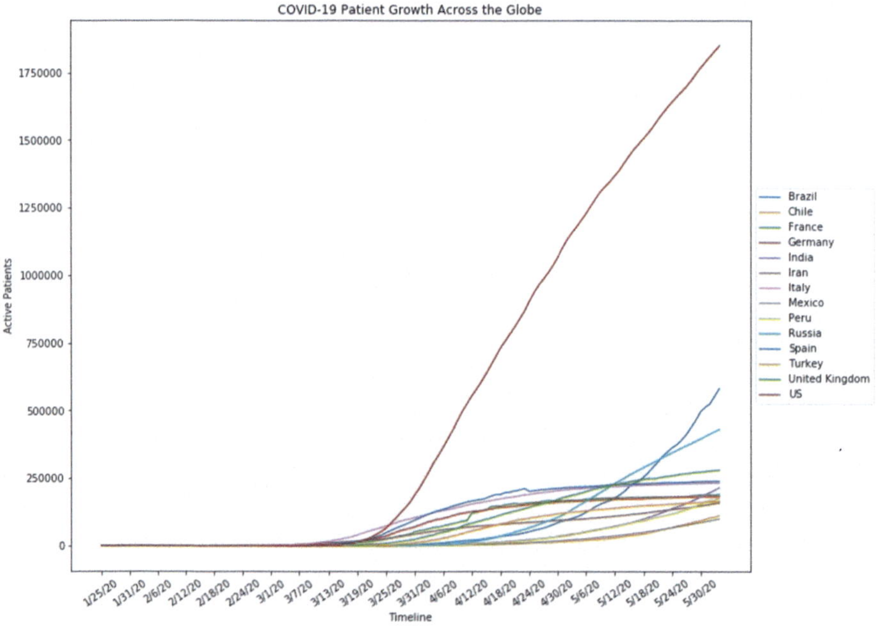

Fig. 5.5 Countries having more than 100,000 active patients

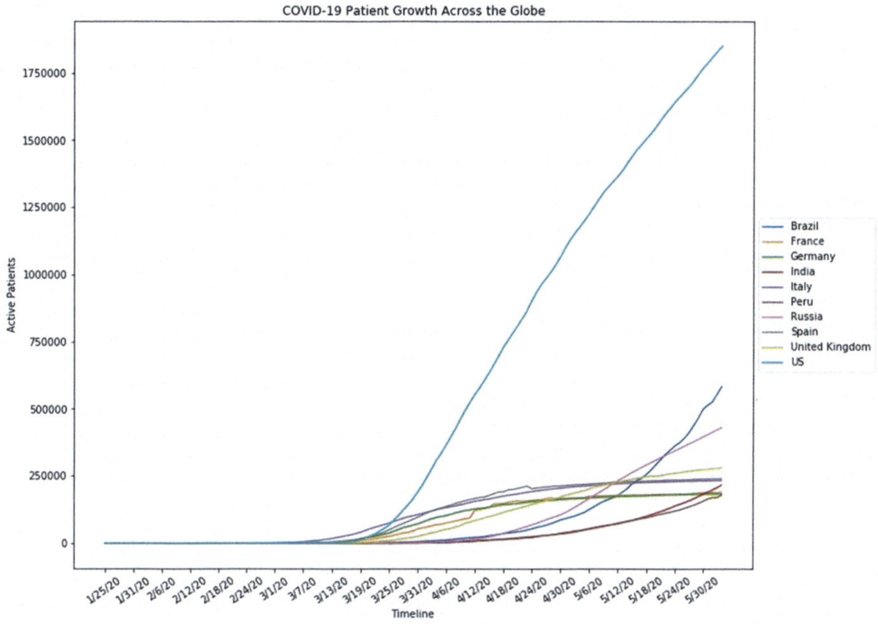

Fig. 5.6 Top ten countries with most COVID-19 active patients

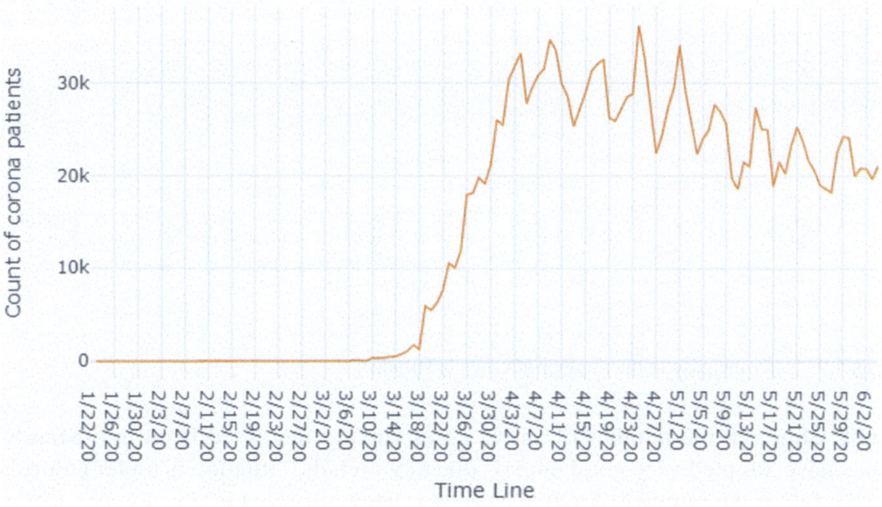

Fig. 5.7 Daily increase in number of cases in the USA

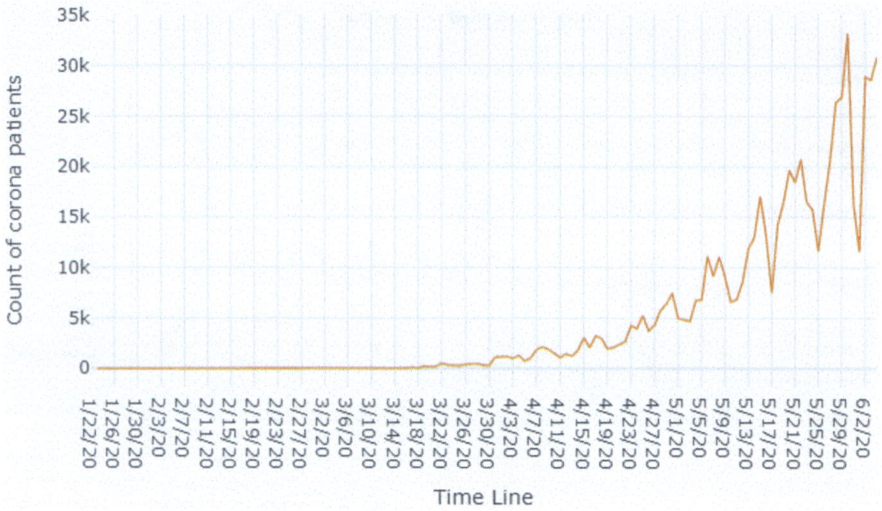

Fig. 5.8 Daily increase in the number of cases in Brazil

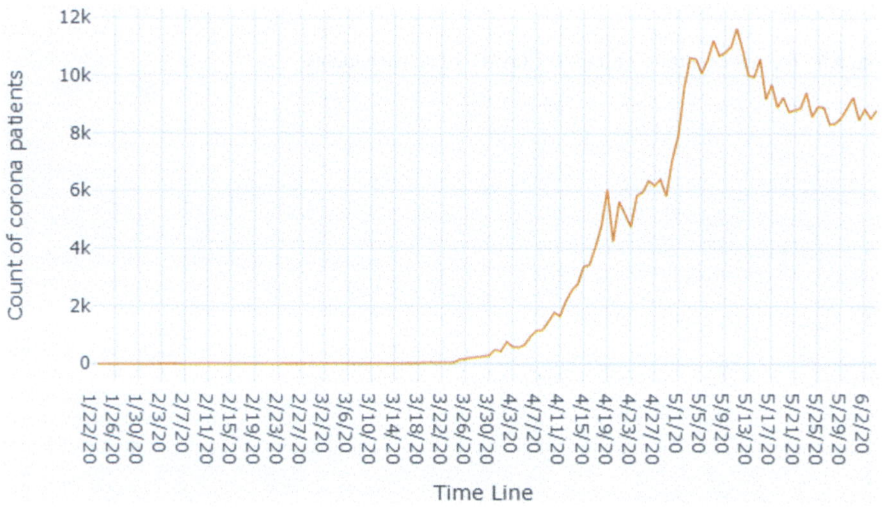

Fig. 5.9 Daily increase in the number of cases in Russia

Italy, although the number of active cases steeply increased from mid-March, they have adopted very good models due to which the situation is under control, and a fall in the number of active cases has been observed in this country (refer to Fig. 5.10).

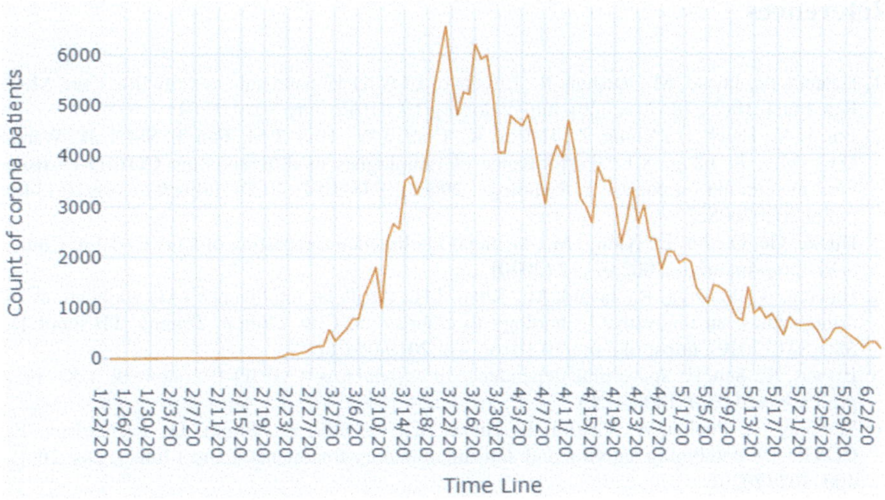

Fig. 5.10 Daily increase in the number of cases in Italy

5.5 Conclusions and Future Scope

In the present work, a critical review on the applications of artificial intelligence and Internet of Things for detection and future directions to fight against COVID-19 has been presented in view of identifying the high-risk areas and individuals and to adopt the safety measures consequently. The major outcomes of the study can be summarized as follows:

The artificial intelligence and machine learning tools are significantly beneficial to identify the infections caused by COVID-19 and could be helpful to monitor the state of infected people in a region. The Internet of Things is a novel tool which can remotely control and monitor the health measures like ventilators, drone sanitization/surveillance, resource management, etc., in a very effective and efficient manner.

These tools can abruptly upgrade the curing frequency and decision-making for the patients with the help of very fast algorithms. These are very useful in the treatment and cure of active COVID-19 cases and also in monitoring their health posttreatment.

These tools can facilitate to inform and alert the people regarding the spread of the virus by investigating the available data and are helpful in predicting, forecasting, and monitoring the health conditions.

The society can be made aware of this contagious virus and the ways to prevent/fight against COVID-19.

The work can further be extended to track the pandemic spread at various levels such as molecular, medical history, and epidemiological claims by using various other artificial intelligence and forecasting techniques. Further, the study can be effective to overcome the major tremor caused at different scales of economic, social, healthcare, and psychological prevalence in the society.

References

1. Haleem, A., Javaid, M., Vaishya, R.: Effects of COVID 19 pandemic in daily life. Curr. Med. Res. Pract. **10**(2), 78–79 (2020). https://doi.org/10.1016/j.cmrp.2020.03.011
2. Bai, H.X., Hsieh, B., Xiong, Z., Halsey, K., Choi, J.W., Tran, T.M., Pan, I., Shi, L.B., Wang, D.C., Mei, J., Jiang, X.L.: Performance of radiologists in differentiating COVID-19 from viral pneumonia on chest CT. Radiology. **296**(2), E46–E54 (2020). https://doi.org/10.1148/radiol.2020200823
3. Hu, Z., Ge, Q., Jin, L., Xiong, M.: Artificial intelligence forecasting of COVID-19 in China. arXiv preprint arXiv:2002.07112 (2020)
4. Haleem, A., Vaishya, R., Javaid, M., Khan, I.H.: Artificial intelligence (AI) applications in orthopaedics: an innovative technology to embrace. J. Clin. Orthop. Trauma. **11**(Suppl 1), S80–S81 (2019). https://doi.org/10.1016/j.jcot.2019.06.012
5. Biswas, K., Sen, P.: Space-time dependence of coronavirus (COVID-19) outbreak. arXiv preprint arXiv:2003.03149 (2020)
6. Stebbing, J., Phelan, A., Griffin, I., Tucker, C., Oechsle, O., Smith, D., Richardson, P.: COVID-19: combining antiviral and anti-inflammatory treatments. Lancet Infect. Dis. **20**(4), 400–402 (2020)
7. Cao, Y., Li, L., Feng, Z., Wan, S., Huang, P., Sun, X., Wen, F., Huang, X., Ning, G., Wang, W.: Comparative genetic analysis of the novel coronavirus (2019-nCoV/SARS-CoV-2) receptor ACE2 in different populations. Cell Discov. **6**, 11 (2020). https://doi.org/10.1038/s41421-020-0147-1
8. Fang, L., Karakiulakis, G., Roth, M.: Are patients with hypertension and diabetes mellitus at increased risk for COVID-19 infection? Lancet Respir. Med. **8**(4), e21 (2020). https://doi.org/10.1016/S2213-2600(20)30116-8
9. Ge, Y., Tian, T., Huang, S., Wan, F., Li, J., Li, S., Yang, H., Hong, L., Wu, N., Yuan, E., Cheng, L., Lei, Y., Shu, H., Feng, X., Jiang, Z., Chi, Y., Guo, X., Cui, L., Xiao, L., Li, Z., Yang, C., Miao, Z., Tang, H., Chen, L., Zeng, H., Zhao, D., Zhu, F., Shen, X., Zeng, J.: A data-driven drug repositioning framework discovered a potential therapeutic agent targeting COVID-19. bioRxiv (2020). https://doi.org/10.1101/2020.03.11.986836
10. Gozes, O., Frid-Adar, M., Greenspan, H., Browning, P.D., Zhang, H., Ji, W., Bernheim, A., Siegel, E.: Rapid AI development cycle for the coronavirus (COVID-19) pandemic: initial results for automated detection & patient monitoring using deep learning CT image analysis. arXiv2003.05037 (2020)
11. Metsky, H.C., Freije, C.A., Kosoko-Thoroddsen, T.-S.F., Sabeti, P.C., Myhrvold, C.: CRISPR-based COVID-19 surveillance using a genomically-comprehensive machine learning approach. bioRxiv (2020). https://doi.org/10.1101/2020.02.26.967026
12. Ong, E., Wong, M.U., Huffman, A., He, Y.: COVID-19 coronavirus vaccine design using reverse vaccinology and machine learning. bioRxiv (2020). https://doi.org/10.1101/2020.03.20.000141
13. Randhawa, G.S., Soltysiak, M.P.M., El Roz, H., de Souza, C.P.E., Hill, K.A., Kari, L.: Machine learning using intrinsic genomic signatures for rapid classification of novel pathogens: COVID-19 case study. bioRxiv (2020)
14. Senior, A.W., Evans, R., Jumper, J., Kirkpatrick, J., Sifre, L., Green, T., Qin, C., Žídek, A., Nelson, A.W.R., Bridgland, A., Penedones, H., Petersen, S., Simonyan, K., Crossan, S., Kohli, P., Jones, D.T., Silver, D., Kavukcuoglu, K., Hassabis, D.: Improved protein structure prediction using potentials from deep learning. Nature. **577**, 706–710 (2020). https://doi.org/10.1038/s41586-019-1923-7
15. Wang, Y., Hu, M., Li, Q., Zhang, X.-P., Zhai, G., Yao, N.: Abnormal respiratory patterns classifier may contribute to large-scale screening of people infected with COVID-19 in an accurate and unobtrusive manner. arXiv2002.05534 (2020)
16. Arora, R., Kaushik, S.C., Kumar, R., Arora, R.: Multi-objective thermo-economic optimization of solar parabolic dish Stirling heat engine with regenerative losses using NSGA-II and decision making. Int. J. Electr. Power Energy Syst. **74**, 25–35 (2016)

17. Arora, R., Kaushik, S.C., Kumar, R., Arora, R.: Soft computing based multi-objective optimization of Brayton cycle power plant with isothermal heat addition using evolutionary algorithm and decision making. Appl. Soft Comput. **46**, 267–283 (2016)
18. Arora, R., Arora, R.: Multiobjective optimization and analytical comparison of single-and 2-stage (series/parallel) thermoelectric heat pumps. Int. J. Energy Res. **42**(4), 1760–1778 (2018)
19. Arora, R., Arora, R.: Multicriteria optimization based comprehensive comparative analyses of single-and two-stage (series/parallel) thermoelectric generators including the influence of Thomson effect. J. Renew. Sustain. Energy. **10**(4), 044701 (2018)
20. Arora, R., Kaushik, S.C., Kumar, R.: Multi-objective optimization of solar powered Ericsson cycle using genetic algorithm and fuzzy decision making. In: 2015 International Conference on Advances in Computer Engineering and Applications, pp. 553–558. IEEE (2015)
21. Arora, R., Kaushik, S.C., Kumar, R.: Multi-objective optimization of an irreversible regenerative Brayton cycle using genetic algorithm. In: 2015 International Conference on Futuristic Trends on Computational Analysis and Knowledge Management (ABLAZE), pp. 340–346. IEEE (2015)
22. Maputi, E.S., Arora, R.: Design optimization of a three-stage transmission using advanced optimization techniques. Int. J. Simul. Multidiscip. Des. Optim. **10**, A8 (2019)
23. Maputi, E.S., Arora, R.: Multi-objective spur gear design using teaching learning-based optimization and decision-making techniques. Cogent Eng. **6**(1), 1665396 (2019)
24. Arora, R., Kaushik, S.C., Kumar, R.: Multi-objective thermodynamic optimization of solar parabolic dish Stirling heat engine with regenerative losses using NSGA-II and decision making. Appl. Solar Energy. **52**(4), 295–304 (2016)
25. Kumar, R., Kaushik, S.C., Kumar, R., Hans, R.: Multi-objective thermodynamic optimization of an irreversible regenerative Brayton cycle using evolutionary algorithm and decision making. Ain Shams Eng. J. **7**(2), 741–753 (2016)
26. Hyndman, R.J., Koehler, A.B., Snyder, R.D., Grose, S.: A state space framework for automatic forecasting using exponential smoothing methods. Int. J. Forecast. **18**(3), 439–454 (2002)
27. Taylor, J.W.: Exponential smoothing with a damped multiplicative trend. Int. J. Forecast. **19**(4), 715–725 (2003)
28. Makridakis, S., Andersen, A., Carbone, R., Fildes, R., Hibon, M., Lewandowski, R., et al.: The accuracy of extrapolation (time series) methods: results of a forecasting competition. J. Forecast. **1**(2), 111–153 (1982)
29. Petropoulos, F., Makridakis, S.: Forecasting the novel coronavirus COVID-19. PLoS One. **15**(3), e0231236 (2020)
30. Liu, D., Clemente, L., Poirier, C., Ding, X., Chinazzi, M., Davis, J.T., Vespignani, A., Santillana, M.: A machine learning methodology for real-time forecasting of the 2019–2020 COVID-19 outbreak using Internet searches, news alerts, and estimates from mechanistic models. arXiv preprint arXiv:2004.04019 (2020)

Chapter 6
COVID-19 Under Origin and Transmission: A Data-Driven Analysis for India and Bangladesh

Ajantha Devi and Hashnayne Ahmed

Abstract The coronavirus disease 2019 (COVID-19) is an exceptionally contagious and pathogenic viral disease brought about by the SARS-CoV-2 infection that was first detailed at Wuhan, China, and later it spreads everywhere throughout the world. It was a severe acute respiratory syndrome (SARS)-like virus, and the primary host of this virus is bats, revealed through genome analysis. The intermediate medium between human and bats is still unknown, and it is quite contagious, resulting in rapid spreading of this disease. All things considered, there are no clinically endorsed medications or antibodies for this sickness, yet a few precautions and staying away from close contacts are suggested. The number of COVD-19 confirmed cases is rapidly increasing with higher mortality rates, more than other epidemics that occurred in the last century although it still fluctuates. We will analyze the COVID-19 outbreak situation considering confirmed cases, recoveries, mortality rate percentages, etc. India and Bangladesh are two geographically important countries, and we will also analyze the COVID-19 situation for these two countries either with similarities or differences.

Keywords SARS-CoV-2 · Coronavirus · COVID-19 · Transmission · Comparison · India · Bangladesh

A. Devi (✉)
Research Head, AP3 Solutions, Chennai, Tamil Nadu, India
e-mail: ap3solutionsresearch@gmail.com

H. Ahmed
Department of Mathematics, University of Barishal, Barishal, Bangladesh

© The Author(s), under exclusive license to Springer Nature Switzerland AG 2021

F. Al-Turjman et al. (eds.), *Emerging Technologies for Battling Covid-19*, Studies in Systems, Decision and Control 324,
https://doi.org/10.1007/978-3-030-60039-6_6

6.1 Introduction to COVID-19

An infectious disease called coronavirus disease 2019 (COVID-19) was first recognized in December of 2019 in Wuhan City of Hubei territory, China [1]. The disease is brought about by severe acute respiratory syndrome coronavirus 2 (SARS-CoV-2). The principal confirmed instance of COVID-19 was on November 17, 2019, in Hubei, China, and till July of 2020, about 15 million people all over the world have been reported with some shocking statistics of about 616,000 deaths. This communicable disease has basic side effects incorporating fever, weakness, cough, loss of smell and taste, and windedness [2]. Be that as it may, in most of the cases, mild indications are seen with the beginning time presentation of 5 days, ranging from 2 to 14 days. The SARS-CoV-2 spread through close contact and most often through small droplets produced by sneezing, coughing, etc. [3]. It is most contagious at the first 3 days of onset of symptoms, and gradually it loses its contagiousness. Real-time reverse transcription polymerase chain reaction (rRT-PCR) is the most standard diagnosis process for this contagious virus although it gives false negatives sometimes [4]. Chest CT can also be used to diagnose this infectiousness of this virus, but rRT-PCR gives a much better result than chest CT. To prevent the infection, wearing a mask, hand washing, maintaining physical distance from others, maintaining quarantine, etc., are some recommended tasks. Since July 2020, no vaccines have been recommended, so prevention is the one way left, although about four vaccines are in phase III trial in different territories of the world [5].

The World Health Organization (WHO) declared COVID-19 as a world pandemic on March 11, 2020 [1]. It spread in over about 168 countries or territories of the world, shifting its epicenter from China and Italy to Europe and the USA. In South Asia, its fatality rate is low than the other regions of the world. In India, the first case of confirmed COVID-19 was on January 30, 2020, and till July 2020, about 1.2 million cases have been confirmed [5]. The fatality rate is about 2.8% where the global fatality rate is 4.3%, and about half of the confirmed cases are from the popular cities of this country [6].

On another side, Bangladesh got the news of its first case confirmed on March 8, and till July, this virus has spread over the country with many about confirmed 215,000 COVID-19 cases and 2750 deaths [7]. To prevent the spread of this SARS-CoV-2 virus, both the neighboring countries India and Bangladesh followed the most appeared options like other countries of the world, to lock down the most possible epicenters of these countries. Also, a few additions of lockdown time and places results in around 3–5 months lockdown, in certain location as yet continuous and lockdown over the nation. Since there are no pharmaceutical interventions, prevention is the way to keeping a lower transmission, and that is the reason behind choosing lockdown.

The goal of this chapter is to analyze the present statistics of COVID-19 transmissions in these two neighboring countries, India and Bangladesh.

6.2 Literature Review

At the end of December 2019, the World Health Organization (WHO) was informed by China's health authority about some cases of pneumonia of unknown etiology. All the cases were from Wuhan City in Hubei Province and around a local seafood market called Huanan [8]. On January 7, 2020, the novel coronavirus was identified, and the WHO renamed the virus as severe acute respiratory syndrome coronavirus 2 (SARS-CoV-2) and the disease as coronavirus disease 2019 (COVID-19) [9, 10]. On Jan 30, the WHO declared the COVID-19 outbreak situation as a Public Health Emergency of International Concern (PHIEC) since it spread to about 19 countries with a mortality rate of 2.1% [11, 12].

The new infection is from the group of *Coronaviridae* and order *Nidovirales* [13]. It is a pathogenic infection that is encompassed with spike and named a positive-sense abandoned RNA (+ssRNA) infection [14]. Utilizing the genome groupings of SARS-CoV-2, contemplates propose that bats may be the first host of this infection [15]. Be that as it may, bats are improbably liable for the transmission of the infection to people since the Huanan Seafood Wholesale Market does not sell bats, and in the past cases, there was a middle of the road have each time [16, 17].

For example, the Nipah infection in Bangladesh was communicated through bats shedding into crude date palm sap [18]. In another genomic study and bunches of contaminated relatives, clinical specialists affirmed the nearness of individual-to-individual transmission [19, 20]. It happens for the most part through close contacts and little beads created by a tainted individual through hacking or wheezing [2]. The normal side effects that happen for this disease are fever, hack, weakness, windedness, and loss of smell and taste [21, 22]. The asymptomatic transmission likewise identified later with mellow manifestations and now and again, no indications [23].

An investigation establishes the mean hatching time frame was 5.2 days [17] with the most elevated number of 19 or 24 days, albeit the greater part of 14 days [24, 25]. The essential generation number R_0 (shows the job of spreading) for this sickness has been determined as 3.28 [26]. The ailment frequently happens in grown-up male patients with the middle period between 34 and 59 years [12]. It is additionally risky for individuals with incessant comorbidities, for example, cardiovascular and cerebrovascular illnesses and diabetes [27]. Nearly less cases are found in youngsters under 15 years of age [12].

Surveillance is significant for such an infectious SARS-CoV-2 infection to watch its future host variation, viral development, infectivity, contagiousness, and pathogenicity. Auxiliary examination proposes that SARS-CoV-2 may utilize receptor angiotensin-converting enzyme 2 (ACE2) to enter the cells [12, 28]. Promptly, after tying to the open receptor, SARS-CoV-2 enters the cells and appearances the sheltered response [12], and patients face the referenced most basic indications. Some more uncommon indications are migraine, dazedness, stomach torment, looseness of the bowels, queasiness, and spewing [29].

To control the spreading of COVID-19, an enormous measure of testing is required, and for the finding, a constant real-time reverse transcription polymerase chain reaction (rRT-PCR) process is utilized. Be that as it may, case definitions change after some time and in nations [12]. For the patients meeting indicative models are tried for COVID-19 and test, examples are gathered from the upper respiratory plot (nasopharyngeal and oropharyngeal swab) and if conceivable, lower respiratory lot (sputum, tracheal suction or bronchoalveolar lavage) [30]. Since there is no particular antiviral treatment for COVID-19, seclusion and steady consideration incorporating oxygen treatment, liquid administration, and antimicrobials for auxiliary bacterial diseases are suggested [31].

Currently, no immunization is accessible, yet around four antibodies are in stage III trials and are expected to come in the market before 2021 [32]. Albeit, an antibacterial medication named remdesivir (produced for Ebola virus) has been utilized to treat COVID-19 cases in the USA [33]. To control the spread of COVID-19, unique methodologies ought to be actualized in medicinal services settings. Applying emergency and right disease control measures, segregating the cases, and contact tracing are the ways to restrict spreading [34]. Confining contaminated individuals is the essential measure to interfere with transmission. Locking down is one of the prompt activities taken by various nations which eased back the worldwide spread of COVID-19 [35].

The first case of COVID-19 in India was detected in January 30, 2020, which originated from China. In July there are about 1.2 million confirmed cases, the largest number in Asia and the third highest in the world after the USA and Brazil. India's case fatality rate is 2.41% in July, lower than the other countries of the world, and is steadily declining. The recovery rate for India is about 63.18%, and this progress occurred as a result of several locking down steps. Although from June, they started unlocking the country [6].

On account of Bangladesh, the initial three cases were affirmed on March 8, 2020, by the Institute of Epidemiology, Disease Control, and Research (IEDCR). From that point the pandemic spread step by step over the nation, and in July, there are a sum of 2.12 million confirmed cases with 115,000 recuperations and 2700 deaths. Bangladesh is the third most influenced nation in South Asia and seventeenth in over the world. Clinical specialists questioned about insufficient testing here in Bangladesh and extra death of patients with COVID-19 manifestations. Bangladesh announced to shut down from 23rd March 2020 and it proceeds over July. Bangladesh faces noteworthy difficulties to confront the COVID-19 as it is a thickly populated nation and is furthermore a place of a million stateless Rohingya outcasts. It additionally has a critical transient populace living in Italy, an extreme COVID-19-infected nation [7].

6.3 Analysis of COVID-19 and Discussions

At the beginning of this outbreak, the number of confirmed cases doubled every 7.5 days approximately [17]. The virus spread over the Chinese provinces through New Year migration, and as Wuhan is a transport hub, there was major rail interchange [36]. On January 31, Italy had its first confirmed case from China, and on March 13, Italy and Europe were the active center of this pandemic [37]. The first case of COVID-19 in the USA was confirmed on January 15, and on March 26, the confirmed cases reach on the peak than any other countries [38]. The epicenter of this COVID-19 pandemic moved in several places across the world since it started.

The information clearly states the pandemic outbreak situation of COVID-19 disease: spreading, transmutability, characteristics, etc. More than 20 million people had been confirmed COVID-19 positive with a huge case of about 0.7 million deaths till July 25. Figure 6.1 describes the outbreak trend all across the world, specifically the rising amount of confirmed cases. The curve is smoothly increasing concerning the time which points out that the total confirmed cases of COVID-19 across the world are increasing from the start of this outbreak. And it may now follow a linearly increasing trend.

This pandemic occurred in China, and then it moved its epicenter from China to Europe. A huge amount of patients were confirmed through Europe and later in the USA. Although it started in China, it is now out of the top ten countries of the confirmed list with the highest number of active COVID-19 cases in the world. The USA still keeps the peak position of confirmed cases with several actions taken by the US government. Brazil holds the second highest position of confirmed cases, following the USA. And India is very close to Russia, the third highest confirmed case holder across the world. Besides these four countries, the UK, Peru, Chile, South Africa, Mexico, and Iran are the other countries from the top ten with most COVID-19 confirmed cases as on July 27, 2020. Figure 6.2 displays the top ten countries with most COVID-19 confirmed cases.

Active cases are the reduced number of confirmed cases by death and recoveries. Active case comparison shows the situation of the pandemic in any country. In the case of active patients, the USA, Brazil, the UK, Russia, and India hold the same situation in confirmed lists, but Pakistan, Canada, France, and Bangladesh are the new faces here, as shown in Fig. 6.3.

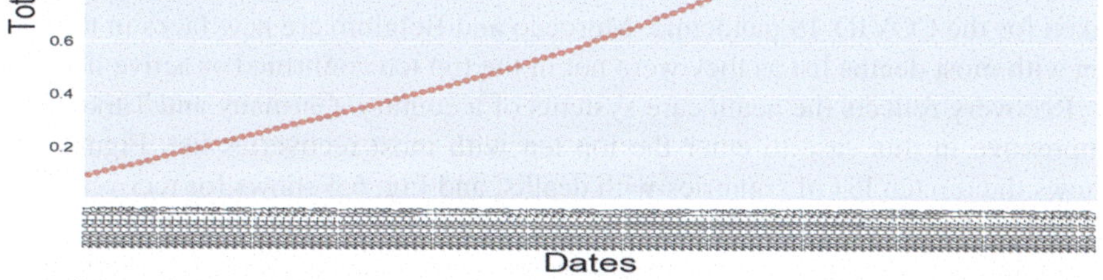

Fig. 6.1 Worldwide confirmed cases over time

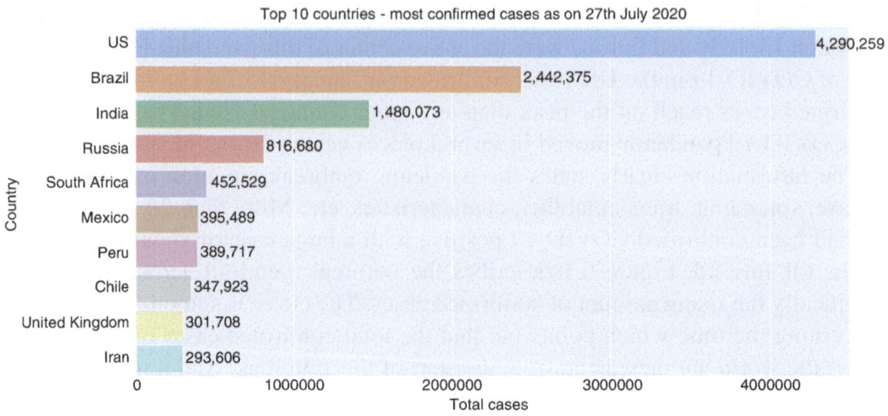

Fig. 6.2 Most confirmed cases across the world

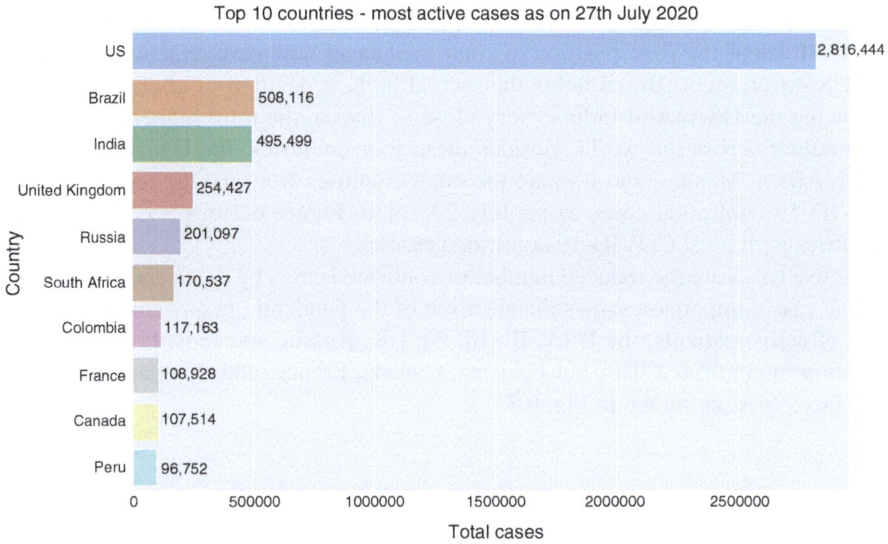

Fig. 6.3 Most active cases across the world

Most deaths occur in the USA as confirmed. India is relatively slower in case of deaths than other countries in the confirmed list which shows the effective initiative taken for the COVID-19 pandemic. Morocco and Belgium are new faces in the top ten with most deaths list as they were not in the top ten confirmed or active list.

Recovery reflects the healthcare systems of a country. Germany and Turkey are impressive in this case to enter the top ten with most recoveries list. Figure 6.4 shows the top ten list of countries with deaths, and Fig. 6.5 shows for recoveries of COVID-19 patients across the world.

Sometimes, the total number of deaths could not express the real scenario of a pandemic as population size and geographical area are different for different

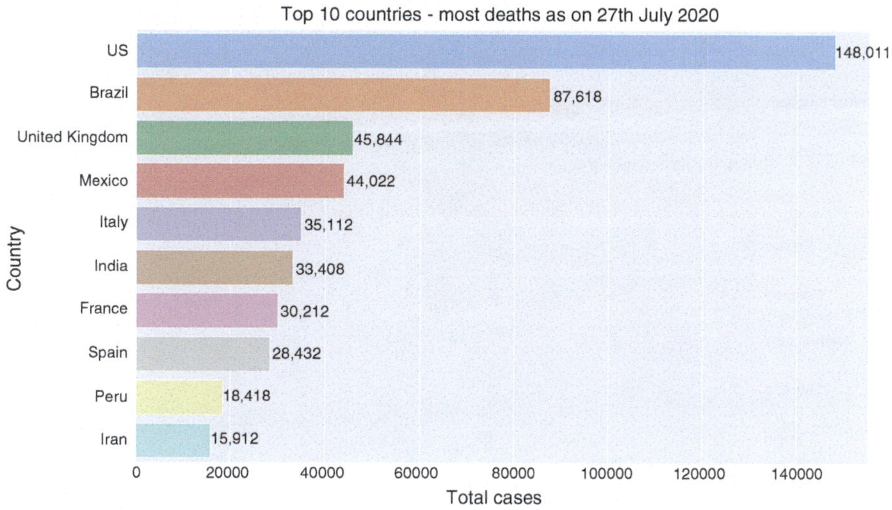

Fig. 6.4 Most death cases across the world

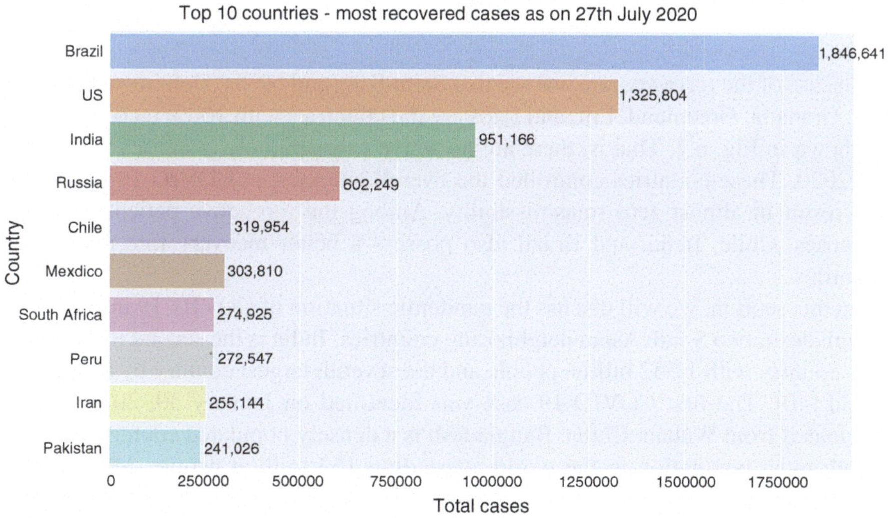

Fig. 6.5 Most recovered cases across the world

countries. And that is the reason to consider a scaled size of the population with per unit of time. The measurement of the number of deaths is called the "mortality rate" or "death rate" [39]. As shown in Fig. 6.6, Yemen has a mortality rate of 36% which is almost more than double than other close countries in terms of mortality rate. Belgium, France, Italy, the UK, Hungary, the Netherlands, Mexico, Antigua and Barbuda, and Spain have a mortality rate of 10–15%. There are no countries here from the top ten with most deaths.

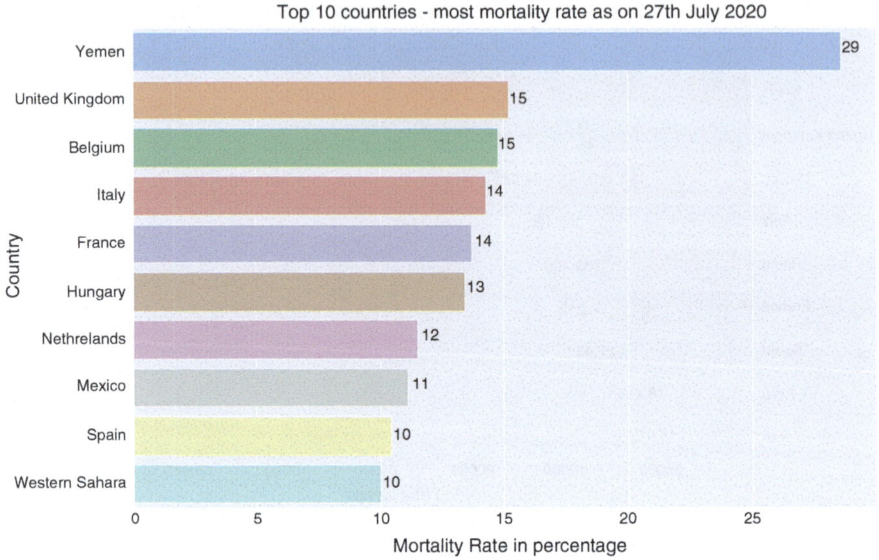

Fig. 6.6 Most mortality rates across the world

In case of the recovery rate, we see that Saint Kitts and Nevis, Dominica, the Holy See, Granada, Greenland, Fiji, and Laos are the countries with 100% recovery rates, as shown in Fig. 6.7. That is, there are no active cases in these countries as of June 25, 2020. These countries controlled the overall situation of COVID-19 pandemic and result in almost zero transmissibility. Among the top active patients holding countries, Chile, India, and Brazil also possess a better recovery rate than other countries.

In this section, we will discuss the pandemic situation of COVID-19 in India and Bangladesh, two South Asian neighboring countries. India is the second most populous country with 1.352 billion people and the seventh largest country by area in the world [40]. The first COVID-19 case was identified on January 30, 2020, which originated from Wuhan, China. Bangladesh is a densely populated country with the eighth most population in the world, exceeding 162 million people. Maintaining social distance to prevent virus transmission is tough in such a populous country. The literacy rate of Bangladesh is about 74%, and population density is 1265 people per square kilometer [41], which is much high. India's literacy rate is almost similar to Bangladesh, but it has a lower population density of 464 people per square kilometer as of 2020 [41]. Besides these, the transmissibility rate mostly depends on social awareness, reactions, and steps taken by governments, etc. In this paper, we are keen to discuss the overall COVID-19 case situations between these two neighboring countries rather than discuss the geographical situations and other measurements. We will take January 30 as the first day of the confirmed case for India and March 8 as the first day of the confirmed case for Bangladesh.

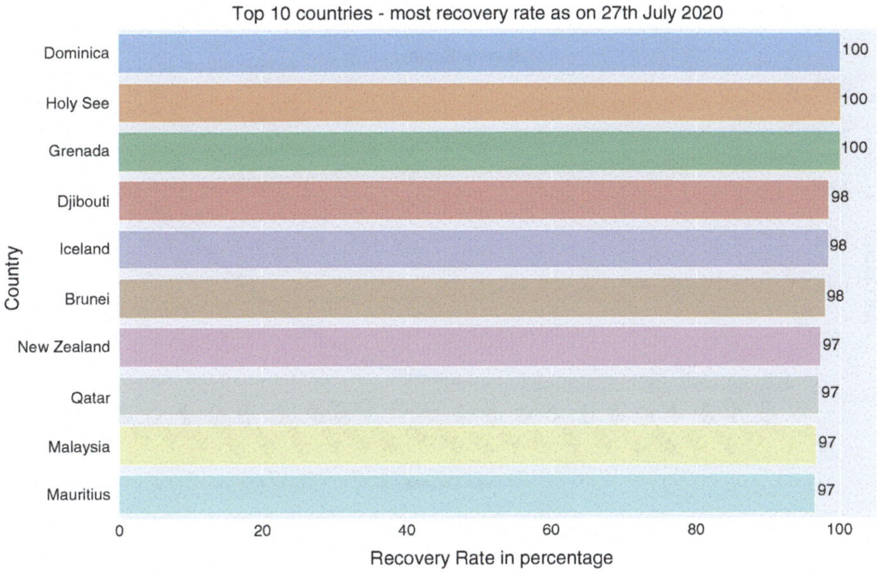

Fig. 6.7 Most recovery rates across the world

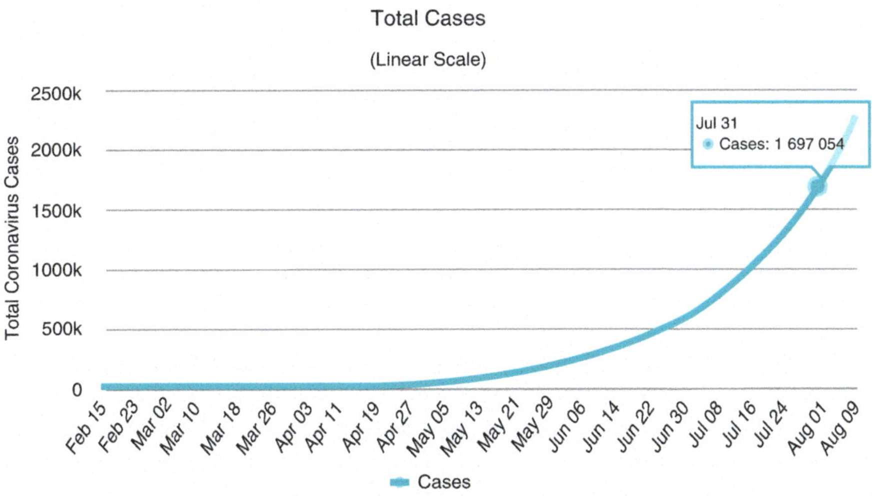

Fig. 6.8 Confirmed cases in India

Figures 6.8 and 6.9 show the curve for confirmed cases with COVID-19 in India and Bangladesh, respectively. The confirmed case rate was very low for both countries at first till the mid of April for India and mid of May for Bangladesh, but it increased very fast afterward. And it continues for both graphs. Figure 6.10 shows a comparative confirmed case graph for both countries.

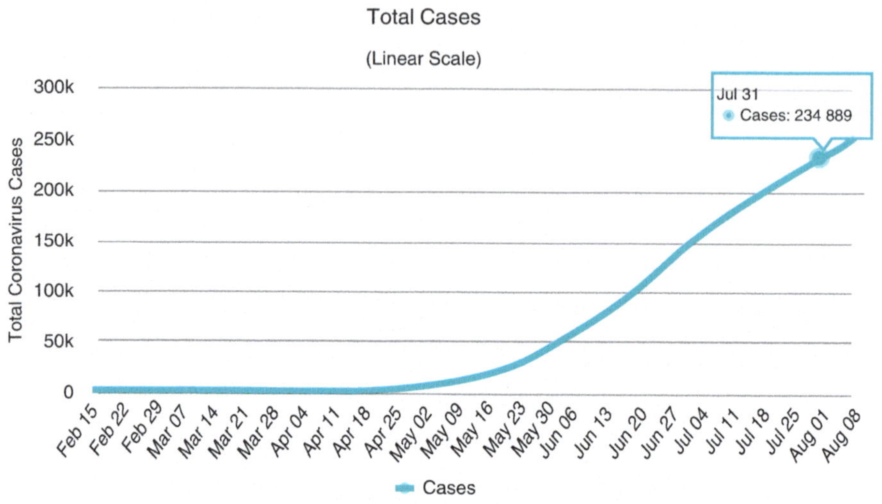

Fig. 6.9 Confirmed cases in Bangladesh

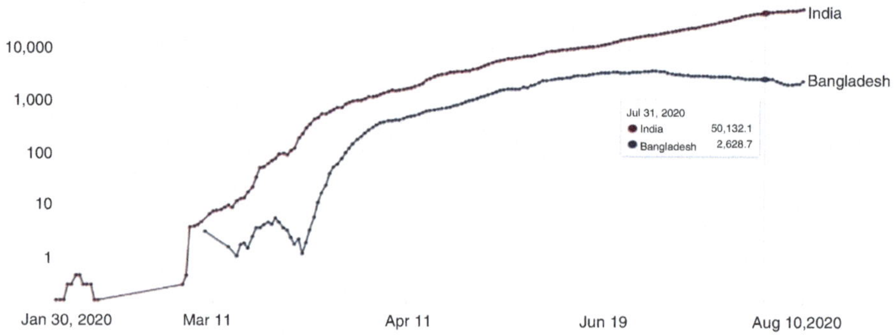

Fig. 6.10 Comparison for total confirmed cases for India and Bangladesh

Here, Figs. 6.11 and 6.12 display the daily new cases for COVID-19 patients in India and Bangladesh, respectively. We see that for India, the number of new cases is equal or increasing, but in the case of Bangladesh, there is some decreasing scenario. Figures 6.13 and 6.14 show the currently active cases, that is, confirmed reduced by recovery and deaths for India and Bangladesh, respectively. Although new cases are downfalling for Bangladesh, active cases are increasing, and it is almost similar to India. We also see a sudden breakpoint in case of Bangladesh's active cases. It was for some combined recoveries entry in the national systems in early June.

Figures 6.15 and 6.16 represent the death cases with time for India and Bangladesh, respectively. Both the graph indicates that the number of death cases for both countries is increasing. Figure 6.17 shows the comparative death cases for India and Bangladesh where we see that the number of deaths is following the same

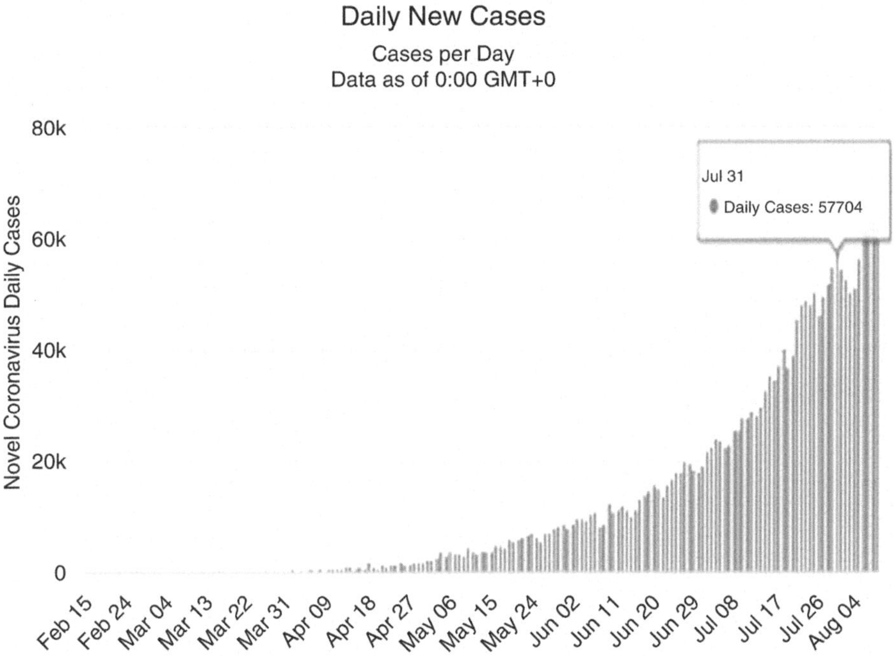

Fig. 6.11 Daily new cases for India

pattern for both countries. Figure 6.18 represents the case fatality rate of deaths with red and indigo curves for India and Bangladesh, respectively.

Although the case fatality rate was very high for Bangladesh in the beginning as now in July, Bangladesh is in a much better situation than India in case of a fatality rate. But India's case fatality curve is much stable, whereas Bangladesh's one not. The case fatality rate for India is also decreasing. However, we know from the previous epidemic that the case fatality rate gives the actual scenario after all populations being recovered or died, and before that, it shows lesser values (Table 6.1).

6.4 Conclusions

This research paper presents the current trend of COVID-19 outbreak from the beginning to June 25, 2020, and more specifically for two South Asian countries: India and Bangladesh. A modified literature review has been introduced considering the origin, transmission, prevention, precautions, vaccines, etc. for the noble SARS-CoV-2 virus. We also analyzed the overall pandemic situation of the world through worldwide data analysis, recovery percentage, active patient percentage, mortality rate percentage, etc. COVID-19 is a contagious disease with unpredictable

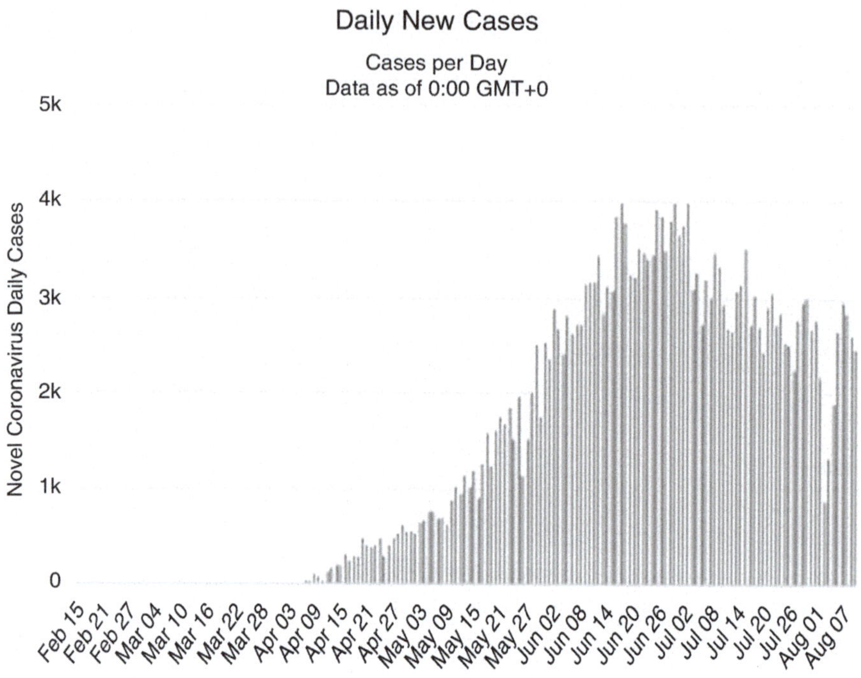

Fig. 6.12 Daily new cases for Bangladesh

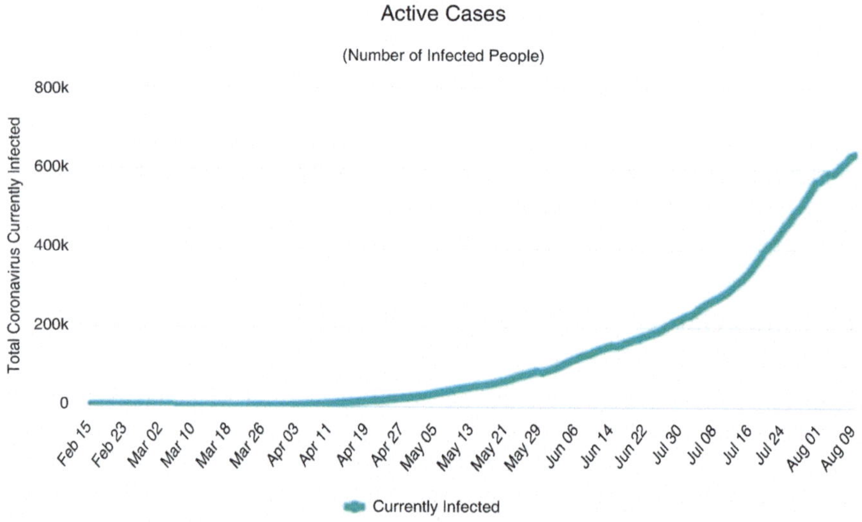

Fig. 6.13 Active cases in India

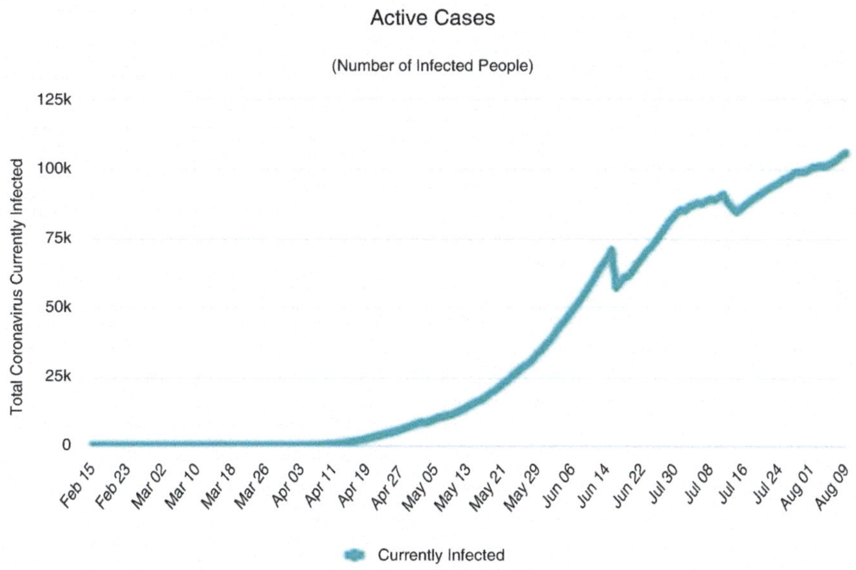

Fig. 6.14 Active cases in Bangladesh

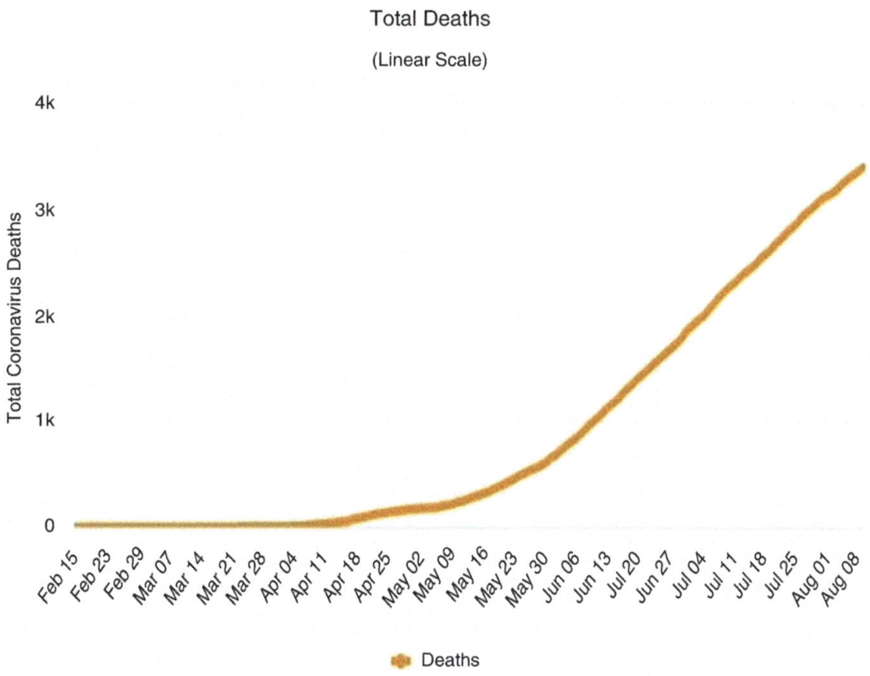

Fig. 6.15 Death cases in Bangladesh

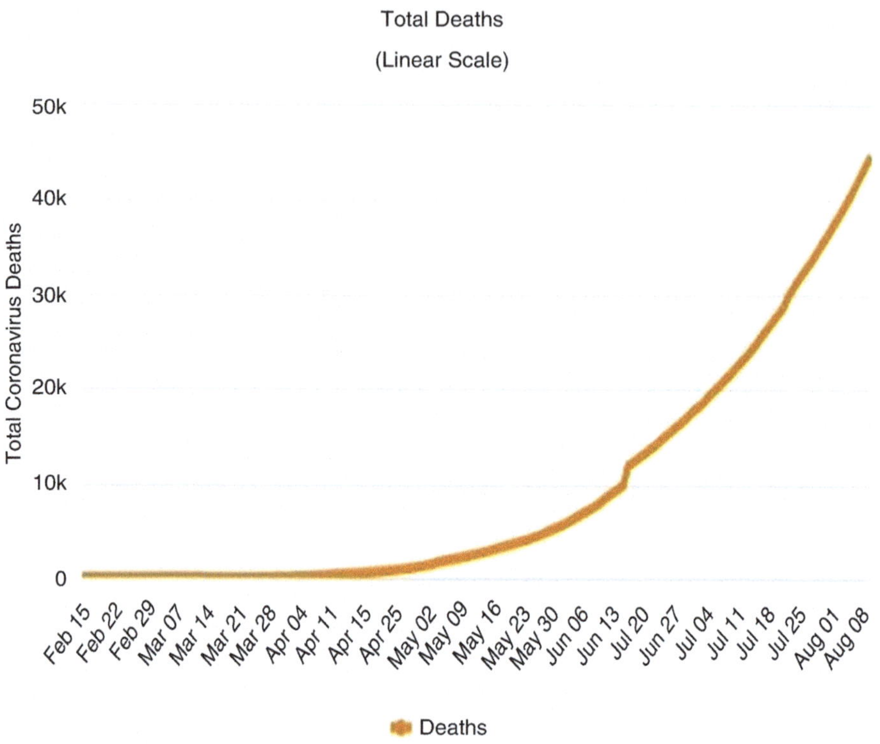

Fig. 6.16 Death cases in India

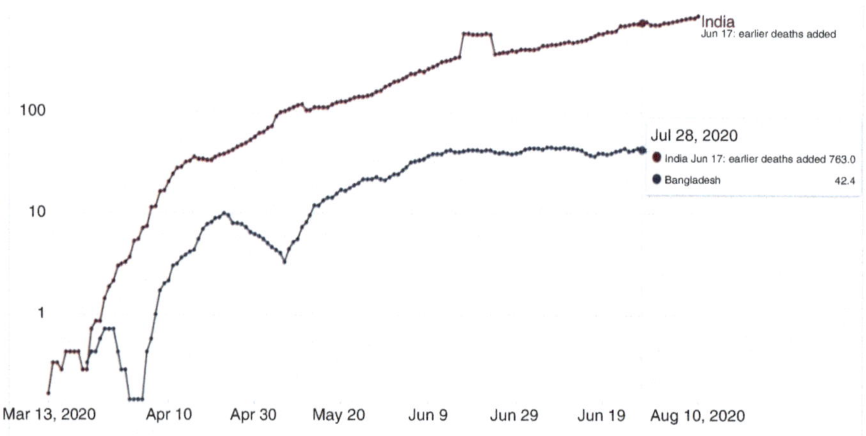

Fig. 6.17 Comparison for death cases

properties, which indicates that still model prediction is tough until it has been successfully contained, and that is the reason for the importance of data-driven analysis. In a pandemic like this, providing information to the public is paramount. For India and Bangladesh, both countries' data for this pandemic situation has been analyzed for confirming cases, active cases, and death cases. These two countries are facing almost similar situations, and the pandemic situations are blooming here day by day. Proper steps and actions can make the transmissibility slower.

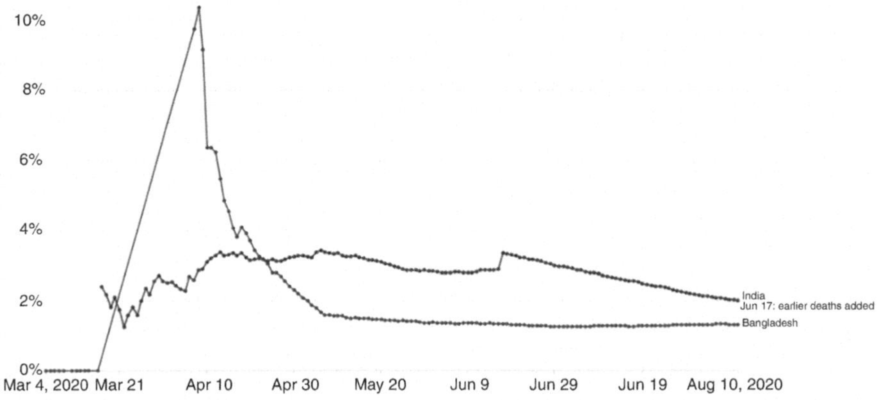

Fig. 6.18 Comparison of fatality rates

Table 6.1 Comparative analysis of COVID-19 transmission between India and Bangladesh

Features	India	Bangladesh	References
First case	January 30, 2020	March 8, 2020	[6, 7]
Area of emergence	Mumbai, Delhi, Ahmedabad, Chennai, Pune, Kolkata, etc.	At the early stage, mainly in Dhaka city and Narayanganj. Later it spreads mainly in all divisional cities	[1, 6, 7]
Origin	China	Italy	[42, 43]
Entry receptor in humans	ACE2	ACE2	[12, 28]
Sign and symptoms	Fever, cough, fatigue, shortness of breath, loss of smell and taste	Fever, cough, fatigue, shortness of breath, loss of smell and taste	[1, 6, 7, 21, 22]
Asymptomatic transmissions	Yes	Yes	[1, 5–7, 23]
Total infected	[a]1,435,453 patients	[a]226,225 patients	[1, 5–7, 25, 41]
Total recovered	[a]917,568 patients	[a]125,683 patients	
Total death	[a]32,771 patients	[a]2965 patients	
Mortality rate	[a]2.49%	[a]1.30%	[44, 45]

[a]As on July 27, 2020

The outbreak spreads are largely influenced by each country's policy and social responsibility [46] to avoid close contacts as prevention is the better cure until the arrival of the COVID-19 vaccine.

References

1. Coronavirus disease (CoVID-19) pandemic. World Health Organizations (WHO). https://www.who.int/emergencies/diseases/novel-coronavirus-2019. Accessed 27 Jul 2020
2. Bouaziz, J.D., et al.: Vascular skin symptoms in COVID-19: a French observational study. J. Eur. Acad. Dermatol. Venereol. **34**, e451–e452 (2020). https://doi.org/10.1111/jdv.16544
3. Paul, A., Chatterjee, S., Bairagi, N.: Prediction on Covid-19 epidemic for different countries: focusing on South Asia under various precautionary measures. medRxiv (2020)
4. Williams, T.C., et al.: Sensitivity of RT-PCR testing of upper respiratory tract samples for SARS-CoV-2 in hospitalized patients: a retrospective cohort study. medRxiv (2020)
5. Coronavirus disease 2019. Wikipedia. https://en.wikipedia.org/wiki/Coronavirus_disease_2019. Accessed 22 Jul 2020
6. COVID-19 pandemic in India. Wikipedia. https://en.wikipedia.org/wiki/COVID-19_pandemic_in_India. Accessed 22 Jul 2020
7. COVID-19 pandemic in Bangladesh. Wikipedia. https://en.wikipedia.org/wiki/COVID-19_pandemic_in_Bangladesh. Accessed 22 Jul 2020
8. Lu, H., Stratton, C.W., Tang, Y.-W.: Outbreak of pneumonia of unknown etiology in Wuhan, China: the mystery and the miracle. J. Med. Virol. **92**(4), 401–402 (2020)
9. Hui, D.S., et al.: The continuing 2019-nCoV epidemic threat of novel coronaviruses to global health—the latest 2019 novel coronavirus outbreak in Wuhan, China. Int. J. Infect. Dis. **91**, 264–266 (2020)
10. Baker, S.C., et al.: Severe acute respiratory syndrome-related coronavirus: the species and its viruses–a statement of the Coronavirus Study Group (2020)
11. Burki, T.K.: Coronavirus in China. Lancet Respir. Med. **8**(3), 238 (2020)
12. Harapan, H., et al.: Coronavirus disease 2019 (COVID-19): a literature review. J. Infect. Public Health. **13**(5), 667–673 (2020)
13. Kramer, A., Schwebke, I., Kampf, G.: How long do nosocomial pathogens persist on inanimate surfaces? A systematic review. BMC Infect. Dis. **6**(1), 130 (2006)
14. Shang, J., et al.: Structure of mouse coronavirus spike protein complexed with receptor reveals the mechanism for viral entry. PLoS Pathog. **16**(3), e1008392 (2020)
15. Zhou, P., et al.: A pneumonia outbreak associated with a new coronavirus of probable bat origin. Nature. **579**(7798), 270–273 (2020)
16. Lu, R., et al.: Genomic characterization and epidemiology of 2019 novel coronavirus: implications for virus origins and receptor binding. Lancet. **395**(10224), 565–574 (2020)
17. Li, Q., et al.: Early transmission dynamics in Wuhan, China, of novel coronavirus–infected pneumonia. N. Engl. J. Med. **382**, 1199–1207 (2020)
18. Hughes, J.M., et al.: Transmission of human infection with Nipah virus. Clin. Infect. Dis. **49**(11), 1743–1748 (2009)
19. Chan, J.F.-W., et al.: A familial cluster of pneumonia associated with the 2019 novel coronavirus indicating person-to-person transmission: a study of a family cluster. Lancet. **395**(10223), 514–523 (2020)
20. Yu, W.-B., et al.: Decoding the evolution and transmissions of the novel pneumonia coronavirus (SARS-CoV-2/HCoV-19) using whole genomic data. Zool. Res. **41**(3), 247 (2020)
21. Han, C., et al.: Digestive symptoms in COVID-19 patients with mild disease severity: clinical presentation, stool viral RNA testing, and outcomes. Am. J. Gastroenterol. **115**(6), 916–923 (2020). https://doi.org/10.14309/ajg.0000000000000664

22. Wang, H.-Y., et al.: Potential neurological symptoms of COVID-19. Ther. Adv. Neurol. Disord. **13**, 1756286420917830 (2020)
23. Bai, Y., et al.: Presumed asymptomatic carrier transmission of COVID-19. JAMA. **323**(14), 1406–1407 (2020)
24. Chu, D.K.W., et al.: Molecular diagnosis of a novel coronavirus (2019-nCoV) causing an outbreak of pneumonia. Clin. Chem. **66**(4), 549–555 (2020)
25. World Health Organization. Global Surveillance for humans with the human with coronavirus (2019-nCoV): interim, 31 January 2020. No. WHO/2019-nCoV/SurveillanceGuide/2020.3. World Health Organization (2020)
26. Liu, Y., et al.: The reproductive number of COVID-19 is higher compared to SARS coronavirus. J. Travel Med. **27**(2) (2020). https://doi.org/10.1093/jtm/taaa021
27. Chen, N., et al.: Epidemiological and clinical characteristics of 99 cases of 2019 novel coronavirus pneumonia in Wuhan, China: a descriptive study. Lancet. **395**(10223), 507–513 (2020)
28. Wan, Y., et al.: Receptor recognition by the novel coronavirus from Wuhan: an analysis based on decade-long structural studies of SARS coronavirus. J. Virol. **94**(7), e00127-20 (2020)
29. Wang, D., et al.: Clinical characteristics of 138 hospitalized patients with 2019 novel coronavirus–infected pneumonia in Wuhan, China. J.A.M.A. **323**(11), 1061–1069 (2020)
30. Patel, A., Jernigan, D.B.: Initial public health response and interim clinical guidance for the 2019 novel coronavirus outbreak—United States, December 31, 2019–February 4, 2020. MMWR Morb. Mortal. Wkly. Rep. **69**(5), 140 (2020)
31. Habibzadeh, P., Stoneman, E.K.: The novel coronavirus: a bird's eye view. Int. J. Occup. Environ. Med. **11**(2), 65 (2020)
32. Coronavirus Vaccine Tracker. The New York Times. https://www.nytimes.com/interactive/2020/science/coronavirus-vaccine-tracker.html. Accessed 24 Jul 2020
33. Holshue, M.L., et al.: First case of 2019 novel coronavirus in the United States. N. Engl. J. Med. **382**(10), 929–936 (2020)
34. Chan, J.F.W., et al.: Middle East respiratory syndrome coronavirus: another zoonotic betacoronavirus causing SARS-like disease. Clin. Microbiol. Rev. **28**(2), 465–522 (2015)
35. Heymann, D.L., Shindo, N.: COVID-19: what is next for public health? Lancet. **395**(10224), 542–545 (2020)
36. World Health Organization. Report of the WHO-China joint mission on coronavirus disease 2019 (COVID-19) (2020)
37. Fredericks, B.: WHO says Europe is the new epicenter of coronavirus pandemic. New York Post (2020)
38. McNeil, D.G.: The US now leads the world in confirmed coronavirus cases. New York Times (2020)
39. Porta, M., et al.: Mortality Rate, Morbidity Rate; Death Rate; Cumulative Death Rate; Case Fatality Rate. A Dictionary of Epidemiology. Oxford University Press, Oxford (2014)
40. World Population prospects—Population division. https://www.population.un.org. United Nations Department of Economic and Social Affairs, Population Division. Accessed 9 Nov 2019
41. Coronavirus Update—Worldometer. Worldometer. https://www.worldometers.info/coronavirus/#countries. Accessed 22 Jul 2020
42. India most infected by Covid-19 among Asian countries, leaves Turkey behind. Hindustan Times (2020). Accessed 30 May 2020
43. IEDCR asks returnees from virus-affected countries to avoid public transport. The Daily Star (2020). Accessed 8 Apr 2020
44. India's COVID-19 fatality rate drops below 2.5%. Anadolu Agency. https://www.aa.com.tr/en/asia-pacific/indias-covid-19-fatality-rate-drops-below-25-/1915934#. Accessed 8 Aug 2020
45. COVID-19: Bangladesh overview. Corona Tracker. https://www.coronatracker.com/country/bangladesh/. Accessed 8 Aug 2020
46. Binti Hamzah, F.A., et al.: CoronaTracker: worldwide COVID-19 outbreak data analysis and prediction. Bull. World Health Organ. **1**, 32 (2020)

Chapter 7
Robotics and Drone-Based Solution for the Impact of COVID-19 Worldwide Using AI and IoT

Rachna Jain, Meenu Gupta, Kashish Garg, and Akash Gupta

Abstract Coronavirus disease 2019 (COVID-19) is an infectious disease caused by the SARS-CoV-2 virus. The disease causes a respiratory illness with symptoms like cough and fever and, in more severe cases, causes difficulty while breathing. COVID-19 spreads primarily through contact with an infected person when they sneeze or cough or by touching a surface that has that virus on it and then touching our mouth, nose, or eyes. The disease was first observed in the central Chinese city of Wuhan at the end of 2019. The outbreak has been declared a global pandemic. The novel coronavirus is already reorienting our lives, but the crisis moments also present an opportunity for more sophisticated and flexible use of technology. The epidemic is impacting the global population as the number of cases is increasing rapidly, and there is an urgent need to stop the virus from spreading. The outbreak has triggered massive demand for digital health solutions, and for this, the drones and robots present an excellent method for automation of manual activities. Drones and robots can be used to provide services to the patients and those who are quarantined and are the most desirable and safe way to fight against the outbreak and limit contamination and spread of the virus. The following chapter will discuss the various solutions based on drones and robots in the field of AI and IoT, such as drones being used for social distancing and robots for sanitization. Further, analysis has been made about the total number of cases and deaths around the world and also how it has affected humanity and what measures have been taken to control this deadly disease.

Keywords COVID-19 · Disease · Drones · Robots · Artificial intelligence (AI) · Internet of Things (IoT) · Technology

---

R. Jain · A. Gupta
Bharati Vidyapeeth's College of Engineering, New Delhi, India

M. Gupta (✉) · K. Garg
Chandigarh University, Gharuan, Punjab, India
e-mail: meenu.e9406@cumail.in

© The Author(s), under exclusive license to Springer Nature Switzerland AG 2021

F. Al-Turjman et al. (eds.), *Emerging Technologies for Battling Covid-19*, Studies in Systems, Decision and Control 324,
https://doi.org/10.1007/978-3-030-60039-6_7

7.1 Introduction

The outbreak of COVID-19 seems to be unstoppable, as the virus has already affected millions of people around the world. The peoples are continuously facing problem due to this deadly virus, which required a cure, but as the number of mortalities is rising, it does not seem to come down. So far, there is no special treatment for coronavirus, and efforts to control its spread have failed. Despite the lockdown in different countries, the number of active cases in the world is only rising. Therefore, there is an urgent need for the surveillance of those who are affected by the virus. The introduction of a digital system may prove beneficial in the coming time in controlling the disease [1].

A wealth of new technologies such as artificial intelligence (AI) and the Internet of Things (IoT) is gaining worldwide attention and becoming very beneficial in these times of crisis. These new technologies possess a great resource in the time of coronavirus. Such techniques are regularly used by doctors and other healthcare staff to communicate with others for manufacturing and making the vaccine for COVID-19 for checkup, surveillance, and deciding the next steps with lesser human contact and involvement [2]. Also, the advanced technologies are used to gather the proper updates and keeping the data well maintained and secured. The machines used under these technologies, such as robots and drones, are supported by wireless connectivity and sensors. The sensors installed inside them help them to visualize and monitor the activities that are happening around them and then correspond to them accordingly [3].

AI is a powerful tool used to develop robots that can help the medical staff and in undertaking sanitization jobs. It is also beneficial to manufacture the healthcare equipment. IoT is proving to be very helpful during COVID-19 with its application of drones, which is continuously being used for monitoring people on the road and ensuring the implementation of quarantine and mask wearing. A drone can also be used by doctors in remote monitoring of in-home patients [3, 4].

7.2 Literature Review

Kamel Boulos et al. discussed the supports of health databases from different technological products. They also talked about the database, which gives a provision for more accurate, efficient, complete, and real-time information on outbreaks and their distribution; this helps to make better decisions about urban fabric risk management. Weber and Podnar Žarko suggest that the IoT devices which support open protocols are much beneficial, and data integrity and safety during communication and transmission should be ensured by the device provider. But this is not at all carried out as explained by Vermesan and Friess, who say that most of the service providers in the city use proprietary solutions that could only be understood by them and often create chaos, and the information is fragmented into pieces. Lawpoolsri et al. suggest that for continuous monitoring, accurate assessment of data, issues like sharing, access, and quality of data should be supported. People's movement from one place to another place has been recorded in public places before lockdown was imposed. As stated by Li et al., there were sensors installed in such locations that can receive and deliver data in real time to the network's digital infrastructure, and their network interconnection makes them extremely successful in providing real-time alerts on various issues [5].

Chun described in the *South China Morning Post* that infrared cameras had been installed at train stations and airports across China. These cameras scan the temperature of the people when gathered in crowds. These cameras also have a special feature of facial recognition, which helps to identify those who are not obeying the self-quarantine orders [6].

Allam and Jones also suggest that for better global understanding and management of urban health, the use of AI data sharing standardization protocols could be used and will be beneficial for the society [7].

The effectiveness of a chatbot based on cognitive behavioral therapy and positive psychological interactions in the nonclinical population has been displayed by Ly et al. The study showed that the people having a "digital relationship" with the chatbot were impacted with good well-being and perceived stress better [8].

Breazeal [9] and Lazzeri et al. (2013) say that robots are now being equipped with "social intelligence" that would help them to react like a normal human being [10]. In [11], authors discuss the problem encountered by charity people in China that relates to crises occurred in tech industry. In this work, authors used Blockchain and Artificial tool for implementation and analysis about handing these crises happened due to COVID-19. Next in [12], author discuss the role of drone in monitoring human emotions. The use of drone is also seen in agriculture for monitoring crops and farming. The main focus of the authors in this paper was to discuss the functionality of drones in social interaction. Drones can also play a vital role in measuring social distancing. Further in [13], the authors focus on mobile-based web survey for identifying COVID-19. They apply machine learning algorithm for further analysis. They propose a method which helps in reducing the spread of viral disease. In [14], the authors propose a novel model using deep Q-learning network that helps in finding drugs to reduce SARS-cov-2-based diseases. Further in [15], they consider the COVID-19 data set of individual patients who died in Hubei, mainland China. The main focus of this study was to analyze the total number of deaths and recovery rate of COVID-19-infected people. Different technologies that have been used in fighting against COVID-19 are discussed in [16]. In this, they discuss the different levels of crises happened due to COVID-19 and medical image processing. The role of AI-based big data in analyzing epidemic outbreaks and the role of smart cities in enhancing the decision by looking policy maker are discussed in [17]. Next in [18], the authors discuss the loss of manpower and economic crisis due to the COVID-19 pandemic. In this work, they discuss the role of wireless communication in COVID-19 and showed how this technology can help in monitoring the spread of viral diseases.

7.3 Critical Event Management

In coping with an unpredicted virus and in the time of such crises, accurate and actionable information is necessary for everyone to take their next step appropriately. There has never been such a pandemic as COVID-19 situation, so researchers around the world are continuously looking for new technologies to fight against this deadly virus. Still, the deployment of such techniques may take a much longer time to impact our lives and save the world from getting diminished. In case of a critical event such as the COVID-19 pandemic, access to information is very important. It has been observed from previous situations that the information in such times is often broken into pieces and cannot provide actionable intelligence. The larger the happening, the more difficult and complicated it is to collect accurate information and assess it to take the necessary next steps.

There are many tools available to solve this complexity and find a more accurate, rapid, and effective response for the pandemic and minimize its impact on society. There are generally four stages of any response management. In the first stage, the data is gathered from various resources about the current situation of COVID-19. This step helps the response team to use the needed analytics tool to use to understand what is happening now and what could happen in the future. A second stage includes the location of required assets, employees, and other vital equipment that could be needed if the situation becomes worse. In the next step, such systems offer large organizations and emergency responders the necessary tools to act for informing people about the actions to be taken and releasing mass scale notifications in severely affected areas and calling up different teams to collaborate if needed. The last stage enables the concerned authorities to review and evaluate all the happenings that occurred during the event so that if something the same happens in the future, the impact may be minimized [19].

7.4 Artificial Intelligence and Internet of Things in Critical Event Management

Internet of Things (IoT) is a well-defined scheme for interconnected computing devices and mechanical devices that possess the capability of transmitting the data over a network without any human or physical involvement at any stage [20]. During lockdown period, it has been observed that IoT systems and devices have been recognized and being used regularly by concerned authorities and responders. These devices help to connect directly those who are affected by an emergency affected by COVID-19. There are several use cases in which IoT can be utilized, such as emergency calling, public warning systems, surveillance systems, and a communication system for situational awareness, proving beneficial in any critical event [19]. It provides a method for all the social workers, patients, doctors, civilians, etc., to get connected and communicate with each when necessary. It is also used to predict the upcoming situation of COVID-19 with the help of data stored in the database. The COVID-19-affected person can use an IoT device for proper monitoring of his or her heart rate, blood pressure, and other personalized activities. The most significant application of this technology in current time is that it can be used to track the real-time location of medical equipment for a hassle-free process without any delay, and the companies can use this technology to detect fraud claims. This improves treatment flow and is helpful in decision-making [20] (Fig. 7.1).

Artificial intelligence is a very powerful tool that can be used to predict the outbreak and help in minimizing its spread [3]. AI has been applied widely to our different lives in several ways and is also regularly contributing to fighting against the coronavirus. This technology is being used to diagnose, respond, or predict the deadly virus spread [19]. AI can be used along with deep learning to enhance the detection and diagnosis of the COVID-19 virus in a person. It can also be used to alleviate the clinical load of patients by enabling an online medical "chatbot," which could help patients recognize the early symptoms of the virus and also help in educating them for taking the next steps. A phone-based software could be used for avoiding hospital consultations, as it will store and detect the patient's data. This data could be developed in AI algorithms for COVID-19 [22]. Further, AI can also contribute to making robots that will assist the doctors and patients in the time of need and could also be used for other purposes such as sanitization (Fig. 7.2).

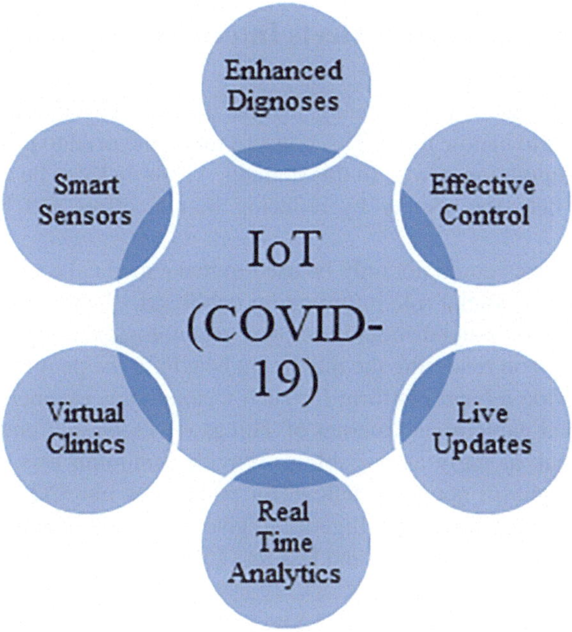

Fig. 7.1 Role of IoT in COVID-19 [21]

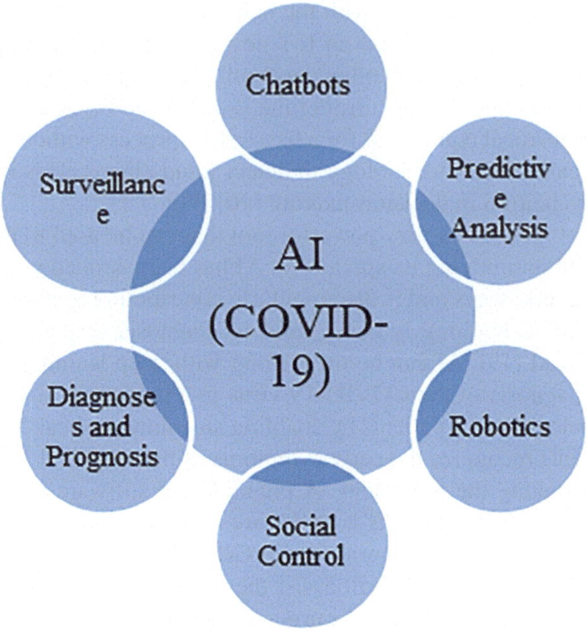

Fig. 7.2 Role of AI in COVID-19 [23]

7.5 Artificial Intelligence Meets Internet of Things (IoT)

Persistently the Internet is transforming, and the datasets present are huge, and it is becoming difficult to handle them. This concern raises the need to process this huge data with the computation power. In this domain, AI and IoT can be a breakthrough [24]. This will help the society by reducing human effort and building some smart things.

These technologies could not only be used to make medical tools and in laboratories but can play a crucial role in providing public safety and such similar situations. Smart city professionals could use these technologies to make collaborative strategies and work on rendering the maximum benefit to the people of the country. Cities could provide a huge platform for such technologies to emerge as per their potential. Thermal cameras or Internet of Things (IoT) sensors could be used to detect the outbreak as early as possible to provide minimum loss to people. But these sensors alone will not be beneficial for pandemics like COVID-19, so they have to integrate with artificial intelligence to give significant benefits. It will result in better management of resources and less loss [5].

7.6 Robots in COVID-19

The outbreak of COVID-19 has now become a pandemic, and therefore global effort is required to fight against it. Robots have the potential to help humans in the current situation. They could be deployed for various purposes and thus serving humanity. These could be used for disinfecting areas, delivering supplies, and many other activities. As seen in the current situation, there is an extensive opportunity and developments available in the field of robotics. This pandemic could prove beneficial for this domain of science to flourish to its full extent. Hence, it develops fully automated robotic systems that could be deployed to serve humanity today and in the upcoming time by providing remote access and avoiding the humans to travel up to the frontlines [25].

7.6.1 Delivery Robots

These community robots ensure the necessary supply of food and medicines and other vital materials, such as masks, face shields, PPE kit, etc., in the community [10]. The robots are used for the delivery of food and medicines to the people who have been quarantined during the COVID-19 period. These robots have been given a special cart-like shape, which brings food to people isolated in a 16-story hotel. Delivery robots are also being used to transport infectious samples to the laboratory for testing so that human interaction can be avoided [26]. Also, these are used to collect transmissible waste from the hospitals and then put it in the dustbins [27]. Robots have become an important part of delivering essential items.

7.6.2 Mobile Robots (Chatbots)

Various healthcare units and hospitals have been regularly updating their digital tools and technologies to provide their best to the patients. AI-based chatbot system has proven very beneficial in the COVID-19 crisis [8]. Chatbots are a computer application that stimulates conversation via chat [28]. These chatbots are natural language processing systems that act as a virtual conversational agent that promotes health and inform and potentially contributes to changes in human behavior. During COVID-19, chatbots could be used to answer the health inquiries, while people look for a specific symptom of the disease such as cough or cold. As many of the countries have been locked down due to the disease, it may have a bad effect on someone's mental health. Chatbots could also be used under this domain to develop therapeutic and preventative interventions [8, 29]. Chatbots help people to recognize the early symptoms and simultaneously educate them on hand hygiene [22]. These bots are a great way to consult about some small health issues which may not require consulting to a doctor in physical and hence maintaining social distancing and avoiding the spread and, in return, could also save us some precious time.

7.6.3 Sterilization Robots

Coronavirus not only spread from direct contact with the infected person or via the respiratory droplets but can also spread via contaminated surfaces. If an infected person touches any surface, then the virus stays over the surface for a certain amount of time, depending upon the material of the surface. So, for this purpose, a special type of robot-controlled noncontact ultraviolet (UV) disinfection is being used in many hospitals. UV light devices have been proven effective in reducing the contamination from such surfaces in the hospitals. This is a good method to disinfect such surfaces with the help of a robot, as it reduces the risk for cleaning personnel, and robots could do this work faster than humans and more effectively. Robots could be made in different sizes for sterilization, depending upon the surface to disinfect [25]. Robots are also being equipped with sprays to clean public areas [10] (Fig. 7.3).

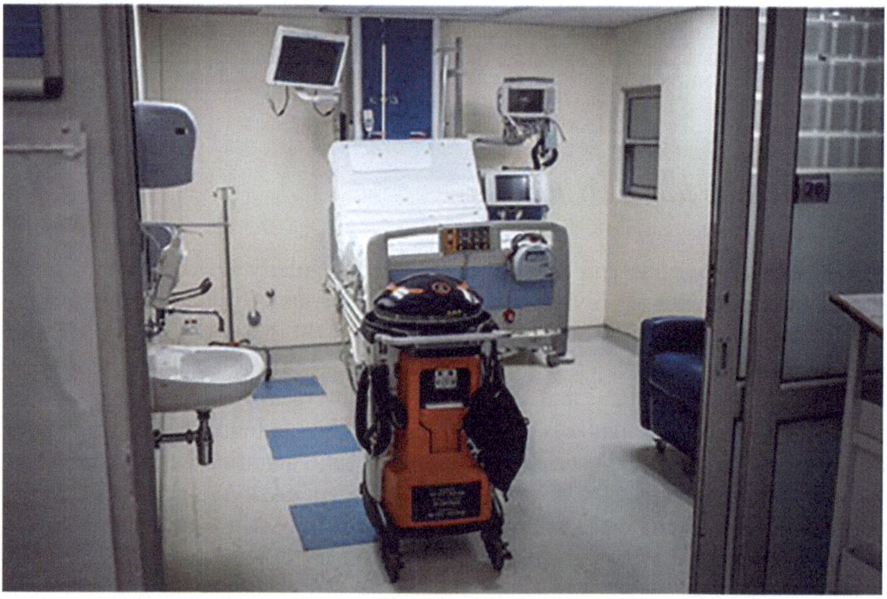

Fig. 7.3 A robot using ultraviolet light to disinfect a hospital room [30]

7.6.4 *Telemedicine Robots*

These are the special robots to help, specifically the patients. These robots have cameras and sensors embedded in them. The video screen helps the doctors to chat with the patients remotely, avoiding the risk of the disease. These robots help healthcare workers to provide treatment to the patients while not being near them. The robots could take the temperatures of the patients and measure the blood pressure [26] (Fig. 7.4).

7.7 Drones in COVID-19

Drones have been playing a very crucial role in the case of this massive pandemic. These are being used for several purposes, such as supplying essential items, monitoring social distancing, or spraying disinfectants around public spaces. Drones allow the fast distribution of essentials in a short time and could also be used by the people post-epidemic event through the use of artificial intelligence, GPS, and large delivery system anywhere and anytime without any need of operator [32] (Fig. 7.5).

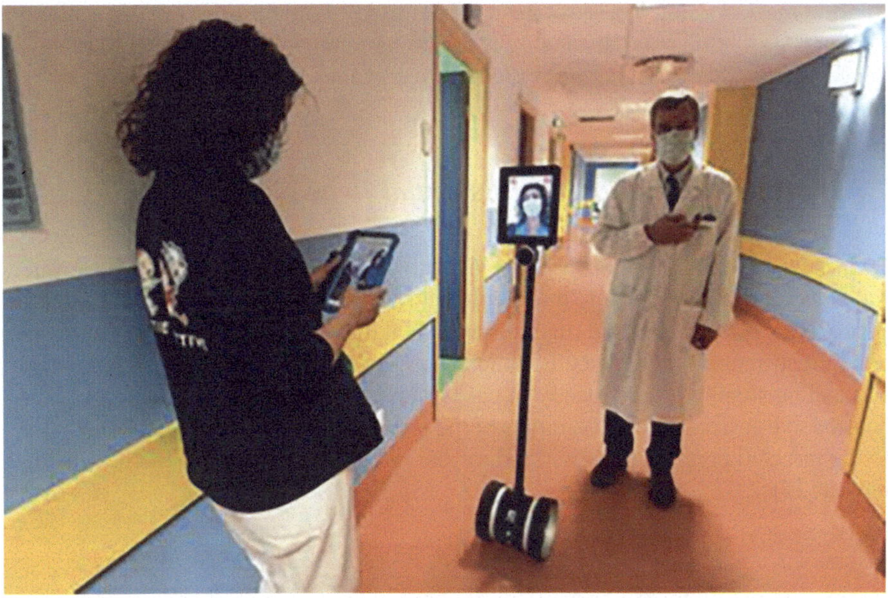

Fig. 7.4 A nurse using the robot to interact with the COVID-19 patient [31]

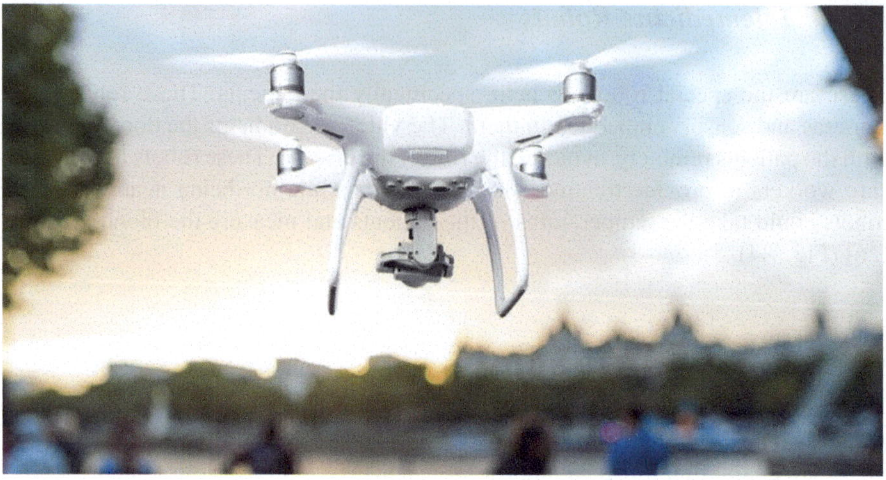

Fig. 7.5 Detection of virus in crowded places with pandemic drone [12]

7.7.1 Traffic and Social Distance Monitoring Through Drones

Artificial intelligence along with IoT is being used to make drones with a special feature of facial recognition, which can identify whether the people on the street are wearing masks or not. These drones are also used to monitor the regular traffic on the roads so that if social distancing is not being maintained or people are roaming unnecessarily, then strict action could be taken against them [6].

7.7.2 Drones for Supplying Essential Items

Drones have been continuously being used to supply essential items such as water, food medicines, lights, etc., to the people who are infected with the COVID-19 virus or are home quarantined and maintaining social distancing. For this purpose, a special infrastructure should be built, which can store all these basic and essential items and can be supplied to the needy in case of an emergency [32]. Drones could also be used to transfer the blood samples of the patients and for providing the medicines to the infected persons. This will reduce the risk of the disease for the doctors and nurses [25].

7.7.3 Drones in Disinfecting Public Areas

Drones are continuously being used to disinfect large public areas. This requires less human interaction and could be done more efficiently while obeying the social distancing norms [26] (Fig. 7.6).

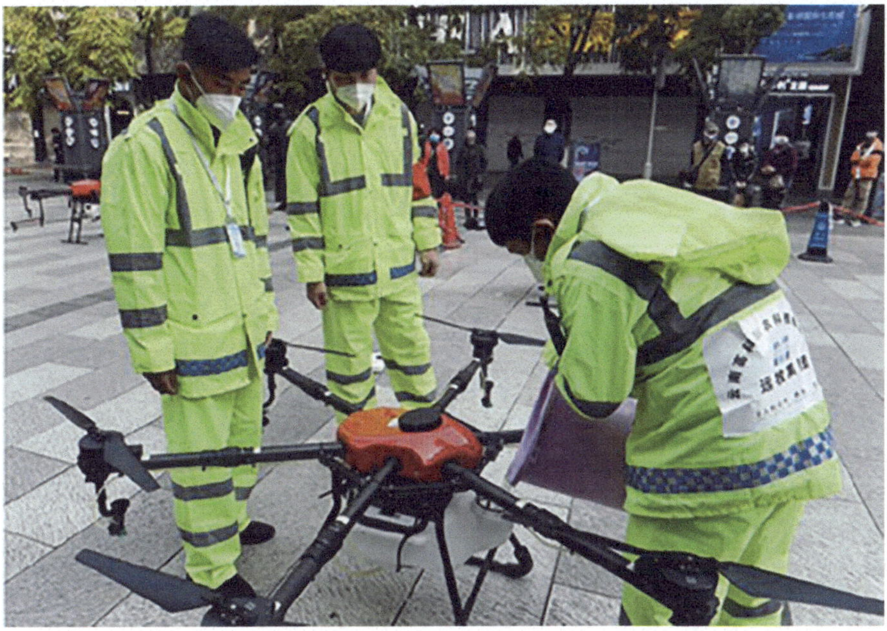

Fig. 7.6 Workers refilling the drone with disinfectant [26]

7.8 Analysis of COVID-19 Impacts on the World

The following section will give an insight into the number of COVID-19 cases around the world and how the different counties are handling this critical situation and coping with the same.

7.8.1 Analysis of the Top Ten Countries with the Highest Number of COVID-19 Cases

The deadly coronavirus has already affected more than 200 countries across the planet. The number of affected cases has been increasing regularly in most of the countries. As of June 2, 2020, 05:55 GMT, there are total 3,089,191 active COVID-19 cases worldwide [33]. Table 7.1 shows the top ten countries which have the highest number of coronavirus cases and are continuously fighting against it (Figs. 7.7 and 7.8).

As the number of cases of COVID-19 is continuously rising, many national and international measures have been taken by different governments of different countries [34]. Most of the governments across the globe placed "lockdown" in their respective countries as "social distancing" plays a very important role in eradicating

Table 7.1 Top ten countries with the highest number of COVID-19 cases and deaths [33]

S. no	Country	Total cases	Active cases	Deaths
1	USA	1,859,323	1,136,982	106,925
2	Brazil	529,405	288,279	30,046
3	Russia	414,878	234,146	5027
4	Spain	286,718	62,633	27,127
5	UK	276,332	N/A	39,045
6	Italy	233,197	41,367	33,475
7	India	198,706	97,344	5608
8	France	189,220	91,344	28,833
9	Germany	183,765	9247	8618
10	Peru	170,039	96,898	4630

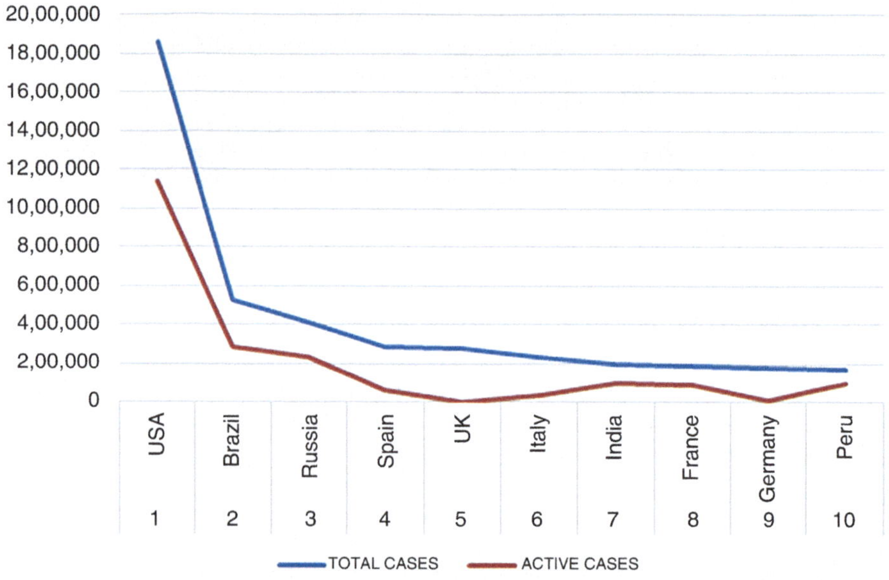

Fig. 7.7 Graphical representation of total and active cases of the top ten most affected countries

this deadly disease. All the public places and private companies were shut down to prevent the virus from spreading [5]. However, many protocols have been applied for the last few months. The countries with the best medical facility such as the USA, Brazil, the UK, and many others failed in providing facilities to their citizens in the time of crisis. The Indian government has recognized the COVID-19 threat in the earlier stage. After analyzing this threat, they imposed lockdown, which resulted in a slower death rate in India. The people in many countries, such as America, were not following the social distancing and self-quarantine norms, which resulted in a high death rate [35].

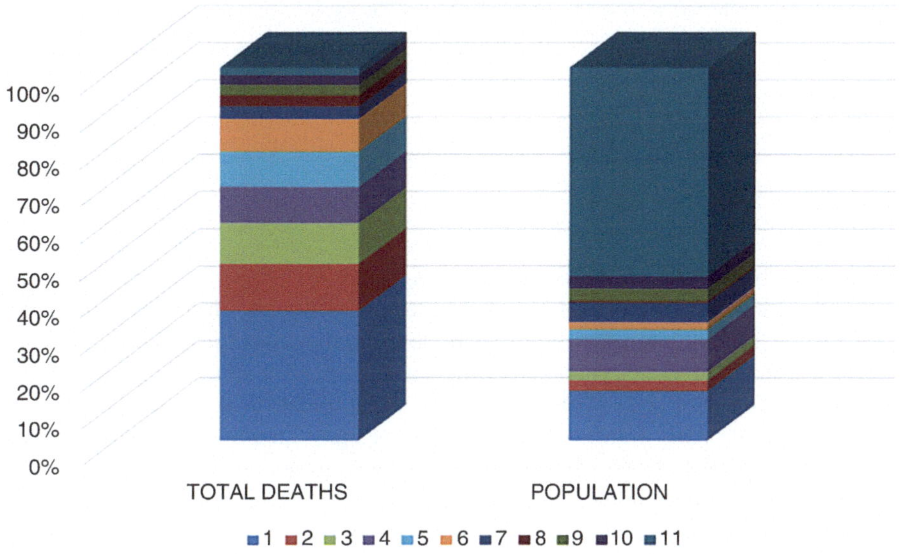

Fig. 7.8 Pictorial representation of deaths in the top ten most affected countries

The Indian government imposed the lockdown in four different phases keeping in mind the different strategies for each stage to be followed so that the citizens could remain calm and follow the self-quarantine norms and maintain social distancing.

7.8.2 Analysis of the Top Five Most Populated Countries Worldwide

Today, the world is suffering from COVID-19, which spread across the globe in a short time. Every country is putting efforts to prepare a vaccine to overcome the impact of this disease, but no one has succeeded. Table 7.2 shows the total infected, recovered, and overall death cases of the top five most populated countries, namely, China, India, the USA, Indonesia, and Pakistan. The impact of COVID-19 on these five most populated countries can be understood by the following analysis.

7.8.2.1 China Case Analysis

China is the most populated country across the globe, with a population of about more than 1.4 billion people. This deadly disease was spread from the Hubei Province of China itself, hence having the highest number of cases initially throughout the world [36]. Approximately 83,017 people were infected from this deadly

Table 7.2 Total infected, recovered, and death cases of the top five most populated countries

Countries	Population	Infected	Recovered	Deaths
China	1,438,656,995	83,017	78,307	4634
India	1,378,364,845	198,317	95,415	5603
USA	330,769,230	1,846,123	601,049	106,033
Indonesia	273,173,742	26,940	7637	1641
Pakistan	220,367,900	72,460	26,083	1543

disease in China in which 4634 lost their lives, and 78,307 got recovered from it. Early detection and timely isolation help them to get rid of this deadly disease. China's government had taken proper actions to fight against this virus [37]. They timely restricted all the international borders and suspended all the flights and train operations. The people of Wuhan district were confined in their houses around 2 months and properly followed all the guidelines provided by the government to get rid of this virus [38]. Finally, the things get back normal in Wuhan, and China's case proves that with the combined efforts of the local public and the government authorities, it became possible to fight against this virus.

7.8.2.2 India Case Analysis

India is the second most populated country across the globe, with a population of about more than 1.35 billion people. In India, this disease was initially identified in a Kerala student who returned from Wuhan on January 30, 2020, and currently, there are about 197,808 cases of COVID-19 recorded in India, among which 5603 people lost their lives, and 95,415 people got recovered from it. Till now, four phases of lockdown had been employed in India. Lockdown 1.0 and Lockdown 2.0 are somewhat successful, and most of the Indian states showed a positive response by reducing the number of infected cases in those states [39]. But after April 30, when Lockdown 3.0 starts, most of the states in India show exponential growth in the infected cases. Till April 30, there are about 33,000 cases only, and it became around six times higher in just a month. Because of different population density, culture, and diversity of the Indian states, it is difficult to analyze the impact of COVID-19 on the whole of India simultaneously [40].

7.8.2.3 USA Case Analysis

The USA is the third most populated country across the globe, with a population of about 33 million people. The USA has the highest number of COVID-19 cases of around more than 1.8 million and reported the highest number of deaths of about more than 100,000 people. The first case of COVID-19 was published on January 20, 2020, in a 35-year-old man of Washington. The primary reason for having such a high number of cases is the delay showed off in the testing [41]. Also, the US government initially refused to relax the regulations, which does not allow the health departments and the states to develop their testing kits based on WHO guidelines. All the COVID-19-infected samples were being sent to the headquarters of the CDC (Centers for Disease Control and Prevention) in Atlanta [42]. After that, the delay increases because of the faulty test kit sent by the CDC. These primary factors are responsible for the considerable increase in COVID-19 cases in the USA.

7.8.2.4 Indonesia Case Analysis

Indonesia is the fourth most populated country across the globe, with a population of about 267 million people. Indonesia is having the lowest infected to total population ratio of around 0.000098 in the five most populated countries in the world. Currently, Indonesia has 26,940 active cases of COVID-19, and approximately 1641 people lost their lives due to this deathly disease. The first cases of COVID-19 were observed in a dance instructor and her mother, who was infected by a Japanese person. Then this virus spread among 34 provinces of the country by April 9, 2020. Although the country has a minimum number of cases as compared to other most populated countries mentioned above, it still has the second highest number of cases in Southeast Asia after Singapore and also has the fifth highest number of deaths recorded in Asia [43]. The highest number of recoveries (i.e., more than 500) was observed on May 30, 2020.

7.8.2.5 Pakistan Case Analysis

Pakistan is the fifth most populated country across the globe, with a population of about 212 million people. Currently, as on 1 June 2020, Pakistan has 72,460 active cases of COVID-19, and around 1543 people lost their lives because of this deathly disease, while about 26,000 people got recovered from it in the country. The virus was first observed in a Karachi student who returned from Wuhan on February 26, 2020, and spread among four provinces by March 18, 2020. According to a report [44], 27% of COVID-19-infected cases were increased due to religious gatherings that took place in Lahore. Till now, the maximum number of cases was recorded in Sindh state, and the highest numbers of deaths were observed in Punjab. The Pakistani government employed various phases of lockdown from April 1 to May 9, after which the lockdown was somewhat eased in the different provinces [45]. Not following social distancing rules leads to an increasing number of COVID-19 cases as compared to the earlier number of cases.

Hence, after analyzing the COVID-19 impacts on the five most populated countries, we can conclude that the population factor is not responsible for the increase in the COVID-19 cases in any country. Instead, it depends upon various other factors like population density, rules and regulations, norms, culture, diversity, and the medical facilities of that country. Along with government initiatives, the attitude of the public toward the government actions also matters. After all, it is the people themselves who can save the country from such type of deadly pandemic.

7.9 Conclusion and Future Scope

Such technologies quite have the potential to change the delivery of healthcare systems around the globe and serve cost-effective health services and narrow the path of well-being gap, but this certainly requires deeper research. Many people may not believe that such technologies could not solve their problems, such as in the case of chatbots, people may hesitate to put in their personal information to get started with the service. They may be uncertain about their quality, or they may think that conversation in this way might lead to some misunderstanding. So there is a need to make the society aware of these upcoming trending technologies, which could help them shortly, so that they can take the maximum benefit out of them for themselves and their families. These technologies could certainly enhance the public health education and communication. The COVID-19 pandemic could prove to be a catalyst for emerging technologies such as artificial intelligence, the Internet of Things, and robotics. The robots and drones have not replaced the human workforce, but these give humanity a chance to operate these technologies by applying their expertise. The world could have any natural calamity at any time, so we should be prepared for any time of situation or pandemic that might hit us. This critical situation of COVID-19 requires unity of people. Every people must follow social distancing and hand sanitization as a solution to fight against this pandemic and work in the concern of every individual on this planet. These analyses help in the future, and people can avoid those things that can harm them. In the future, this analysis can also help a country to take precautions for these critical diseases.

References

1. Rahman, M.S., Peeri, N.C., Shrestha, N., Zaki, R., Haque, U., Ab Hamid, S.H.: Defending against the novel coronavirus (COVID-19) outbreak: how can the internet of things (IoT) help to save the world? Health Policy Technol. **9**(2), 136–138 (2020)
2. Capobussi, M., Moja, L.: 3d Printing technology and internet of things prototyping in family practice: building pulsoximeters during COVID-19 pandemic. Preprints 2020, 2020050163. https://doi.org/10.20944/preprints202005.0163.v1 (2020)
3. Javaid, M., Haleem, A., Vaishya, R., Bahl, S., Suman, R., Vaish, A.: Industry 4.0 technologies and their applications in fighting COVID-19 pandemic. Diabetes Metab. Syndr. Clin. Res. Rev. **14**(4), 419–422 (2020)
4. Behar, J.A., Liu, C., Tsutsui, K., Corino, V.D., Singh, J., Pimentel, M.A., et al.: Remote health monitoring in the time of COVID-19. arXiv preprint arXiv:2005.08537 (2020)
5. Allam, Z., Jones, D.S.: On the coronavirus (COVID-19) outbreak and the smart city network: universal data sharing standards coupled with artificial intelligence (AI) to benefit urban health

monitoring and management. Healthcare. **8**(1), 46 (2020) Multidisciplinary Digital Publishing Institute
6. Naudé, W.: Artificial intelligence against COVID-19: an early review. IZA Discussion Paper No. 13110, Available at SSRN: https://ssrn.com/abstract=3568314 (2020)
7. Nguyen, T.T.: Artificial intelligence in the battle against coronavirus (COVID-19): a survey and future research directions. Preprint (2020)
8. Nadarzynski, T., Miles, O., Cowie, A., Ridge, D.: Acceptability of artificial intelligence (AI)-led chatbot services in healthcare: a mixed-methods study. Digit. Health. **5**, 2055207619871808 (2019)
9. Breazeal, C.: Toward sociable robots. Robot. Auton. Syst. **42**(3–4), 167–175 (2003)
10. Zeng, Z., Chen, P.J., Lew, A.A.: From high-touch to high-tech: COVID-19 drives robotics adoption. Tour. Geogr. **22**(3), 1–11 (2020)
11. Johnstone, S.: A viral warning for change. COVID-19 versus the red cross: better solutions via blockchain and artificial intelligence. In: COVID-19 Versus the Red Cross: Better Solutions Via Blockchain and Artificial Intelligence (February 3, 2020). University of Hong Kong Faculty of Law Research Paper (2020/005) (2020)
12. Malliaraki, E.: Social interaction with drones using human emotion recognition. In: Companion of the 2018 ACM/IEEE International Conference on Human-Robot Interaction, pp. 187–188 (2018)
13. Rao, A.S.S., Vazquez, J.A.: Identification of COVID-19 can be quicker through artificial intelligence framework using a mobile phone–based survey when cities and towns are under quarantine. Infect. Control Hosp. Epidemiol. **41**(7), 826–830 (2020)
14. Tang, B., He, F., Liu, D., Fang, M., Wu, Z., Xu, D.: AI-aided targeted covalent inhibitors design against SARAS-COV-2. bioRxiv. https://doi.org/10.1101/2020.03.03.972133 (2020)
15. Verity, R., Okell, L.C., Dorigatti, I., Winskill, P., Whittaker, C., Imai, N., et al.: Estimates of the severity of coronavirus disease 2019: a model-based analysis. Lancet Infect. Dis. **20**(6), 669–677 (2020)
16. Kumar, A., Gupta, P.K., Srivastava, A.: A review of modern technologies for tackling COVID-19 pandemic. Diabetes Metab. Syndr. Clin. Res. Rev. **14**(4), 569–573 (2020)
17. Inn, T.L.: Smart city technologies take on COVID-19. World Health (2020)
18. Saeed, N., Bader, A., Al-Naffouri, T.Y., Alouini, M.S.: When wireless communication faces COVID-19: combating the pandemic and saving the economy. arXiv preprint arXiv:2005.06637 (2020)
19. Shi, F., Wang, J., Shi, J., Wu, Z., Wang, Q., Tang, Z., et al.: Review of artificial intelligence techniques in imaging data acquisition, segmentation and diagnosis for Covid-19. IEEE Rev. Biomed. Eng. 1–13 (2020)
20. Singh, R.P., Javaid, M., Haleem, A., Suman, R.: Internet of things (IoT) applications to fight against COVID-19 pandemic. Diabetes Metab. Syndr. Clin. Res. Rev. **14**(4), 521–524 (2020)
21. Chakraborty, S., Bhatt, V., Chakravorty, T.: Impact of IoT adoption on agility and flexibility of healthcare organization. Int. J. Innov. Technol. Explor. Eng. **8**(11), 2673–2681 (2019) ISSN: 2278-3075
22. Ting, D.S.W., Carin, L., Dzau, V., Wong, T.Y.: Digital technology and COVID-19. Nat. Med. **26**(4), 459–461 (2020)
23. Singh, V.K., Chandna, H., Kumar, A., Kumar, S., Upadhyay, N., Utkarsh, K.: IoT-Q-Band: a low cost internet of things based wearable band to detect and track absconding COVID-19 quarantine subjects. EAI Endorsed Trans. Internet Things. **20**(21), 163997 (2020)
24. Ghosh, A., Chakraborty, D., Law, A.: Artificial intelligence in internet of things. CAAI Trans. Intell. Technol. **3**(4), 208–218 (2018)
25. Yang, G.Z., Nelson, B.J., Murphy, R.R., Choset, H., Christensen, H., Collins, S.H., et al.: Combating COVID-19—the role of robotics in managing public health and infectious diseases. Sci. Robot. **5**(40), eabb5589 (2020)

26. Murphy, R.R., Adams, J., Gandudi, V.B.M.: Robots are playing many roles in the coronavirus crisis- and offering lessons for future disasters (2020). https://gcn.com/articles/2020/04/24/robots-pandemic-response.aspx
27. Drones for sanitising, robots in isolation wards, special stethoscope—innovations to fight corona. https://economictimes.indiatimes.com/news/science/drones-for-sanitising-robots-in-isolation-wards-special-stethoscope-innovations-to-fight-corona/articleshow /75105576.cms?utm_source=contentofinterest&utm_medium=text&utm_campaign=cppst. Accessed 30 Apr 2020
28. Weißensteiner, A.A.A.: Chatbots as an approach for a faster enquiry handling process in the service industry. Signature. **12**, 04 (2018)
29. Kapoor, A., Guha, S., Das, M.K., Goswami, K.C., Yadav, R.: Digital healthcare: the only solution for better healthcare during COVID-19 pandemic? Indian Heart J. **72**(2), 61–64 (2020)
30. Tavakoli, M., Carriere, J., Torabi, A.: Robotics, smart wearable technologies, and autonomous intelligent systems for healthcare during the COVID-19 pandemic: an analysis of the state of the art and future vision. Adv. Intell. Syst. **2**(7), 2000071 (2020)
31. Yang, T., Gentile, M., Shen, C.F., Cheng, C.M.: Combining point-of-care diagnostics and internet of medical things (IoMT) to combat the COVID-19 pandemic. Diagnostics. **10**(4), 224 (2020)
32. Ruiz Estrada, M.A.: The uses of drones in case of massive epidemics contagious diseases relief humanitarian aid: Wuhan-covid-19 crisis. Available at SSRN 3546547 (2020)
33. Worldometer. Coronavirus updates. https://www.worldometers.info/
34. Deshwal, V.K.: COVID 19: a comparative study of Asian, European, American continent. Int. J. Sci. Res. Eng. Dev. **3**(2), 436–440 (2020)
35. Singhal, N., Prakash, S.: A fight against COVID-19: major IT trends. Available at SSRN 3601504 (2020)
36. Zhou, F., Yu, T., Du, R., Fan, G., Liu, Y., Liu, Z., et al.: Clinical course and risk factors for mortality of adult inpatients with COVID-19 in Wuhan, China: a retrospective cohort study. Lancet. **395**(10229), 1054–1062 (2020)
37. Lin, B., Wu, S.: COVID-19 (coronavirus disease 2019): opportunities and challenges for digital health and the internet of medical things in China. OMICS. **24**(5), 231–232 (2020)
38. Hernández, J.C.: As China cracks down on coronavirus coverage, journalists fight back—The New York Times. Nytimes.com. Accessed 6 Apr 2020
39. Singh, R., Adhikari, R.: Age-structured impact of social distancing on the COVID-19 epidemic in India. arXiv preprint arXiv:2003.12055 (2020)
40. Ghosh, P., Ghosh, R., Chakraborty, B.: COVID-19 in India: state-wise analysis and prediction. medRxiv (2020)
41. Pilkington, E., McCarthy, T.: The missing six weeks: how Trump failed the biggest test of his life. The Guardian. ISSN 0261-3077 (2020). Accessed 28 Mar 2020
42. Wang, J., Huth, L., Umlauf, T., Wang, E., McKay, B.: How the CDC's restrictive testing guidelines hid the coronavirus epidemic. Wall Street J (2020). Archived from the original on 22 Mar 2020. Accessed 23 Mar 2020
43. Setiati, S., Azwar, M.K.: COVID-19 and Indonesia. Acta Med. Indones. **52**(1), 84–89 (2020)
44. Chaudhry, A. Tableeghi Jamaat in hot water in Pakistan too for Covid-19 spread. DAWN (2020). Archived from the original on 8 Apr 2020. Accessed 8 Apr 2020.
45. Coronavirus pandemic: Pakistan to extend lockdown for 2 more weeks as death toll reaches 31 Archived 8 Apr 2020, at the Wayback Machine, The Statesman, 2 Apr 2020
46. Nguyen, C.T., Saputra, Y.M., Van Huynh, N., Nguyen, N.T., Khoa, T.V., Tuan, B.M., et al.: Enabling and emerging technologies for social distancing: a comprehensive survey. arXiv preprint arXiv:2005.02816 (2020)

Chapter 8
Wearable Devices and COVID-19: State of the Art, Framework, and Challenges

Rajalakshmi Krishnamurthi, Dhanalekshmi Gopinathan, and Adarsh Kumar

Abstract In the current century, the novel coronavirus has presented itself as a serious threat to the global human population. However, constructively, with the intervention of the latest computing technology such as the Internet of Things, distributed cloud computing, and artificial intelligence, the COVID-19 pandemic can be effectively handled. From this aspect, the main objectives of this chapter are to study and present various wearable devices as part of the healthcare system toward combating the COIVD-19 pandemic. First, this work aims to review the different wearable devices and their usage to combat COVID-19 by patients, healthcare professional, frontliners, and global citizens. Hence, the major objectives of these wearable devices include device tracking, information sharing, and awareness creation to minimize the risk of coronavirus infection. Second, the chapter addresses a generalized framework toward the implementation of wearable devices to handle the COVID-19 pandemic. Next, this chapter aims to review monitoring techniques and various mechanisms used to analyze the data gathered from wearable devices in order to extract useful and critical information pertaining to users in the COVID-19 scenario. This chapter involves reviewing efficient techniques and algorithms that exist in literature for data analysis based on vital body signals from the wearable sensor devices. This effort enhances the patient/healthcare staff monitoring mechanism and helps to uncover preventive solutions in the COVID-19 scenario. Particularly, the data processing and analysis mechanisms such as data denoising, data aggregation, data outlier detection, and missing data imputation are emphasized. Finally, the chapter addresses various challenges associated with wearable devices in the COVID-19 scenario such as real-time processing, heterogeneity, interoperability, security, and privacy.

R. Krishnamurthi (✉) · D. Gopinathan
Jaypee Institute of Information Technology, Noida, India
e-mail: k.rajalakshmi@jiit.ac.in

A. Kumar
University of Petroleum and Energy Studies, Dehradun, India

© The Author(s), under exclusive license to Springer Nature Switzerland AG 2021

F. Al-Turjman et al. (eds.), *Emerging Technologies for Battling Covid-19*, Studies in Systems, Decision and Control 324,
https://doi.org/10.1007/978-3-030-60039-6_8

Keywords Wearable devices · COVID-19 · Identification · Collaboration · Monitoring · Crowdsourcing

8.1 Introduction

The coronavirus disease, abbreviated as COVID-19, is a virulent disease instigated by a novel virus, nCOVID, also termed severe acute respiratory syndrome coronavirus 2 (SARS-CoV-2). As of 12 April 2020, the World Health Organization (WHO) reported that approximately 1,700,000 people were infected by this coronavirus. In addition, more than 100,000 people were reported dead due to this novel virus infection. Keeping this in mind, the recent studies exhibit that efficient solutions for handling the COVID-19 pandemic can be achieved with the intervention of emerging computing technologies such as wearable devices, the Internet of Things (IoT), cloud computing, fog computing, and big data, which play vital roles in empowering the global citizens [1–3]. Hence, this work aims to explore how wearable devices can provide efficient solutions regarding identification, monitoring, collaborating, and crowdsourcing to tackle the effects of COVID-19. The wearable devices are smart sensor-based electronic devices that can be worn by a person and carried easily. These wearable devices are capable of sensing vital body signals. Additionally, these devices are able to gather, transmit, store, process, and analyze data to extract information from these sensor signals [4, 5].

Wearable devices are quite popular in critical healthcare systems due to their user-friendliness, light weight, and accuracy. In recent years, the IoT-based smart healthcare system has impacted greatly on the rising demand of wearable devices [6, 7]. The benefit of IoT-enabled wearable healthcare devices is that they provide individuals with the knowledge they need to gain greater control over their health outcomes. Wearable devices and the IoT would support and reduce the human interference in healthcare, allowing context-based automation. In many works, IoT healthcare systems have been built for various reasons, including rehabilitation, diabetes control, assisted ambient living (AAL) for elderly people, and more [8, 9]. Although these systems have been developed for many different objectives, they are each intricately connected by their use of common enabling technologies. Such applications include fall detection, quantification of physical activity, study of human habits, and monitoring elderly people care. Electrochemical accelerometer sensors are commonly used to monitor human physical activity. These sensors are capable of measuring the speed of any moving object. With respect to human physical activity monitoring, the accelerometer sensors provide information regarding individual activities and the number of footsteps for quantitative evaluation [10, 11]. Most wearable devices are non-invasive nanomaterial-based biosensors that measure the vital signs by being put on the body or near the body.

Another aspect of wearable devices is general human movement tracking or motion tracking. The human motion tracking mechanism has several useful applications in the medical field, sports, and in other domains. Wearable biological sensors include watches, shoes, bandages, glasses, contact lenses, and rings conveniently attached to the body of a person and functioning in terms of portability, ease of use, and adaptability [12–14]. A wide range of wearables have been available in recent years on the market offering rising functionalities and wear options. Several different wearable devices have been developed by various companies: fitness trackers, smart watches, headsets paired, smart glasses, wristbands, etc. Wearable devices can sense, capture, and store physiological data and improve the quality of human life. They carry out several micro-level activities such as checking incoming messages and immediate processing of urgent data. Figure 8.1 shows various wearable smart devices available for users. These wearable devices are equipped with sensors (e.g., accelerometer, gyroscope), network ports, camera, data processor, etc., which are a successful candidate for tracking the everyday behavior of users (hiking, jogging, smoking, etc.) [1]. The sensors measure temperature, humidity, motion, heartbeat, etc. Wearable devices are currently used in several domains such as healthcare, sports, and navigation systems.

During the COVID-19 pandemic, wearable sensors and nano-biosensors have gained considerable publicity due to the contactless-based healthcare diagnosis.

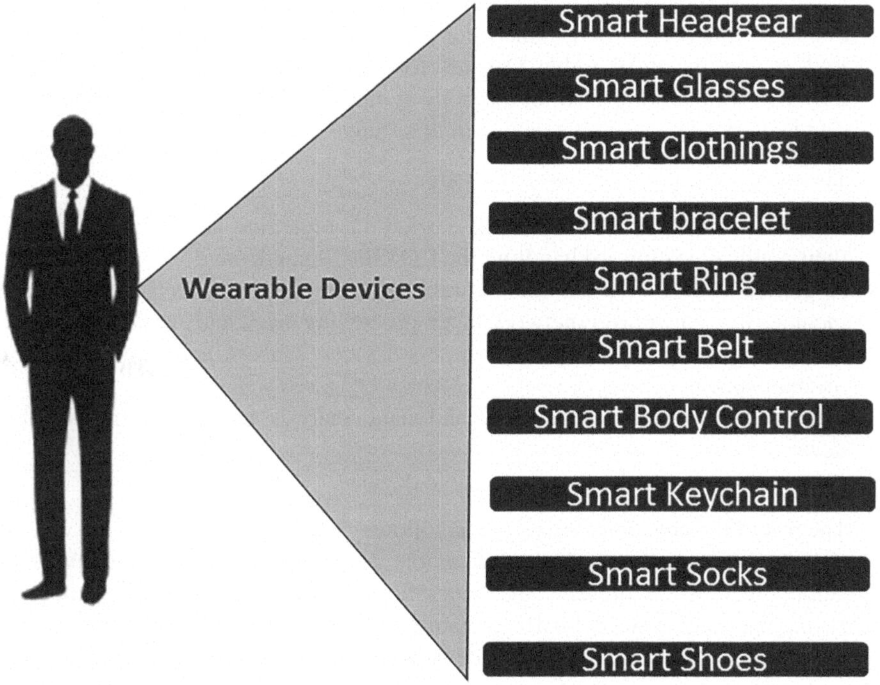

Fig. 8.1 Wearable smart devices

The wearable sensors are capable of measuring vital signals of the human physical body such as heart rate, blood pressure, skin coloration, body temperature, respiratory rate, sleep duration, and body motion. These measured quantities are clinically important and can also be obtained through contactless processes [15–17]. Various surveys and studies have been conducted based on the usage of wearable devices to handle the COVID-19 pandemic as follows.

- *Stanford Covid-19 Detection Study* addresses the fitness of users through tracing their activities. The wearable devices considered for this study are Fitbit, Apple Watch, Garmin, and the Oura ring. The study focuses on the prediction of infectious disease onset, including COVID-19. The wearer's vital health data is collected through wearable devices and is processed for further analysis and predictions.
- *Duke Covidentify* aims to study wearable devices and to determine the ability of wearable devices to identify COVID-19 and influenza-like symptoms. This daily-based survey aims to measure the severity of viral infection through wearable devices. The study involves wearable devices such as Fit bit and Garmin.
- *Scripps Detect Study* involves the study and analysis of various human body vital information, such as heart rate, sleep length, and fitness activities. The study uses wearable devices such as Apple Watch, Fitbit, Beditt, Oura, and Garmin, which are capable of sharing data with remote cloud servers.
- *UCSF TemPredict* works according to the principle of measuring the body temperature and identifying any changes in the temperature from the baseline threshold. The Oura ring is used as the wearable device in this study.
- *RNI Feasibility* of Wearable Devices for Covid Monitoring aims to forecast COVID-19 infection based on the body symptoms and mind signals. The Oura ring is used as the wearable device in this study.

The major objectives of this chapter are:

1. A review of several research works carried out regarding wearable devices and their applications toward handling the COVID-19 pandemic.
2. A generalized framework for wearable devices in the COVID-19 situation includes the sensor layer, network layer, processing layer, and applications layer.
3. Comprehend and study various wearable devices, sensors, and data monitoring mechanisms.
4. Data gathering, data processing, and data analysis techniques in wearable devices.
5. Address various challenges in wearable devices.

The rest of the chapter is organized as follows. Section 8.2 elaborates the various existing works related to IoT-based wearable devices for handling the COVID-19 situation. Section 8.3 presents the generalized framework on wearable devices regarding handling the COVID-19 pandemic and Sect. 8.4 discusses the sensing and monitoring mechanisms in wearable devices that involve device identification and user identification. Section 8.5 presents the detailed mechanisms such as data processing, data analysis, and artificial intelligence incorporated by IoT-based wearable device toward handling COVID-19. Section 8.6 discusses various challenges associated with wearable devices in COVID-19. Finally, Sect. 8.7 concludes the chapter with future scope.

8.2 Related Works

The Chinese Sina-microblog [3] discussed the effect of information dynamics related to how the information regarding COVID-19 propagates among the citizens in Provinces of China. For this study, the Sina-microblog was considered. The data dissemination model permits the user to discuss topics from two different news platforms, namely CCTV and China Daily. The CCTV is a broadcasting channel based on several general topics. While China Daily aims at specific new information. The users of Sina microblog could instantiate multiple instances of microblogging picked from both CCTV and Chain daily. The data dissemination pattern from this perspective model was analyzed to provide insight regarding the multilevel diffusion of COVID-19 related information. Hence, the authors claimed that a serious lack of analysis models regarding information and fake information diffusion could lead to chaos, aggression, and serious health emergencies among citizens of China.

Hence, it is critical to understand the characteristics of the coronavirus and to find efficient ways to handle the pandemic situation.

The coronavirus takes 14 days to show symptoms, and during this period, asymptomatic patients can infect large numbers of people [18–20]. Hence, it is necessary and critical to have an observation system that determines the highly infectious regions and all the people in contact with the patients who have tested positive. To obtain the direct contact of the infected person is easy, but all the other people who had contact with the infected person also have to be identified.

In Singapore, under the "Smart Nation" initiative, the government aims to enhance protection and security for its citizens through a "Contact Tracing" application on mobile devices. As of 5 June 2020, there were approximately 37,000 confirmed cases of COVID-19 among the 5.7 million population of the country. A three level care system has been developed to provide support for oneself, relatives, and the community. The contact map is generated for any COVID-19 patient within a 14-day span. The wearable device-based digital footprints are used to carry out the tracing process. The digital signature through ATM, video recordings of public spots, and private buildings are used to implement the efficient contact tracing map.

In [21], the authors propose an IoT-based solution to determine the precise paths of infected persons (exact coordinates labeled with time). The system is deployed in smartphones. The application collects the required geo-localization data along with the time and sends it to the analysis layer. The analysis layer observes both the location and health data of the infected person. The system has an authorities' interface which offers functionalities to the authorities such as government, health officials, and other organizations who are responsible for monitoring and controlling the outbreak.

This section discusses (1) various types of sensors that exists in the literature and (2) various wearable device-based solutions for combating the COIVD-19 pandemic. First, there are various healthcare monitoring sensors that can be attached to belts, clothes, and fixed on the skin [18, 20, 22–24]. Commonly used healthcare wearable sensors are temperature sensors, pressure sensors [24, 25], acoustic sensors [18, 20, 26], humidity sensors [19], oximetry sensors [27], and multimodal sensing platforms [22].

- Temperature sensors [27]—The temperature sensors are used in a wide variety of applications such as the human body temperature sensor, robot skin temperature measurement, and machines/appliances temperature monitoring. Regarding COVID-19, the human body temperature measurement can be obtained using LM 35, SMT 160-30, and DS 1820. Table 8.1 below shows the characteristics of these sensors.
- Pressure sensors—These sensors are based on the diaphragm contraction and relaxation. This sensor is designed as a belt [24] and an electromechanical film (EMFit), which is a capacitive pressure sensor that has a thin porous polypropylene film structure with a sensitivity of 30–170 pC/N. During the respiration process, the expansion of the chest exerts a force on the sensor and produces a voltage change proportional to this motion. The second type of pressure sensors is [25] designed as a facemask and used effectively during respiration when in contact with inhaled and exhaled air. The EMFit sensor performed well regarding the detection of respiratory rate. This sensor is suitable only for still or modest moving patients [24] because measurement accuracy depends on body movements.
- Acoustic sensors—Acoustic sensors are used to monitor lung sounds and placed near the nose, mouth, throat, and suprasternal notch [18, 20, 26] to obtain the acoustic signals related to breathing. It is a user-friendly wearable device placed next to the nose using tape [18]. It measures the respiratory rate during sleep and sends the signals through wireless communication to a smartphone. The normal and abnormal lung sounds monitored and evaluated by the sensors are used to detect asthma attacks [28].
- Humidity sensors—Humidity sensors for breathing analysis [19] are based on a porous graphene network, which is a chemical structure capable of detecting moisture. This sensor senses the rhythm of human respiration, apnea, speech, and whistle. The sensors are attached to the body with a facemask. The disadvantage of using this sensor is that long time use is also uncomfortable. It still needs some improvements to further commercialization.

Table 8.1 Characteristics of temperature sensors

Sensor	Temperature		Voltage (V)
	Min (°C)	Max (°C)	
LM35	−55	+150	4–30
SMT160	−45	+130	450–700
DS1820	−50	+125	2.5–5

- Oximetry sensors—Oximetry sensors measure oxygen saturation [27]. This sensor can be worn on different body parts such as wrist, finger, head, ear, thigh, and ankle. It measures the absorption of light according to the levels of oxygenated and deoxygenated blood. Oximetry monitors respiratory problems and blood oxygen levels.
- Multimodal sensing platforms—It is a monitoring platform consisting of a chest-patch, wristband, and handheld spirometer [22]. The objective of this sensor is to track health and environmental factors for respiratory diseases such as asthma. The spirometer assesses lung functionality; the chest-patch monitors ECG, skin impedance, photoplethysmography (PPG), wheezing, and motion; and the wristband measures temperature, humidity, PPG, ozone concentration, and motion.

According to the author in [29], COVID-19 has influenza-like symptoms. This includes an average increase in heartbeat rate to 8.5 beats per minute, a body temperature increase of 1 °C and shortened sleep duration. The Huami wearable device can measure the resting heart rate (RHR) and sleep duration of the user. Two types of sensors, namely photoplethysmography and accelerometer sensors, are used for this purpose. The continuous monitoring of flu-like illness is provided through Huami wearable devices. During these observation periods, the physiological anomalies such as RHR and sleep duration are further analyzed through predicting algorithms to narrow down the possibility of COVID-19 infection. Figure 8.2 illustrates the basic parameters that need to be measured from the human user through wearable devices when COVID-19 is suspected.

In 2020, the authors in [30] proposed a wearable device "EasyBand" to handle user mobility depending on the safety parameters during the COVID-19 pandemic situation. EasyBand is based on the programmable microcomputing on chips with

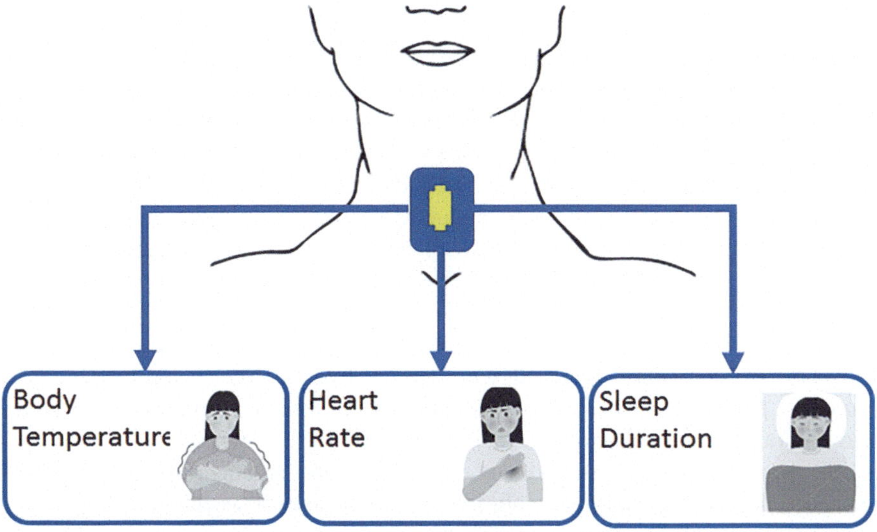

Fig. 8.2 Basic parameters measured through wearable device for COVID-19

IoT technology, and is also capable of performing smart functions such as identifying and establishing communication with similar peer devices. Further, the proposed device can gather information regarding the nearby contacts, and store the relevant information for almost 15 days. The device is also capable of providing users with safety alerts, with three status levels: safe zone, moderate safe zone, and high infectious zones.

In [31], the authors proposed a smart helmet to combat the exposure effect of COVID-19 in public places. This wearable smart helmet has two inbuilt types of sensing cameras: optical and thermal camera. First, the thermal camera senses the body temperature of passerby within the detection zone. If any passerby body temperature exceeds the minimal threshold temperature, the optical camera captures an image and performs digital image processing to fetch the information regarding the person. Further, the details of the person such as image and temperature are recorded and intimated to the concerned health care officials through mobile GSM communication module.

The authors in [32] discuss the nano material-based biosensor for healthcare monitoring and diagnosis of COVID-19 in suspected patients. The nano biosensors include the geno sensor and immuno sensor that are embedded on-chip to perform assessment of COVID-19 patients. The data gathered from the sensors are further analyzed through AI supported data processing and analysis algorithms. Interfacing of nano sensor-based bio chip with the IoT is known as the Internet of Bio-Nano Things (IoBNT). This IoBNT can be used in several ways such as data sharing with other medical and healthcare centers across the globe, faster assessment of COIVD-19 infection, contact tracing, quarantine management, and targeted COIVD-19 patient sensing.

The authors in [33] proposed a wearable bracelet named iBand that performs information exchange between users and the persons in their close contact. Whenever the iBand user comes in close contact with their relatives, the handshake and proximity are detected through the infrared detector. The iBand functionality is similar to the social media and networking platforms, where the main objective is to connect humans and share information. However, in the case of iBand, the added advantage is that the users can use their bio vital signals and senses such as touch. Google Glass promises to be efficient and the most popular wearable computing device. The advantages of Google Glass include being lightweight, user friendly, all day wearable, and supporting virtual display through augmented reality. Table 8.2 illustrates the summary of various wearable devices that have proved popular during the COVID-19 pandemic.

The wearable devices such as Lovegety, groupwear, Synchro.beat, Digital Proxies, and Smart-Its Friends disseminate the information of similar interested groups of people [37–40]. These wearable devices initiate communication within wireless range and exchange sensor readings. Similarly, SwissMarte SpotMe is a secure wearable RFID-based device used in event organization and provides enhanced security and privacy solutions to event control worldwide. It provides solutions to analyze audience performance and behavior, and to understand the audience's intent to buy, participate, learn, or perform their activities.

Table 8.2 Summary of wearable device during the COVID-19 pandemic in literature

S.n	Authors	Products	Measuring parameters	Focus
1	Tripathy et al. (2020) [30]	EasyBand	• Proximity • Peer device networking and communications • Alert system	Mobility during COVID-19
2	Mohammed et al. (2020) [31]	IOT based smart helmet	• Body temperature • Facial recognition	COVID-19
3	Mujawar et al. (2020) [32]	Nano-enabling biosensing systems	• Glucose, coagulation, blood gas, electrolytes, cholesterol	COVID-19
4	Chamberlain et al. (2020) [34]	Smart thermometers	Body temperatures	COVID-19
5	Nittas et al. (2020) [35]	Healthcare device	• Audiovisual cues • Skin color changes using video recordings • Vital signs using wearable device	Telehealth
6	Tayal, et al. (2020) [36]	Remote monitoring device	Body vital signals	Fitness during COVID-19
7	Kanis et al. (2020) [33]	iBand	Body vital signals	Social networking during COVID-19

Under "Future Travelling," a leading initiative project called Guide2Wear deals with various public transportation services through wearable devices based on different user mobility types. The main objective of Guide2Wear is to enhance and optimize the intermodal behaviors of passengers based on their mobility pattern. The passengers are provided with fast, accurate, and suitable services and information based on those mobility patterns and recommended an appropriate environment friendly mode of transportation. The information dissemination involves representation of data about mobility pattern, driver supportive or traffic information regarding a specific transportation mode.

8.3 Framework for Wearable Devices as a Monitoring Mechanism for COVID-19

Wearable devices are gaining popularity because of their lightweight design and their continuous tracking capabilities to improve the quality of life of users. These devices are the basic building block of the Wearable IoT (WIoT). A wearable IoT device collects data from the sensors, processes and analyses the data using some intelligent algorithms and sends valuable information to the wearers. A robust technological framework offered by IoT facilitates data collection and storage by integrating the prominent technologies such as cloud computing [41] and big data [42].

The WIoT framework connects the medical infrastructure, including doctors and hospitals, to assess the patient's condition regardless of their location [43].

The framework for WIoT as a monitoring mechanism for COVID-19 consists of (1) data collection and monitoring from remote locations (2) virtual management of the collected data (3) analyzing the collected data and controlling data (4) following up the report obtained. The overall impact of this framework includes a better tracing of contacts, identification of clusters, and acquiescence of isolation. The devices in this framework use various applications to meet the important requirement of lessening the effects of the COVID-19 pandemic. It predicts the forthcoming condition with the help of appropriate collected data. The tracking of bio-vital signs such as heart beat rate, blood pressure, glucometer, and other activities improves the personalized attention.

The wearable devices perform tasks such as to sense, analyze, store, transmit, and apply. The processing may happen either on the wearer or at a distant location. Personalized information processing is required for each scenario, which transforms the sensory data to knowledge to respond to the situation efficiently. A prominent area where the wearables are used is the health sector, which enables doctors to capture the activity of long-term patients and exercising compliance, provide efficient delivery of pharmaceutical items for chronic patients, and provide availability of tools for evaluating and recommending their ability to carry out complex motor tasks using remedial approaches.

The basic processes involved in wearable device-based health monitor systems can be divided into three layers, namely perception, service, and API layer as shown in Fig. 8.3. The perception layer contains various sensors to collect data in real time.

The service layer contains various application programs to analyze the data and suggest a method to improve the activity. The API layer contains various APIs that store a new profile of the wearer or retrieve the existing information of previously registered wearers.

The wearable devices can be placed inside the body, on the body, and around the body. Inside-body wearable devices are placed inside the human body (for example, a Pacemaker). On the body wearable devices are worn on the body and include accessories such as smart watch, smart band, smart jewelries, and smart clothing. Around the body devices work within proximity of the users. These devices collect data around the users such as environment data. The two devices involved in the wearable device framework are (1) wearable device and (2) host device. Wearable

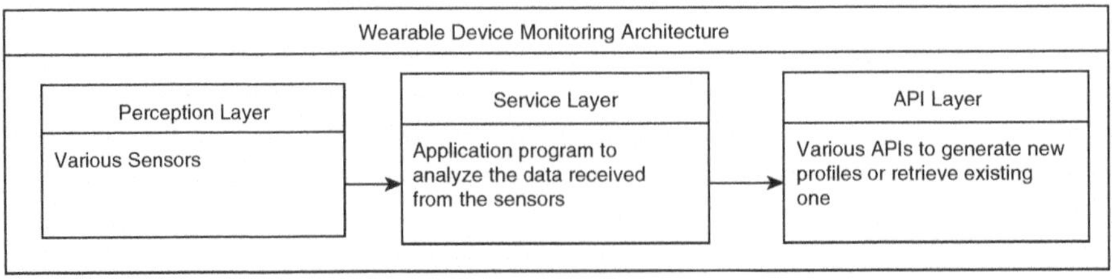

Fig. 8.3 Wearable device-based health monitoring process

devices sense data for the activity generation, and they have limited storage, low computation, and low battery power, whereas the host device has more computation power, larger storage capacity, and larger battery power.

The wearable device collects the sensor data and can apply some pre-processing techniques to reduce the volume of data that can be transmitted to the host or can directly send the raw data to the host depending on the design of the device. It then sends the desired data to the host device. In [9], the authors propose a daily activity monitoring wearable IoT device where some computation is performed at the wearable device before sending data to the host device. User's activities are collected using a 9-axis wristband. The data is pre-processed and segmented at the device level prior to sending to the host. However, the potential problem that needs to be addressed here is that it requires strong authentication and access control mechanisms to support the wearable devices and the data associated with them. An authentication is required to identify the authorized user of the device. An authentication based on the biometric parameters can provide an efficient solution to this.

Thus, a generalized WIoT framework with four functional layers includes a sensing layer, networking layer, processing layer, and applications layer.

- *Sensing layer:* The first layer collects the monitored data from the wearable sensors such as on-body and near-body sensors, which capture physical parameters such as heart activity, blood pressures, respiratory rate, and physical movement. These data are preprocessed to prepare it for analysis [44–46]. In general, the wearable devices are application dependent. Most of these devices are integrated with communication abilities, limited on-board power management, and embedded computing facilities with a small storage support. The limited storage and computing facilities in the sensing devices and the limitations in communication bandwidth and battery power makes the wearable devices insufficient to work in an independent manner. Hence, the integration of these sensing devices with the IoT infrastructure provides a better platform for data aggregation, storage, and transmission, which provides a better analysis framework.
- *Networking Layer:* The network layer configures the wearable devices using a standard or hybrid topology to provide interoperability, energy efficiency, network management, and QoS requirement. In addition, it should also maintain security and privacy of the user data from the personalized healthcare applications [8, 47, 48].
- *Processing layer:* The data processing layers suggested in [29, 43, 45, 49] use different intelligent algorithms, such as the supervised, unsupervised, semi-supervised approaches; knowledge-based approaches, which includes semantic reasoning and modeling; or using hybrid approaches.
- *Application layer:* The application layer of the WIoT architecture provides high quality services to healthcare providers as well as individuals [50, 51]. A user-friendly interface provides a better way to access these solutions to people who are typically not familiar with using intricate technological interfaces.

Figure 8.4 illustrates the general framework of various layers involved in the WIoT for the COVID-19 scenario. The main challenge in developing applications is

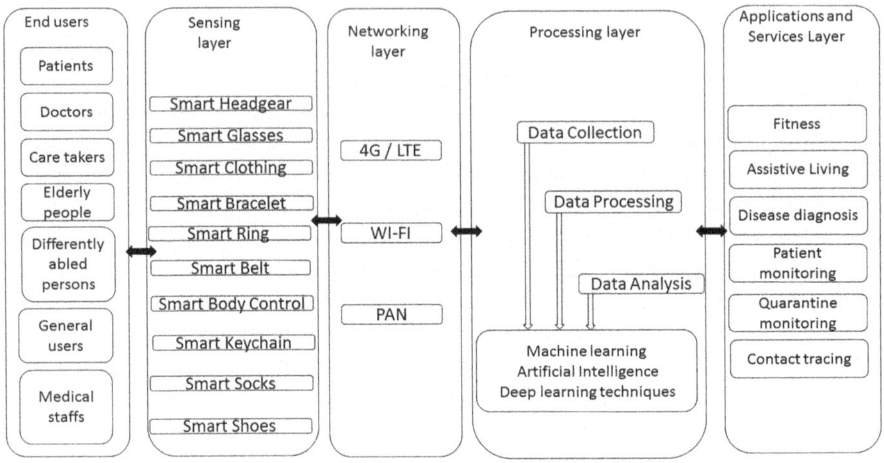

Fig. 8.4 Generalized framework for the wearable device-based health monitoring system

that they should abstract the details that are irrelevant to patients or users and summarize the details appropriately to healthcare professionals to help them make appropriate decisions from their end. Data fusion is involved in monitoring mechanisms for wearable devices.

8.4 Sensing and Monitoring Mechanisms in Wearable Device Made for COVID-19

The IoT on a day-to-day basis is viewed as the utility of products or apps serving people's real-life requirements in different ways, such as home protection, intelligent lighting, and other tasks that are easily controllable with devices such as smartphones and smart voice recognizers. In the current pandemic situation, every country battling against COVID-19 is looking for a genuine and productive solution to face the multiple complications arising. The number of infected persons increases daily globally; the technology behind the IoT well supports data exchange and collection, especially because it is already used in various domains of healthcare.

The major benefits of the IoT for the COVID-19 pandemic is that it guarantees effective control, better diagnostics, and better treatment with lower cost and fewer mistakes. During quarantine, the infected persons can be monitored better. The IoT network can track high-risk patients using vital signs such as blood pressure, heartbeat, and glucose level [31, 52].

In general, the WIoT personal healthcare can be broadly classified as (1) physical activity monitoring, which monitors physical parameters such as motion, breathing, and heart activity; (2) self-monitoring application, which concentrates on improving the quality of life of an individual; (3) clinical decision support for diagnosis and treatment, and emergency health services. This application works according to health data of the individual. It automatically analyzes the data and should be able to predict the diseases, monitor the responses of the treatment provided by the patient, and (4) provide assisted living solutions for the elderly and differently abled [44, 53]. For patients suffering from disorders such as stroke, chronic pain, and heart failure, it gives assistance to the elderly people who live independently.

The types of sensors depend on the output signals they generate that include the underlying concepts and technological capabilities. There are multiple types of sensors, such as contact sensors, accelerometers, audio and motion detectors, available for activity monitoring. They are generally classified into two categories as per the way in which they are placed all through status monitoring, namely action tracking sensors and sensors for mobility monitoring.

- *Action monitoring sensors: The* action monitoring sensors are wearable sensors [4–6] that are attached directly or indirectly to the monitored person or object. These sensors produce a signal when some form of action is performed by the monitored entity. The sensors can be placed in clothing, footwear, heels, mobile devices, etc. They can also be placed directly onto the body. To monitor various temperature, sound, vibration, light, pressure, pollutants, etc., parameters, different sensors, such as thermal, acoustic, vibration, and pressure, should be implemented [2].
- *Mobility monitoring sensors:* The second type of wearable sensors are GPS sensors. These types of sensors are useful when monitoring activities are in mobile environments or when involved in location changes [7].

Recent advances in sensor technology, wearable computing, the IoT, and wireless networking have led to research in healthcare and remote monitoring of the health and behaviors of people. Wearable device monitoring such as health monitoring systems encompass data processing and analysis of data that is retrieved from wearable devices such as smartphones, smart watches, wristbands, along with the various connected devices [8]. These systems continuously monitor the patient's health conditions and activities by sensing and transmitting different parameters such as heart rate, ECG, body temperature, blood pressure, and respiratory rate. The data collected are then fused and analyzed for the diagnosis and treatment of patients with chronic diseases such as hypertension and diabetes.

The monitoring function is helpful for health officials to remotely monitor in-home patients. It also provides innovative methods regarding the quarantine of infected patients, which will dramatically reduce the high risk of mortality and improve the treatment process and care. In addition, it also guarantees better crowd management, transportation management, and safety for the public. Hence, the important objective of the monitoring mechanism in wearable devices is pattern identification of users.

The patterns of interactions between individuals play an important role in determining potential routes for infectious transmission pathways. Hence, awareness of these patterns is very much relevant to identify infectious pathways, to inform about the epidemic spread, and to take effective control measures to adopt prevention strategies or interventions [54–58]. The common methods for pattern identification are contact-based pattern and spatiotemporal-based pattern identification of individuals.

Contact Pattern: In the monitoring mechanism of wearable devices, the contact pattern plays a vital role in the spread of infection among the people in the population. The relationship between the disease spread and contact pattern information is useful to identify the activities such as where the disease is most likely to be transmitted and to take most effective interventions such as wearing a mask, vaccination, hand-wash, etc.

Spatiotemporal Pattern: Recent technological developments such as mobile and wearable sensors have made it likely to be able to measure human beings with high spatiotemporal resolutions in a variety of contexts. It is believed that transmission of disease involves the spatiotemporal proximity of people regarding several infectious diseases, including some of the diseases with the greatest pandemic potential, such as influenza and COVID-19. Spatiotemporal proximity is usually approximated by social relations where social interactions (family, friends, colleagues, etc.) are assumed to catch most of the potential disease transmission.

In [59], the authors describe the infrastructure for data collection from wearable devices. These devices exchange radio-packets in peer-to-peer fashion to track the location and proximity of individuals. The radio-packets are exchanged between the devices located within 1–1.5 m of one another. The sensors are also calibrated while the face-to-face closeness of two people carrying them can be measured over a period of 20 s with a likelihood approaching 99%. Therefore, contact data is obtained in a temporal resolution of 20 s: two persons are considered to be in contact over a 20 s time period if at least one packet is exchanged between their sensors within that time; and the contact event is considered completed, if the sensors do not exchange packets during a 20 s interval as described in (see http://www.sociopatterns.org) [59, 60]. The machine senses the close-up experiences through which an infectious disease transmission may be communicated, e.g., by coughing, sneezing, or handshaking [60].

8.5 Data Gathering, Data Processing, and Data Analytics for Wearable Devices in COVID-19

The monitoring functions of IoT includes data collection, data transfer, data analytics, and data storage.

- *Data Gathering*: The data is collected through various sensors, smartphones, etc.
- *Data transfer*: The collected data is then transferred for analytics to the central cloud server for decision-making. In the current COVID-19 pandemic situation, the IoT is immensely helpful. This technology uses drones for surveillance to confirm the implementation of isolation and mask wearing.

- *Data Analytics:* It is used to trace the contact patterns in the social network and is helpful to trace the outbreak; and track the patients who break the quarantine.

8.5.1 Data Gathering Mechanisms for Wearable Devices

The wearable devices have a receiver, a signal processer, and battery power that enables them to work as a microcomputer. They can also connect to other smart devices and communicate through Bluetooth, infrared, RFID, etc. Furthermore, the data generated from the sensors can be handled either by the platform of dedicated servers that is responsible for collecting and processing the information from the sensors or rely on cloud computing services [3]. In general, most IoT applications bank on cloud computing services that provide remote access through the internet.

Physical parameters include movement, stress, vibration, temperature, heart rate and acceleration, neurological or cardiovascular diseases such as seizures or hypertensions, and pulmonary diseases such as asthma or chronic pulmonary obstructive disease. Temperature measurements on the human body can provide a lot of useful information regarding health conditions such as stroke, heart attack, pulmonary shock, and infections.

To achieve the objective of effective monitoring, first it is necessary to monitor the quality of movement and detect reduced or weakened movement and also estimate the important physical parameters that affect movement. Accelerometers are commonly used sensors for activity tracking, which is used to detect falls, motion, and analysis of body movement and orientation of posture.

8.5.2 Data Processing Mechanisms for Wearable Devices

The unprecedented growth of wearable devices, including smart bands, wristwatches, smartphones, has resulted in the collection of a massive amount of sensor data regarding people's daily life activities. These collected data can be used in various applications in activity tracking, remote monitoring of health, location tracking, etc. The increase in the volume of heterogeneous data necessitates a stronger data processing ability. The conventional methods of data processing will not meet the requirements of new applications. For this scenario, artificial intelligence (AI) technologies have been applied to the data processing with wearable devices. In the current pandemic health crisis of COVID-19, the medical community is seeking new technology to control and monitor COVID-19's spread. AI is one such technology that can easily monitor the virus spread and identify high-risk persons and thus control infections in real-time. It helps predict the probability of mortality by examining prior patient data. It also helps counter this virus by screening individuals and providing warnings and recommendations to contain the infection [61–63].

The main advantage of using AI during the COVID-19 pandemic includes

1. *Primary detection and diagnostics*—a physician can identify and match a COVID-19 symptom with AI support. Samples can be taken from the infected person to confirm the infection and can be analyzed to provide faster decision-making that is cost-effective and diagnostic.
2. *Treatment monitoring*—An automated monitoring and prediction of the virus spread can be established. A neural network algorithm can be used to extract the features that provide help to monitor and treat the affected persons. In addition, it can provide a daily count of the patients and the steps to be implemented during the COVID-19 pandemic situation.
3. *Contact pattern detection*—AI can help assess infection rates by recognizing clusters and "hot spots" with this virus, and can effectively track and control the contacts of individuals. One can predict the future course of this disease and its likely reappearance.
4. *Predict the cases and mortality*—It can trace and predict the type, risk, and likely spread of infection from the available data. In addition, it helps to identify the most susceptible areas, individuals, and nations and take actions accordingly.
5. *Minimizing the workload of healthcare employees*—The AI techniques can also reduce the heavy workload of healthcare professionals. The significant rise in the number of COVID-19 patients also can be reduce by employing AI techniques [64–69].

There are different data processing models for processing the sensor data from the wearable devices. The unprecedented and continued growth of wearable devices has generated and continues to generate a huge volume of data. The data collected from these wearable devices needs to be properly analyzed to provide an insight to users to make an appropriate decision. Because of the wearable devices' limited processing and storage space, the big data analysis and storage is done in remote locations such as the cloud. In [70], the authors propose a model that uses big data analysis to update the knowledge base to provide a tailored recommendation based on the analysis of the data. They propose a three-layer data analysis model. The first layer is data collection and management, the second layer is a customized adaptive analysis layer, and the third layer is a personalized adaptive service layer. The first layer collects the raw data from the sensors attached in the wearable devices through the android app and transfers the data to the cloud. The second layer populates a customized knowledge base through trained parameters to help users make decisions. The third layer extracts facts from the custom knowledge base to provide the user with recommendations.

Raw data collected from the wearable sensors often has noise and may contain sensor errors. Hence, pre-processing of data should be done before further processing of data. The pre-processing of data includes (1) filtering irregular artifact removal data, (2) missing value imputation, (3) removing high-frequency noise, and (4) normalizing sensor data.

8.5.3 Data Analysis Mechanisms for Wearable Devices

Precise outbreak prediction models are necessary to obtain insight into the possible spread and consequences of communicable diseases. The prediction models help the Governments and other administrative bodies to propose new plans and assess already executed plans. It has been reported that COVID-19 has infected more than 2.5 million people with more than 170,000 confirmed deaths worldwide. The complexity of population-wide behavior in different geopolitical areas and differences in containment strategies has dramatically increased model uncertainty in addition to the many known and unknown variables involved in the spread.

Since no vaccine has been invented so far, the main focus in the management of the spread of the pandemic is to flatten the epidemic curve. The technologist and researchers are trying to assimilate information and technology in order to understand the behaviors and characteristics of this virus. In [71], the authors propose a mathematical Susceptible, Exposed, Infectious, Recovered (SEIR) and regression model to evaluate the spread of COVID-19 in India. They have performed an empirical study on the dataset provided by John Hopkins University, USA [72].

The four components of SEIR are: Susceptible (S) denotes the fraction of susceptible persons (those capable of contracting the disease), Exposed (E) is the fraction of exposed persons (those that have been infected but have no symptoms), Infected (I) is the fraction of infectious persons (those capable of transmitting the disease), and Recovered (R) is the fraction of the individuals recovered (those who have recovered from the disease). To study the infectious disease spread, this model assumes that no birth or death or new individual are introduced in the population. Everyone in this population of study is assigned one of the states as Susceptible (S_t), Exposed (E_t), Infectious (I_t), or Recovered (R_t) over a period of time t. The total population at time t is denoted by $N_t = S_t + E_t + I_t + R_{t.}$

This model computes a basic reproductive number R_0 as given in Eq. (8.1), which denotes how many people will be affected from a single infected person over a period. R_0 presents a threshold for the stability of the disease-free equilibrium. The R_0 value greater than 1, equal to 1, and less than 1 indicates the spread is increasing in the absence of intervention, the spread is stable or endemic, and the spread is expected to stop, respectively. Thus, the growth of the virus outbreak can be estimated using R_0.

$$R_0 = \alpha * \beta * \frac{1}{\gamma + \mu} * \frac{\varepsilon}{\mu + \varepsilon} \tag{8.1}$$

where

α : denotes the number of contacts per unit time, β : probablity of disease spread per contact

γ : recovery rate

μ : death rate

ε : rate of progression to infectious state

$\frac{1}{\gamma+\mu}$: duration of infection

$\frac{\varepsilon}{\mu+\varepsilon}$: probablity of recovering from exposed stage

In [60], the authors propose a model based on machine learning to predict the sustainability of patients with severe COVID-19. They performed this study on the blood samples of 404 infected patients from Wuhan, China, to identify crucial predictive parameters of disease severity. This study is formulated as a classification problem with input parameters such as basic information, symptoms, blood samples, laboratory tests, including kidney, liver coagulation function, electrolyte and inflammatory factors, which severely increase the risk of associated patients, and outputs the survival rates or death at the end of the Inspection period. They developed a prognostic model based on XGBoost machine learning that predicts the success rates of critical patients with more than 90% accuracy using the last sample and 90% from any other blood sample. This enables COVID-19 patients to detect, intervene early, and potentially reduce mortality.

In [73], the authors propose a machine learning and soft computing model to predict the outbreak of COVID-19. They have considered two scenarios to predict the outbreak. In the first scenario, data of 3 weeks is taken to predict the outbreak on day n and, in the second scenario, 5 days are used to predict the outbreak for day n. The machine learning methods multilayer perceptron (MLP) and adaptive network-based fuzzy inference system (ANFIS) are used to predict the outbreak of five countries: Italy, Germany, Iran, the USA, and China. They have evaluated the performance using root mean square error (RMSE) and correlation coefficient R as shown in Eqs. (8.2) and (8.3), respectively.

$$\text{RMSE} = \sqrt{\frac{1}{N}\Sigma(D-P)^2} \tag{8.2}$$

$$R = \frac{N\Sigma(PD)-\Sigma(D)\Sigma(P)}{\sqrt{\left[N\Sigma D^2\ (\Sigma D)^2\right]\left[N\Sigma P^2\ (\Sigma PD)^2\right]}} \tag{8.3}$$

where N represents the number of samples, P and D represent the predicted output and expected output values, respectively.

8.6 Challenges Associated with Wearable Devices in the COVID-19 Scenario

This section elaborates on various challenges involved with wearable devices regarding COVID-19. Five main challenging factors include quick identification of infection and providing clinical guidelines, accurate predication of infections, efficient algorithms based on recent techniques such as machine learning and deep learning, user centric software applications, security and privacy, and underlying protocol standards.

Quick Identification of the Virus and Clinical Guidelines The COVID-19 pandemic caused an alert on public health surveillance. The popularity of wearable devices allows for a new perspective on infectious disease precautions. The wearable biosensors are recording many signals of physiology. And when paired with advanced analytics, they provide a "huge potential" to identify changes in physiology that signify clinical deterioration requiring medical intervention. The challenges in wearable devices include quick identification of the virus and to get the clinical guidelines from the physicians to track the contact patterns of the infected person.

Accurate Prediction In the current COVID-19 situation, rapid wearable diagnostics are urgently needed to identify and isolate COVID-19 cases and to track and prevent the spread of the virus. The physiological data collected from the wearables should be capable of predicting symptoms of disease; it could open the door to research into tracking and managing other diseases and conditions. The wearables should allow direct implementation of automated vital signs such as temperature, blood, and oxygen/heart rate tracking for the individuals who are in quarantine or the people in isolation at home with alerts sent out.

Efficient Algorithms Wearables should be able to measure the core temperature, which is one of the possible symptoms of Covid-19. Detection of characteristic changes in body temperature and other critical data enables COVID-19 symptoms to be identified early on. Combined use of the detection algorithm and the wearables should help immensely to isolate and avoid further spread of COVID-19. Tracing the origin of an outbreak, quarantining patients who are potentially contaminated, treating critically ill patients, and preventing cross-infection between medical personnel and patients all take enormous human resources; and an intensified epidemic would further strain the systems.

User Centric Applications The WIoT device supporting application software that are developed need to be user-friendly and have user centric interfaces. User experiences play vital roles in the software, hardware components, and physical interfaces. Users include the common public, including the elderly, differently abled persons, young children, adults, community dependent, professionals, and care givers. Therefore, the software development should be simple, efficient, affordable, and long-term applicable.

Security and Privacy In the current COVID-19 pandemic situation, the difficulties of using such wearable devices include the protection and privacy of the data obtained, which is special and crucial from the point of view of patient safety.

Protocol Standards Caution is to be taken when the data network is incorporated into the systems and the protocols involved. Real time processing and offloading into remote cloud servers must be optimized and efficient for underlying network capabilities. Additionally, the wearable devices are resource constrained due to being battery operated. Hence, the protocol standards and networking capability must be energy efficient.

8.7 Conclusion and Discussion

This chapter addressed the important role of wearable devices as part of the healthcare system toward handling the COVID-19 pandemic. The wearable devices are a specialized IoT. Apart from typical sensing and internet connectivity, wearable devices have added features such as being lightweight, worn by users, user friendly, and connected to networks with health professionals. First, the comprehensive overview of existing wearable devices for combating COVID-19 was presented. Next, a generalized framework for wearable devices that includes layers such as sensing, networking, processing, and application layers was demonstrated. Then, the detailed processes of data gathering, data processing, and data analysis were presented. Finally, the challenges associated with wearable devices were presented.

References

1. Ayatollahitafti, V., et al.: Requirements and challenges in body sensor networks: a survey. J. Theor. Appl. Info. Tech. **72**(2) (2015)
2. Johnson, M., et al.: A comparative review of wireless sensor network mote technologies. In: 8th IEEE Conference on Sensors (IEEE SENSORS 2009), Christchurch, New Zealand (2009)
3. Flammini, A., Sisinni, E.: Wireless sensor networking in the internet of things and cloud computing era. Procedia Eng. **87**, 672–679 (2014)
4. Kern, N., Schiele, B., Junker, H., Lukowicz, P., Troster, G.: Wearable sensing to annotate meeting recordings. Pers. Ubiquit. Comput. **7**, 263–274 (2003)
5. Lukowicz, P., Ward, J., Junker, H., Starner, T.: Recognizing workshop activity using body worn microphones and accelerometers. In: Proceedings of Pervasive Computing, pp. 18–23 (2004)
6. Lee, S., Mase, K.: Activity and location recognition using wearable sensors. IEEE Pervasive Comput. **1**, 24–32 (2002)
7. Rodgers, M.M., Pai, V.M., Conroy, R.S.: Recent advances in wearable sensors for health monitoring. IEEE Sensors J. **15**(6), 3119–3126 (2015). https://doi.org/10.1109/JSEN.2014.2357257
8. Uddin, M., Salem, A., Nam, I., Nadeem, T.: Wearable sensing framework for human activity monitoring. In: Proceedings of the 2015 Workshop on Wearable Systems and Applications, pp. 21–26 (2015)
9. Yang, C.-C., Hsu, Y.-L.: A review of accelerometry-based wearable motion detectors for physical activity monitoring. Sensors. **10**(8), 7772–7788 (2010)
10. Mathie, M.J., Coster, A.C.F., Lovell, N.H., Celler, B.G.: Accelerometry: providing an integrated, practical method for long-term, ambulatory monitoring of human movement. Physiol. Meas. **25**, R1–R20 (2004)

11. Zhu, X., Liu, W., Shuang, S., Nair, M., Li, C.-Z.: Intelligent tattoos, patches, and other wearable biosensors. In: Narayan, R.J. (ed.) Medical Biosensors for Point of Care (poc) Applications, pp. 133–150. Woodhead Publishing, Duxford (2017)
12. Khan, Y., Ostfeld, A.E., Lochner, C.M., Pierre, A., Arias, A.C.: Monitoring of vital signs with flexible and wearable medical devices. Adv. Mater. **28**, 4373–4395 (2016)
13. Bandodkar, A.J., Wang, J.: Non-invasive wearable electrochemical sensors: a review. Trends Biotechnol. **32**, 363–371 (2014)
14. Dubey, H., et al.: Fog computing in medical Internet-of-Things: architecture, implementation, and applications. In: Khan, S.U., Zomaya, A.Y., Abbas, A. (eds.) Handbook of Large-Scale Distributed Computing in Smart Healthcare. SCC, pp. 281–321. Springer, Cham (2017). https://doi.org/10.1007/978-3-319-58280-1_11
15. Mukhopadhyay, S.C.: Wearable sensors for human activity monitoring: a review. IEEE Sensors. **15**, 1321–1330 (2015)
16. Rodgers Mary, M., Vinay, P., Conroy Richard, S.: Recent advances in wearable sensors for health monitoring. IEEE Sensors. **15**, 3119–3126 (2015)
17. Fang, Y., Jiang, Z., Wang, H.: A novel sleep respiratory rate detection method for obstructive sleep apnea based on characteristic moment waveform. J. Healthc. Eng. **2018**, 1–10 (2018) https://www.hindawi.com/journals/jhe/2018/1902176/
18. Pang, Y., Jian, J., Tu, T., Yang, Z., Ling, J., Li, Y., et al.: Wearable humidity sensor based on porous graphene network for respiration monitoring. Biosens. Bioelectron. **116**, 123–129 (2018). https://doi.org/10.1016/j.bios.2018.05.038
19. Molinaro, N., Massaroni, C., Lo Presti, D., Saccomandi, P., Di Tomaso, G., Zollo, L., et al.: Wearable textile based on silver plated knitted sensor for respiratory rate monitoring. In: 2018 40th Annual International Conference of the IEEE Engineering in Medicine and Biology Society (EMBC), pp. 2865–2868. IEEE (2018). http://ieeexplore.ieee.org/document/8512958/
20. Dieffenderfer, J., Goodell, H., Mills, S., McKnight, M., Yao, S., Lin, F., et al.: Low-power wearable systems for continuous monitoring of environment and health for chronic respiratory disease. IEEE J. Biomed. Health Inform. **20**(5), 1251–1264 (2016) http://ieeexplore.ieee.org/document/7479442/
21. Benreguia, B., Moumen, H., Merzoug, M.A.: Tracking COVID-19 by tracking infectious trajectories. arXiv preprint arXiv:2005.05523 (2020)
22. Ionescu, C.M., Copot, D.: Monitoring respiratory impedance by wearable sensor device: protocol and methodology. Biomed. Signal Process. Control. **36**, 57–62 (2017). https://doi.org/10.1016/j.bspc.2017.03.018
23. Reinvuo, T., Hannula, M., Sorvoja, H., Alasaarela, E., Myllyla, R.: Measurement of respiratory rate with hig hresolution accelerometer and EMFit pressure sensor. In: Proceedings 2006 IEEE Sensors Applications Symposium, 2006, pp. 192–195. IEEE (2006) [cited 6 Jan 2015]. http://ieeexplore.ieee.org/lpdocs/epic03/wrapper.htm?arnumber=1634270
24. Yuasa, Y., Takahashi, K., Suzuki, K.: Wearable flexible device for respiratory phase measurement based on sound and chest movement. In: 2017 IEEE International Conference on Systems, Man, and Cybernetics (SMC), pp. 2378–2383 (2017)
25. Ejupi, A., Menon, C.: Detection of talking in respiratory signals: a feasibility study using machine learning and wearable textile-based sensors. Sensors. **18**(8), 2474 (2018) www.mdpi.com/1424-8220/18/8/2474
26. Shkel, A.A., Kim, E.S.: Wearable low-power wireless lung sound detection enhanced by resonant transducer array for pre-filtered signal acquisition. In: 2017 19th International Conference on Solid-State Sensors, Actuators and Microsystems (TRANSDUCERS), pp. 842–845. IEEE (2017). http://ieeexplore.ieee.org/document/7994180/
27. McCaughey, E.J., McLachlan, A.J., Gollee, H.: Non-intrusive realtime breathing pattern detection and classification for automatic abdominal functional electrical stimulation. Med. Eng. Phys. **36**(8), 1057–1061 (2014). https://doi.org/10.1016/j.medengphy.2014.04.005
28. Jubran, A.: Pulse oximetry. Crit. Care. **19**(1), 272 (2015) [cited 2 Feb 2019]. http://ccforum.com/content/3/2/R11

29. Nilashi, M., Asadi, S., Abumalloh, R.A., Samad, S., Ibrahim, O.: Intelligent recommender systems in the COVID-19 outbreak: the case of wearable healthcare devices. J. Soft Comput. Decis. Support. Syst. **7**(4), 8–12 (2020)
30. Tripathy, A.K., Mohapatra, A.G., Mohanty, S.P., Kougianos, E., Joshi, A.M., Das, G.: EasyBand: a wearable for safety-aware mobility during pandemic outbreak. IEEE Consum. Electron. Mag. **47**, 777–780 (2020)
31. Mohammed, M.N., Syamsudin, H., Al-Zubaidi, S., Sairah, A.K., Ramli, R., Yusuf, E.: Novel COVID-19 detection and diagnosis system using IOT based smart helmet. Int. J. Psychosoc. Rehabil. **24**(7) (2020)
32. Mujawar, M.A., Gohel, H., Bhardwaj, S.K., Srinivasan, S., Hickman, N., Kaushik, A.: Aspects of nano-enabling biosensing systems for intelligent healthcare; towards COVID-19 management. Mater. Today Chem. **17**, 100306 (2020)
33. Kanis, M., Winters, N., Agamanolis, S., Cullinan, C., Gavin, A.: iBand: a wearable device for handshake augmented interpersonal information exchange. Extended Abstracts Ubicomp 2004 (2004)
34. Chamberlain, S.D., Singh, I., Ariza, C.A., Daitch, A.L., Philips, P.B., Dalziel, B.D.: Real-time detection of COVID-19 epicenters within the United States using a network of smart thermometers. medRxiv (2020)
35. Nittas, V., von Wyl, V.: COVID-19 and telehealth: a window of opportunity and its challenges. Swiss Med. Wkly. **150**(1920), w20284 (2020)
36. Tayal, M., Mukherjee, A., Chauhan, U., Uniyal, M., Garg, S., Singh, A., Bhadoria, A.S., Kant, R.: Evaluation of remote monitoring device for monitoring vital parameters against reference standard: a diagnostic validation study for COVID-19 preparedness. Indian J. Community Med. **45**(2), 235 (2020)
37. Swatch, Synchrobeat. http://www.swatch.com/synchro/index2.html
38. SpotMe. http://www.spotme.ch
39. nTag. http://www.ntag.com
40. Charm Tech Badge. http://www.charmed.com
41. Khan, S., Shakil, K.A., Alam, M.: Cloud-Based Big Data Analytics—A Survey of Current Research and Future Directions. In: Big Data Analytics, pp. 595–604. Springer, Singapore (2018)
42. Qi, J., Yang, P., Min, G., Amft, O., Dong, F., Xu, L.: Advanced internet of things for personalised healthcare systems: a survey. Pervasive Mobile Comput. **41**, 132–149 (2017)
43. Huang, Y., Zheng, H., Nugent, C., McCullagh, P., Black, N., Hawley, M., Mountain, G.: Knowledge discovery from lifestyle profiles to support self-management of chronic heart failure. In: 2011 Computing in Cardiology, pp. 397–400. IEEE (2011)
44. Rafferty, J., Nugent, C., Chen, L., Qi, J., Dutton, R., Zirk, A., et al.: NFC based provisioning of instructional videos to assist with instrumental activities of daily living. In: 2014 36th Annual International Conference of the IEEE Engineering in Medicine and Biology Society, pp. 4131–4134. IEEE (2014)
45. Alwashmi, M.F.: The use of digital health in the detection and management of COVID-19. Int. J. Environ. Res. Public Health. **17**(8), 2906 (2020)
46. Marinsek, N., Shapiro, A., Clay, I., Bradshaw, B., Ramirez, E., Min, J., Trister, A., Wang, Y., Althoff, T., Foschini, L.: Measuring COVID-19 and influenza in the real world via person-generated health data. medRxiv (2020)
47. Behar, J.A., Liu, C., Tsutsui, K., Corino, V.D.A, Singh, J., Pimentel, M.A.F., Karlen, W., et al.: Remote health monitoring in the time of COVID-19. arXiv preprint arXiv:2005.08537 (2020)
48. Capodilupo, E.R., Miller, D.J.: Changes in health promoting behavior during COVID-19 physical distancing: utilizing WHOOP data to examine trends in sleep, activity, and cardiovascular health. medRxiv (2020)
49. Zhu, G., Li, J., Meng, Z., Yu, Y., Li, Y., Tang, X., Dong, Y., et al.: Learning from large-scale wearable device data for predicting epidemics trend of COVID-19. Discret. Dyn. Nat. Soc. Article ID 6152041, 8 pp (2020)

50. Zhang, F., Wang, H., Chen, R., Hu, W., Zhong, Y., Wang, X.: Remote monitoring contributes to preventing overwork-related events in health workers on the COVID-19 frontlines. Precis. Clin. Med. **3**(2), 97–99 (2020)
51. Chung, Y.-T., Yeh, C.-Y., Shu, Y.-C., Chuang, K.-T., Chen, C.-C., Kao, H.-Y., Ko, W.-C., Chen, P.-L., Ko, N.-Y.: Continuous temperature monitoring by a wearable device for early detection of febrile events in the SARS-CoV-2 outbreak in Taiwan, 2020. J. Microbiol. Immunol. Infect. **53**(3), 503 (2020)
52. Vaishya, R., Javaid, M., Khan, I.H., Haleem, A.: Artificial intelligence (AI) Applications for COVID-19 Pandemic. Diabetes Metab Syndr Clin Res Rev. **14**(4), 337–339 (2020). https://doi.org/10.1016/j.dsx.2020.04.012
53. Hussain, S., Kang, B.H., Lee, S.: A wearable device-based personalized big data analysis model. In: International Conference on Ubiquitous Computing and Ambient Intelligence, pp. 236–242. Springer, Cham (2014)
54. Smieszek, T., Salathe, M.: A low-cost method to assess the epidemiological importance of individuals in controlling infectious disease outbreaks. BMC Med. **11**, 35 (2013)
55. Salathe, M., Kazandjieva, M., Lee, J.W., Levis, P., Feldman, M.W., Jones, J.H.: A high-resolution human contact network for infectious disease transmission. Proc. Natl. Acad. Sci. U. S. A. **107**, 22020–22025 (2010)
56. Cauchemez, S., Bhattarai, A., Marchbanks, T.L., et al.: Role of social networks in shaping disease transmission during a community outbreak of 2009 H1N1 pandemic influenza. Proc. Natl. Acad. Sci. U. S. A. **108**, 2825–2830 (2011)
57. Temime, L., Opatowski, L., Pannet, Y., Brun-Buisson, C., Boelle, P.Y., Guillemot, D.: Peripatetic health-care workers as potential superspreaders. Proc. Natl. Acad. Sci. U. S. A. **106**, 18420–18425 (2009)
58. Barrat, A., Cattuto, C., Tozzi, A.E., Vanhems, P., Voirin, N.: Measuring contact patterns with wearable sensors: methods, data characteristics and applications to data-driven simulations of infectious diseases. Clin. Microbiol. Infect. **20**(1), 10–16 (2014)
59. Cattuto, C., Van den Broeck, W., Barrat, A., Colizza, V., Pinton, J.F., Vespignani, A.: Dynamics of person-to-person interactions from distributed RFID sensor networks. PLoS One. **5**, e11596 (2010)
60. Yan, L., Zhang, H.T., Goncalves, J., Xiao, Y., Wang, M., Guo, Y., et al.: A machine learning-based model for survival prediction in patients with severe COVID-19 infection. MedRxiv (2020)
61. Haleem, A., Javaid, M., Vaishya, R.: Effects of COVID 19 pandemic in daily life. Curr. Med. Res. Pract. **10**(2), 78–79 (2020). https://doi.org/10.1016/j.cmrp.2020.03.011
62. Bai, H.X., Hsieh, B., Xiong, Z., Halsey, K., Choi, J.W., Tran, T.M., Pan, I., Shi, L.B., Wang, D.C., Mei, J., Jiang, X.L.: Performance of radiologists in differentiating COVID-19 from viral pneumonia on chest CT. Radiology. **296**(2), E46–E54 (2020). https://doi.org/10.1148/radiol.2020200823
63. Hu, Z., Ge, Q., Jin, L., Xiong, M.: Artificial intelligence forecasting of COVID-19 in China. arXiv preprint arXiv:2002.07112 (2020)
64. Gozes, O., Frid-Adar, M., Greenspan, H., Browning, P.D., Zhang, H., Ji, W., Bernheim, A., Siegel, E.: Rapid AI development cycle for the coronavirus (COVID-19) pandemic: initial results for automated detection & patient monitoring using deep learning CT image analysis. arXiv preprint arXiv:2003.05037 (2020)
65. Pirouz, B., ShaffieeHaghshenas, S., ShaffieeHaghshenas, S., Piro, P.: Investigating a serious challenge in the sustainable development process: analysis of confirmed cases of COVID-19 (new type of coronavirus) through a binary classification using artificial intelligence and regression analysis. Sustainability. **12**(6), 2427 (2020)
66. Ting, D.S., Carin, L., Dzau, V., Wong, T.Y.: Digital technology and COVID-19. Nat. Med. **26**(4), 459–461 (2020)
67. Wan, K.H., Huang, S.S., Young, A., Lam, D.S.: Precautionary measures needed for ophthalmologists during pandemic of the coronavirus disease 2019 (COVID-19). Acta Ophthalmol. **98**(3), 221–222 (2020)

68. Li, L., Qin, L., Xu, Z., Yin, Y., Wang, X., Kong, B., Bai, J., Lu, Y., Fang, Z., Song, Q., Cao, K.: Artificial intelligence distinguishes COVID-19 from community-acquired pneumonia on chest CT. Radiology. **19**, 200905 (2020)
69. Smeulders, A.W., Van Ginneken, A.M.: An analysis of pathology knowledge and decision making for the development of artificial intelligence-based consulting systems. Anal. Quant. Cytol. Histol. **11**(3), 154–165 (1989)
70. Chowel, G., Viboud, C.: A practical method to target individuals for outbreak detection and control. BMC Med. **11**, 36 (2013)
71. Pandey, G., Chaudhary, P., Gupta, R., Pal, S.: SEIR and regression model based COVID-19 outbreak predictions in India. arXiv preprint arXiv:2004.00958 (2020)
72. Dong, E., Du, H., Gardner, L.: An interactive web-based dashboard to track COVID-19 in real time. Lancet Infect. Dis. **20**(5), 533–534 (2020). https://doi.org/10.1016/S1473-3099(20)30120-1. Published online Feb 19
73. Ardabili, S.F., Mosavi, A., Ghamisi, P., Ferdinand, F., Varkonyi-Koczy, A.R., Reuter, U., et al.: Covid-19 outbreak prediction with machine learning. Available at SSRN 3580188 (2020)

Chapter 9
Effectiveness of Big Data in Early Prediction and Measure for COVID-19 Using Data Science

P. Tomar, M. Mann, D. Panwar, C. Diwaker, and P. Kumar

Abstract COVID-19 originates from a group of infections related to severe acute respiratory syndrome (SARS). Through data analysis, frameworks have demonstrated to have the option to approximate how patterns may progress. Data analysis assumes a key role, as does arithmetic, which, together with data science, permits us to have a top to bottom comprehension of the subtleties of nature and how things are made. As in the previous years, the pioneers of data science have had a mind-blowing effect on the reality where information and examination have been utilized to drive critical change throughout the spread of the sickness. One of the primary recorded uses of information examination was in 1852, during a cholera episode in London. John Snow, one of the primary information-driven disease transmission specialists, had the option to geospatially examine the passing that happened in London and in this manner segregate the wellspring of the infection. Depending on his investigation, specialists had the option to focus on their interventions to quickly check the spread of the pandemic. During this pandemic, information can be an exceptional factor as far as quality and consistency. Complexities of this sort incorporate instances of false-positive patients. Large data and data science can be utilized to check consistency with isolate and can be utilized for tranquilizing

P. Tomar (✉)
Gautam Buddha University, Greater Noida, India
e-mail: pradeep.tomar@gbu.ac.in

M. Mann
IIIT, Sonepat, India

D. Panwar
Amity University, Jaipur, India

C. Diwaker
UIET, Kurukshetra University, Kurukshetra, India

P. Kumar
Centre For Railway Information Systems, New Delhi, India

© The Author(s), under exclusive license to Springer Nature Switzerland AG 2021

F. Al-Turjman et al. (eds.), *Emerging Technologies for Battling Covid-19*, Studies in Systems, Decision and Control 324,
https://doi.org/10.1007/978-3-030-60039-6_9

investigation. These are only a portion of the arrangements offered by new advanced innovations in the field of data science to confront the coronavirus crisis. We provide here early prediction and early survey, with the genuine and potential commitment of data science to the battle against COVID-19, just as the present requirements on these commitments. It expects to draw brisk take-away from a quick extending conversation and developing a collection of work, to fill in as a contribution for fast reactions in research, approach, and clinical examination. The expense of the pandemic as far as lives and monetary harm will be horrible; at the hour of composing, incredible vulnerability encompassed appraisals of exactly how awful and of how fruitful both non-pharmaceutical and pharmaceutical reactions can be. Improving data science, one of the most encouraging information expository apparatuses to have been created over the previous decade or something like that, to help decrease these vulnerabilities, is a beneficial interest. Data science isn't yet assuming a huge job in the battle against COVID-19, at any rate from the epidemiological, demonstrative, and pharmaceutical perspectives. Its utilization is compelled by an absence of data and by an excess of noisy data. Enthusiastically, data analysts and researchers have responded to the challenge.

Keywords Deep learning · Breast Cancer Coimbra · Immunotherapy · Attribute selection

9.1 Introduction

COVID-19 originates from a group of infections related to severe acute respiratory syndrome (SARS) [1]. Coronavirus illness (COVID-19) is an aggravation infection from another infection. The illness causes respiratory affliction (like flu) with signs, for instance, cool, hack, and fever, and, in dynamically genuine cases, the issue in relaxing. COVID-19 has been seen as an overall pandemic [2].

As of date affirmed COVID-19 cases across the globe are 1,498,833 and mortality roughly 5.8%. Continuously the death rate is expanding and it's a disturbing component for the entire world. Transmission is ordered into four phases depending on the method of spread and time [3]. Each country forced various systems beginning from remaining in-home, utilizing covers, travel limitations, staying away from parties, regularly washing hands, and cleaning the spots frequently on the account of a typical exertion to battle the flare-up of this ailment. Numerous nations forced a lockdown express that forestalls the development of the residents pointlessly [4].

In India, the flare-up of coronavirus has upset the working of life in general. All were pushed to remain back to the shield from the repulsive transmission. In the underlying stages, the affirmed cases are those that come back from administers followed by transmission using nearby transmission [5].

"Huge information" is a monstrous measure of data that can be unbelievable. For over two decades, it has become a subject of extraordinary enthusiasm given its incredible potential [6]. Various transparent and private corporations produce, store, and study immense knowledge to strengthen their administrations. In the healthcare sector, administrative reports, hospital clinical data, and implications of psychiatric tests and online apps provide various hotspots with massive volumes of knowledge [7]. A significant part of broad knowledge related to open healthcare is also derived from the biomedical examination [8]. The legitimate administration and scrutiny of this information are needed to infer important data. Someone else that is almost identical to finding a needle in the bundle by dissecting enormous information fast. There are various difficulties in each step of the management of extensive information that must be executed by using top-of-the-line registration solutions for an enormous analysis of information [9]. That is why providers of medical care need to be equipped entirely with the correct structure to build and break down tremendous knowledge in a methodical way and provide practical responses and enhance general health.

9.2 Background

There are several promising and life-saving outcomes in the use of broad knowledge analysis in social security. Widespread information refers to the huge amount of data produced by the digitalization of all that is united and explicitly breached by innovations. It uses specific wellbeing details from the community (or from a single person) to assist in the prevention of plagues, fixing illness, capping expenditures, etc. [10], as used in public resources.

Since we live longer, models of treatment have changed, and many of these advances must be driven by information. Specialists must be as much as possible aware of a patient and, from the start, as reasonably expected, to obtain noticed signs of real disorder when emerging—it is unmistakably basic and more affordable to reward any disease at first. In the analysis of knowledge for healthcare, avoidance is preferable to deciding and whether a patient should be identified in a wide-ranging manner to provide security a personalized package. The corporation seeks to resolve the difficulties the knowledge of a patient contains: everywhere it is processed and put in emergency departments, hospitals, surgical treatments, etc., with the inability to interact properly [11].

It has been exorbitant and tedious for quite a long time to collect enormous information measures for clinical use. With the progress made at present, it is simpler not only to gather this information but also to transform it into important basic pieces of knowledge, which could be used to better reflect. The reasons behind the review of information for human services are using information-led findings to anticipate and deal with a problem before the no return is over, but also survey policies and medicines more quickly, monitor stock, incorporate patients further into their welfare, and enable them to take care of themselves.

9.2.1 Big Data Analytics in Healthcare

The need for massive information is also colossal in medicinal services, as expenses in countries such as the United States are increasing. As a survey by McKinsey says, "After over 20 years of consistent builds, medicinal services costs currently speak to 17.6 percent of GDP—almost $600 billion more than the normal benchmark for a country of the United States' size and riches" [12].

Costs are far larger, so to say, than they should be, and for as much as 20 years, they have grown. Here we simply need a shrewd, insightful deduction. Also, the driving forces of today change: Many insurance companies are shifting from administrative charges to schemes that organize lasting results (which use expensive, now and again usually useless medicines and recompensing many patients quickly) [12].

In the past, all the considerations showed no immediate impetus for the suppliers of medicinal services to provide persistent, intensive use of research data to each other. As more get charged based on the interpretation of outcomes, there is a cash-related opportunity for information to be exchanged that can be used to enhance patients' lives and lower costs for defensive companies [13].

Finally, doctoral options have become more and more validated, meaning that they are not solely dependent on tutoring and professional appraisal, but on broad scopes of research and clinical knowledge. As with numerous companies, social information events and the board are growing, and experts need help. This latest research means that there is a greater interest than ever in recent memory in broad knowledge review at medical facilities, and the emergence of SaaS BI devices further suggests that they need to be tested [9].

9.2.2 Effectiveness of Big Data Against COVID-19

Near to COVID-19, which constantly gather data from sites across the world, social security staff, scholars, experts in health communication, and decision-makers are supporting global episode information.

There has been some fascinating information coming about because of GPS investigations of populace development by district, city, and so on, which at last gives a perspective on the populace's consistency—or absence of consistency—with social removing mandates. Moreover, in any event, an advanced thermometer invention follows temperatures reported by their devices, suggesting that, despite approval of a social repression regulation, normal temperatures in some areas have declined [14].

How have advances made it possible to source, aggregate, and synthesize incident data globally in Big Data management and data preparation?

For such cases like these, there are various chances of using Big Data as a general population and an enterprise, while the strength of Big Data for the search of a solution has still not been made viable [15].

For example, considerations of large-scope COVID-19 real-world evidence (RWE) could help to boost medicines' progress in a progressive and patient-friendly manner, drawing information from several true sources—including patient care currently being treated in medical clinic environments [16].

The pandemic of COVID-19 could be seen as an inspiration for determining how to improve access to information. We at Paraxial try to ally with other experts in medication improvement and industry relations to help with this exercise in the United States, but we must move quickly [17].

What can Big Data allow a more data-driven and proactive battle against global pandemics?

As both the general public and industry see more noteworthy progress, we still have to take measures to make viable use of large data intensity in the search for a solution to COVID-19. Progressive examination and sign findings within the framework of social insurance are one of some huge improvements in the computerization of the early pandemic surface. There will be more variations in a regional context. Large data models improved pandemic standards. Our ability to absorb and respond to therapy depends early and on our efforts to use as much exposure knowledge as possible. This will help us to understand contrasts in the introduction, to respond to the various therapeutic modalities, and to codify the drugs that have a better impact.

How does Big Data contribute to clinical trials' efficiency and effectiveness?

During this time, clinical preliminary tasks take full advantage of the information's capacity to interface us with the patients. The result is a faster, more focused access to these significant studies and patient entry while ensuring quiet access [18].

We at Paraxial are investigating approaches to make huge-scope COVID-19 RWE considerations that can pull information from what we are seeing with patients right now under treatment. A portion of the potential advantages incorporates an increasingly understanding-driven and patient-accommodating spotlight on recognizing and creating potential cures [19].

The key advantage is an open door for quicker and close to the constant assessment of dynamic dependent on the information. This will spare lives and result in recognizing viable treatments quicker.

Another thought is to distinguish expected patients at the purpose of testing and afterward quickly populate understanding narratives and track progress by connecting to different genuine sources using tokenization with constrained weight on the patient and the site.

When medicinal services information can be utilized straightforwardly (e.g., engineered control arms) to construct the clinical informational collection for well-being and adequacy examination, fewer patients should be selected and randomized, lessening the complete span of the investigation and the calculated weight on patients.

9.3 The Outbreak of COVID-19 and Exponential Growth of COVID-19 Cases

The ongoing flare-up of coronavirus sickness 2019 (COVID-19) in territory China was described by an unmistakable subexponential increment of affirmed cases during the early period of the plague, appearing differently about an underlying exponential development expected for an unconstrained episode. We show that this impact can be clarified as an immediate result of control approaches that adequately exhaust the powerless population [20].

On the account of COVID-19, exponential development will happen in the ailment rate in people in as much as:

- There is at any rate one tainted individual in the populace pool
- Regular contact among contaminated and uninfected individuals from the populace happens
- There are enormous quantities of uninfected likely among the populace

Coronavirus spreads exponentially instead of straightly. Exponential development inclination makes it difficult for residents to assess the status of the pandemic in their nations remembering the expected results for inevitable days [21]. A significant point in our COVID-19 arrangement of blog entries is to introduce and give intelligent representations and instruments, understandable by the non-master, that will assist in facilitating the exponential development predisposition obstruction and shed some light on patterns and relationships supporting COVID-19 data [21].

When you have a progression of information from date A to date B, we are not fit for imaging the information to come during the next days. All things considered, here comes the guide of prescient displaying! We can take a model that is compelled to comply with exponential development conduct and tune it in an information-driven way (e.g., utilizing the accessible information from date A to date B) to fit them best. This activity is deciphered as follows: among all conceivable exponential development bends (which are interminable), to discover and utilize the one that follows the accessible information as firmly as could reasonably be expected.

Government restrictions have been actively carried out in China on the production of corona viral diseases 2019 (COVID-19) as a result of severe extreme respiratory coronavirus 2 (SARS-CoV-2). The fast increment of emphatically analyzed cases and a resulting ascent of auxiliary flare-ups in numerous nations overall raised worry on a universal scale. The World Health Organization (WHO) in this way reported the COVID-19 episode The Global Public Health Crisis on 31 January, which was eventually declared as a pandemic on 11 March [22].

An underlying exponential development of affirmed cases is conventionally expected for an uncontrolled flare-up, as watched, e.g., during the 2009 flu A (H1N1) pandemic or the 2014 Ebola episode in West Africa [2]. Even though in Hubei the quantity of research facility-affirmed cases $C(t)$ was seen to develop exponentially toward the beginning of January, the ensuing ascent followed a sub-exponential, superlinear, mathematical scaling law $t\mu$ with a type $\mu = 2.3$ (between 24 January and 9 February). For the greater part of the influenced Chinese territories of terrain China, nonetheless, this sort of mathematical ascent happened from the earliest starting point of the case giving an account of 21 January [23]. The examples μ change around a run of the mill estimation of $\mu = 2.1 \pm 0.3$ for the affirmed case bends in other generously influenced territories (affirmed case tallies bigger than 500 on 12 February), showing mathematical development notwithstanding land, socioeconomic contrasts, potential contrasts in control systems, and heterogeneities that may impact and affect how the neighborhood pestilence unfurls. In the end, case checks started to go amiss from the watched scaling laws around 9 February for Hubei and toward the beginning of February for the rest of the territories, moving toward an immersion behavior [23].

9.4 Predicting Survival Chances Using Data Sciences

9.4.1 Finding Who Is Most at Danger from COVID-19

AI has demonstrated to be significant in anticipating dangers in numerous circles.

With clinical hazard explicitly, AI is conceivably fascinating in three key manners.

- Infection chance: What is the danger of a particular individual or gathering getting COVID-19?
- COVID-19 Chapter International Disaster Public Health Warning on 31 January and eventually on 11 March [22] as a pandemic.
- Outcome hazard: What is the hazard that a particular treatment will be incapable for someone in particular or gathering, and how likely would they say they are to bite the dust?

AI can help foresee every one of the three dangers. Also, we can see how AI is used in associated areas and how it could contribute to the COVID-19 chance forecast [24].

9.4.2 Infection Risk Estimation

Early statistics indicate that important risk factors that decide how likely an individual is to get COVID-19 are age, pre-existing conditions, general hygiene habits, social habits, number of human interactions, frequency of interactions, location and climate, and socioeconomic status.

In the early stages, there is still potential analysis for the pandemic ebb and flow. For example, DeCapprio et al. used AI to create an underlying COVID-19 vulnerability index. Avoidance estimates, for example, wearing veils, washing hands, and social separating, are for the most part prone to impact generally speaking danger also. As more and better information opens up and as of now progressing investigations produce results, we will probably observe progressively pragmatic uses of AI for foreseeing contamination risk [25].

9.4.3 Assessment of Who Is at Risk of a Critical Case

If a person or gathering has been contaminated, we need to foresee the risk of that person or collect problems or require propelled clinical consideration. Some people experience only minor side effects, and other individuals cause severe pulmonary disease or serious respiratory disorder (ARDS) that is considered to be harmful. Nonetheless, it is better to begin therapy early if more serious symptoms are expected to occur, as they all need to be properly handled and screened for soft signs [26].

In the *Computers, Materials and Continua* diary, specialists distributed an article demonstrating that AI might anticipate the probability of a patient creating ARDS just as the danger of mortality, just by taking a gander at the underlying side effects. The specialists recognize the restrictions of this examination:

> "An away from this examination is the size of the dataset; 53 patients with some inadequate information just as a restricted range of seriousness."

9.4.4 Predicting Treatment Outcomes

An augmentation of seriousness forecast is anticipating the treatment's result, which is frequently truly a matter of foreseeing life and demise. It is valuable to realize how likely a patient is to endure, given certain side effects. However, on this present, it's critical to remember that not all patients are treated similarly. Given a particular patient or gathering, how compelling is a particular treatment liable to be?

If we can anticipate the results of explicit treatment strategies, at that point specialists can treat patients all the more adequately. Utilizing AI to customize treatment plans isn't explicit to COVID-19, and AI has recently been utilized to anticipate treatment results for patients with epilepsy, as only one model. Scientists have likewise utilized AI to foresee reactions to malignant growth immunotherapy [16].

Since treatment alternatives for COVID-19 are as yet developing, it will probably be some time before we see AI applied to foresee results for explicit medicines. Be that as it may, result expectation stays a significant piece of hazard evaluation, working connected at the hip with the disease and seriousness forecasts we talked about above.

9.5 Fighting COVID-19 Using Big Data and Data Science

COVID-19 has transformed us, how we communicate, our propensities, and even our psyches. It is genuine that we are battling the infection from numerous points of view. Social removing, immunizations, and clinical medicines are the most notable, yet additionally, numerous different methodologies have risen, some of them from the data science and AI people group [27].

One of them is the COVID-19 Mobility Monitoring venture in Italy, which utilizes information gathered from anonymized clients who have been selected to give access to their area information namelessly, through a GDPR-agreeable system. Information is gathered from cell phones with iOS and android utilizing various sensors, for example, GPS, signals, Wi-Fi, and systems. They will probably quantitatively investigate the effect of the imprisonment and social removing measures forced in Italy [28].

Information science is an entirely important instrument that researchers and governments are utilizing to adapt to the impacts of the COVID-19 pandemic, and numerous incredible applications are rising at an extremely quick pace. It is exceptionally compensating to realize that our field is assisting with this worldwide emergency and it can help with numerous different issues of our advanced society [28].

9.5.1 Role of Data Science in Global Health Emergency

The tremendous knowledge strategy should talk of a major development in the area of human resources outreach—promoting the improvement of the instructional frames in treatment and ultimately promoting effective control of individuals to enhance the health of whole communities. The size of the approach increases both the expected dangers and potential benefits. Although the methodology can have the greatest incentive for low-asset settings, it is generally powerless in such settings against discontinuity and abuse. The vulnerability is supposed to be restricted by community-oriented administration, diligent analysis, and specialist organizations.

The dynamics should not be taken for granted. Another opportunity for worldwide wellbeing institutions to provide valuable governance in countries that are low-and-center salaries is the shift from paper to petabyte computerized supplies [29].

A working social insurance framework is essential for the endurance of mankind. Without specialists, medicines, and malady counteraction measures, we'd return to the Dark Ages (and still, after all that, there were specialists). Modern social insurance gear produces a great deal of wellbeing information, and this is the place Big Data applications can help [30].

9.5.2 Virus and Drug Research Using Data Science

It costs up to $2.6 billion and takes 12 years to put up medication for sale to the public. Large information permits researchers to reproduce the response of medication with body proteins and various kinds of cells and conditions, so it has a lot higher probability of picking up the Food and Drug Administration endorsement and restoring assorted patients (e.g., individuals with certain change profiles) [31].

Informatics can use different arrangements for organized and unstructured biomedical information obtained from diverse tests, therapeutic results, contextual studies, online life, etc. Such advanced scientific calculations would then be used to recreate how the medicines will work with body proteins and how the pace of success is anticipated [32].

The recreation can accelerate the procedure making beginning screening adequate to decide the chance of the medication viability. In addition to the fact that it means a tremendous decrease in the expense and time of medication advancement, however, it additionally mitigates the dangers of disappointment.

Information science strategies are likewise ready to incorporate with genomic information in exploration to give exact bits of knowledge into hereditary issues emerging out of explicit medications and sicknesses.

Medication improvement is a tedious and complex excursion, with a high vulnerability that medication will succeed, while the rise of a major information approach has altered our methodologies to handle long-standing difficulties in tranquilizing advancement. The proposition of different high-throughput innovations and an assortment of numerous omics information are quickening the interpretation of essential exploration revelations into clinical practice. The previous decade has seen the interpretation of a few examination results from genomics information to FDA endorsement in facilities, and in the interim, numerous as of late created information-driven methodologies have additionally demonstrated promising potential for clinical practice. An early and surely understand model is headache medicine, which is initially utilized for the absence of pain treatment, while by coordinating the data from the electronic wellbeing records (EHRs) of patients, post-advertising reconnaissance information, and pharmacological investigation, specialists likewise found the capability of anti-inflammatory medicine to treat colorectal disease, and the US Preventive Services Task Force discharged the draft suggestion on ibuprofen to forestall colorectal malignancy in September 2015 [33].

9.5.3 *Analysis and Prediction of Foreign Epidemic in the Future*

Formal, quantitative methodologies are presently broadly used to make expectations about the probability of an irresistible infection flare-up, how the ailment will spread, and how to control it. A few entrenched techniques are accessible, including hazard factor investigation, chance demonstrating, and dynamic modeling [34]. All things considered, prescient demonstrating is particularly the "specialty of the conceivable," which will in general drive research exertion toward certain regions and away from others which might be at any rate as significant. Expanding on the undoubted achievement of quantitative demonstrating of the study of disease transmission and control of human and creature illnesses, for example, AIDS, flu, foot-and-mouth ailment, and BSE, consideration should be paid to building up an increasingly all-encompassing system that catches the job of the basic drivers of ailment dangers, from demography and conduct to land use and environmental change.

None of us can precisely and completely anticipate the results of any pandemic, the all-out disease rates, or the last loss of life as of right now. These are troublesome occasions for all of us, on the account of the concern and the vulnerability of the circumstance. We just don't have the foggiest idea of what will occur, yet with information science, we have a superior possibility of foreseeing it precisely than we ever have had in the past [35].

Yet, even once the pandemic is finished, there will at present be information science work to do. The information assortment may stop because there are no new cases, yet that is an ideal opportunity to ensure that what was gathered is put away and overseen appropriately. Glancing back at the circumstance with the advantage of knowing the past can be agonizing, yet it's the main way we can guarantee that exercises picked up during this time are completely comprehended. After everything closes is likewise an opportunity to take a gander at the frameworks and structures (clinical, logical, social) that worked, and the ones that didn't, with the perspective on progress.

9.5.4 *Future and Roles of Data Science in Prediction and Measurement for COVID-19*

The precision of customary determining to a great extent relies upon the accessibility of information to base its forecasts and gauges of vulnerability. In episodes of pandemics, there is no information at all to start with and afterward constrained over the long haul, making forecasts broadly dubious.

Propelled representation has helped governments and analysts intently watch everyday improvements of COVID-19 and settle on choices successfully. Descriptive insights as well as examining the relationship among different variables are permitting chiefs to think about and comprehend the effect of the pandemic. Different associations are preparing a gigantic measure of information and giving perception to exhibit how the infection got out [36].

Information researchers are anticipating the spread of COVID-19 alongside data on the number of lives it is probably going to influence. Notwithstanding, anticipating with inadequate information can additionally befuddle individuals during these difficult occasions. Existing datasets (on COVID-19) are staggeringly one-sided. For example, while ascertaining the death rate, typically engineers take a gander at the passings per affirmed case. In any case, the supposition that will be that we have caught the entirety of the affirmed cases, which isn't valid [37].

The job of information science is basic to mentioning information-driven objective facts on how the COVID-19 pandemic is spreading. About pandemic, clinical information can be profoundly factor regarding quality just as consistency; complexities of this incorporate instances of bogus positive patients. In any case, governments and specialists are depending progressively on information and forecast models in the plague setting [37].

Information researchers are utilizing huge information for AI calculations fit for creating a large number of restorative antibodies to discover medicines for COVID-19 with a high likelihood of progress. Leading immune response disclosure in a lab regularly takes years; in any case, these calculations recognize antibodies that can battle against the infection in only 7 days. This is only one of the numerous ways information-driven arrangements are quickening the speed at which coronavirus treatments are found, created, and delivered [37].

9.6 Conclusion

The spread of virus is exponential, and the application of data science in optimal measurements for outcomes of exponential model has been gratefully acknowledged in the recent past. This paper suggests how to fit COVID data as an exponential fit model. Different factors responsible for capturing this deadly virus are identified, and corresponding critical case scenarios are discussed in this study. The argumentation on predicting various available treatment and possible outcomes are studied in detail. The study focuses on the recent growth of data science in solving various exponential problems, the capabilities of the field in early prediction, measurement of spread, and its outcomes. Finally the study established an optimistic look toward the capabilities of data science in future outbreak of similar viruses. This study does not reflect an exact solution but suggested many underlying mechanisms through which guided study in data science can be performed on COVID-19 and similar outbreaks.

References

1. Khetrapal, S., Bhatia, R.: Impact of COVID-19 pandemic on health system & sustainable development goal 3. Indian J. Med. Res. **151**, 395 (2020)
2. Surveillances, V.: The epidemiological characteristics of an outbreak of 2019 novel coronavirus diseases (COVID-19)—China, 2020. China CDC Wkly. **2**, 113–122 (2020)
3. World Health Organization. Pandemic influenza preparedness and response. World Health Organization. Accessed 23 Dec 2009 (2010)
4. Sujatha, R., Chatterjee, J.: A machine learning methodology for forecasting of the COVID-19 cases in India 2020. Stoch. Environ. Res. Risk Assess. **34**, 959–972 (2020)
5. Yang, Z., Zeng, Z., Wang, K., Wong, S.-S., Liang, W., Zanin, M., et al.: Modified SEIR and AI prediction of the epidemics trend of COVID-19 in China under public health interventions. J Thorac. Dis. **12**, 165 (2020)
6. Sivarajah, U., Kamal, M.M., Irani, Z., Weerakkody, V.: Critical analysis of big data challenges and analytical methods. J. Bus. Res. **70**, 263–286 (2017)
7. Feldman, B., Martin, E.M., Skotnes, T.: Big data in healthcare hype and hope. Dr. Bonnie. **360**, 122–125 (2012)
8. Bellazzi, R.: Big data and biomedical informatics: a challenging opportunity. Yearb. Med. Inform. **23**, 8–13 (2014)
9. Raghupathi, W., Raghupathi, V.: Big data analytics in healthcare: promise and potential. Heal. Inf. Sci. Syst. **2**, 3 (2014)
10. Baro, E., Degoul, S., Beuscart, R., Chazard, E.: Toward a literature-driven definition of big data in healthcare. Biomed. Res. Int. **2015**, 639021 (2015)
11. Manogaran, G., Thota, C., Lopez, D., Vijayakumar, V., Abbas, K.M., Sundarsekar, R.: Big data knowledge system in healthcare. In: Internet things big data technologies for next generation healthcare, pp. 133–157. Springer (2017)
12. Mezghani, E., Exposito, E., Drira, K., Da Silveira, M., Pruski, C.: A semantic big data platform for integrating heterogeneous wearable data in healthcare. J. Med. Syst. **39**, 185 (2015)
13. Lin, K., Xia, F., Wang, W., Tian, D., Song, J.: System design for big data application in emotion-aware healthcare. IEEE Access. **4**, 6901–6909 (2016)
14. Wang, C.J., Ng, C.Y., Brook, R.H.: Response to COVID-19 in Taiwan: big data analytics, new technology, and proactive testing. J.A.M.A. **323**, 1341–1342 (2020)
15. Duan, K., Liu, B., Li, C., Zhang, H., Yu, T., Qu, J., et al.: Effectiveness of convalescent plasma therapy in severe COVID-19 patients. Proc. Natl. Acad. Sci. U. S. A. **117**, 9490–9496 (2020)
16. Zhou, C., Su, F., Pei, T., Zhang, A., Du, Y., Luo, B., et al.: COVID-19: challenges to GIS with big data. Geogr. Sustain. **1**(1), 77–87 (2020)
17. Ienca, M., Vayena, E.: On the responsible use of digital data to tackle the COVID-19 pandemic. Nat. Med. **26**, 463–464 (2020)
18. Desai, M.A.: Importance of AI & big data in the fight against coronavirus. Tathapi (UGC CARE J.). **19**, 455–466 (2020) ISSN 2320-0693
19. Mayo, C.S., Matuszak, M.M., Schipper, M.J., Jolly, S., Hayman, J.A., Ten Haken, R.K.: Big data in designing clinical trials: opportunities and challenges. Front. Oncol. **7**, 187 (2017)
20. Pocock, S.J., Hughes, M.D., Lee, R.J.: Statistical problems in the reporting of clinical trials. N. Engl. J. Med. **317**, 426–432 (1987)
21. Yuan, J., Li, M., Lv, G., Lu, Z.K.: Monitoring transmissibility and mortality of COVID-19 in Europe. Int. J. Infect. Dis. **95**, 311–315 (2020)
22. World Health Organization. Naming the coronavirus disease (COVID-19) and the virus that causes it. https://www.who.int/emergencies/diseases/novelcoronavirus-2019/technical-guidance/naming-the-coronavirus-disease-(covid-2019)-and-the-virus-that-causes-it
23. Novel CPERE: The epidemiological characteristics of an outbreak of 2019 novel coronavirus diseases (COVID-19) in China. Zhonghua Liu Xing Bing Xue Za Zhi. **41**, 145 (2020)

24. Rao, A.S.R.S., Vazquez, J.A.: Identification of COVID-19 can be quicker through artificial intelligence framework using a mobile phone–based survey when cities and towns are under quarantine. Infect. Control Hosp. Epidemiol. **41**, 826–830 (2020)
25. Covid, C.D.C., Team, R.: Severe outcomes among patients with coronavirus disease 2019 (COVID-19)—United States, February 12–March 16, 2020. MMWR Morb. Mortal. Wkly. Rep. **69**, 343–346 (2020)
26. Daurat, A., Millet, I., Roustan, J.-P., Maury, C., Taourel, P., Jaber, S., et al.: Thoracic Trauma Severity score on admission allows to determine the risk of delayed ARDS in trauma patients with pulmonary contusion. Injury. **47**, 147–153 (2016)
27. Latif, S., Usman, M., Manzoor, S., Iqbal, W., Qadir, J., Tyson, G., Castro, I., Razi, A., Boulos, M.N.K., Weller, A., Crowcroft, J.: Leveraging data science to combat COVID-19: a comprehensive review 2020. https://www.researchgate.net/publication/340687152_Preprint_Leveraging_Data_Science_To_Combat_COVID-19_A_Comprehensive_Review
28. Livingston, E., Bucher, K.: Coronavirus disease 2019 (COVID-19) in Italy. J.A.M.A. **323**, 1335 (2020)
29. Rahimian, F., Salimi-Khorshidi, G., Payberah, A.H., Tran, J., Ayala Solares, R., Raimondi, F., et al.: Predicting the risk of emergency admission with machine learning: development and validation using linked electronic health records. PLoS Med. **15**, e1002695 (2018)
30. Sohrabi, C., Alsafi, Z., O'Neill, N., Khan, M., Kerwan, A., Al-Jabir, A., et al.: World Health Organization declares global emergency: a review of the 2019 novel coronavirus (COVID-19). Int. J. Surg. **76**, 71–76 (2020)
31. Cockburn, I.M., Henderson, R.M.: Absorptive capacity, coauthoring behavior, and the organization of research in drug discovery. J. Ind. Econ. **46**, 157–182 (1998)
32. Kubinyi, H.: 3D QSAR in drug design: volume 1: theory methods and applications, vol. 1. Springer (1993)
33. Murphy, R.F.: An active role for machine learning in drug development. Nat. Chem. Biol. **7**, 327–330 (2011)
34. Li, L., Yang, Z., Dang, Z., Meng, C., Huang, J., Meng, H., et al.: Propagation analysis and prediction of the COVID-19. Infect. Dis. Model. **5**, 282–292 (2020)
35. Abidi, S.S.R., Goh, A.: Applying knowledge discovery to predict infectious disease epidemics. In: Pacific Rim Int. Conf. Artif. Intell., pp. 170–181. Springer (1998)
36. Wynants, L., Van Calster, B., Bonten, M.M.J., Collins, G.S., Debray, T.P.A., De Vos, M., et al.: Prediction models for diagnosis and prognosis of covid-19 infection: systematic review and critical appraisal. B.M.J. **369** (2020)
37. Kraemer, M.U., Yang, C.H., Gutierrez, B., Wu, C.H., Klein, B., Pigott, D.M., Du Plessis, L., Faria, N.R., Li, R., Hanage, W.P.B.J.: The effect of human mobility and control measures on the COVID-19 epidemic in China. Science. **368**, 493–497 (2020)

Chapter 10
COVID-19: Creating a Paradigm Shift in Indian Education System

Kiran Ahuja and Indu Bala

Abstract With the spread of the coronavirus, an unprecedented number of students around the world are not able to go to schools, colleges and universities to stop the spread of pandemic COVID-19. The epidemic is expected to have enormous economic concerns and it is also having devastating effects on global education. With the rapid spread of the coronavirus, educational institutions around the world are making a radical decision to switch from traditional face-to-face course content deliveries to online content delivery. This is a major paradigm shift that will potentially reshape the future of Indian education system with the accelerated adoption of digital technology. The COVID-19 situation is a blessing in disguise to experiment with new tools and technologies to make education delivery meaningful to the students who cannot go to campuses. It's an opportunity to be more knowledgeable and to be more productive while developing new skill sets and accelerated professional skills through online learning and assessment. In this chapter, we have reviewed the educational challenges and opportunities posed by the unexpected outbreak of COVID-19 pandemic followed by the discussion on the recalibration of the Indian educational system after COVID-19. Various readily available platforms for the adoption of digital/online learning are explored and discussed in detail. In the chapter end, some recommendations are made for the betterment of the Indian education system after COVID-19.

Keywords Education disruption · COVID-19 · Online learning · ICT · Digital learning management

K. Ahuja (✉)
DAV Institute of Engineering and Technology, Jalandhar, Punjab, India
e-mail: askahuja2002@gmail.com

I. Bala
Lovely Professional University, Phagwara, Punjab, India

© The Author(s), under exclusive license to Springer Nature Switzerland AG 2021

F. Al-Turjman et al. (eds.), *Emerging Technologies for Battling Covid-19*, Studies in Systems, Decision and Control 324,
https://doi.org/10.1007/978-3-030-60039-6_10

10.1 Introduction

With the existing pandemic situation due to COVID-19 virus, most nations have closed their institutions/universities nationwide, disrupting the learning of billions of students worldwide [1, 2]. The proliferation of COVID-19 and the worldwide lockdown have led to the adoption of digital tools in various fields, including education. Universities, schools, and colleges have switched toward e-learning to continue the uninterrupted flow of knowledge. The closure of institutions/universities has not only interrupted the studies of the students worldwide; it also hampered key evaluation period, and many university exams have been postponed or cancelled. Many schools or educational governing/regulatory bodies have decided to promote students in high standards directly, while in higher education, many institutions/universities have opted for online assessment rather than regular assessments. The COVID-19 has caused a major paradigm shift in the whole education sector and heralded a new era of education for both teachers and students [3, 4]. Thus, the education system today has a dire need to shift regular teaching on distance learning programs and platforms to reach the students at different geographical locations. Schools and governments are exploring processes to permit students to get hold of education at home.

In the current scenario, it is more important than ever that education not be discontinued; otherwise, it can cause serious consequences for the mental well-being and development of students. In the hindsight of this brutal pandemic, the education sector is one of the few sectors that are on the path of being positively transformed. E-learning facilitates young learners to get indulged in studies without losing connection with subjects during lockdown.

Here, it is important to understand that e-learning is not only a platform for distance learning but also an adaptation of new and interesting digital tools to make learning more interesting. UNESCO is also facilitating many developing nations to mitigate the instant consequences of institutions closures, especially the more susceptible and deprived communities [5], and in their efforts to promote continuing education for all through distance education, as shown in Fig. 10.1.

In this chapter, we have discussed the immediate challenges faced by the educational fraternity to shift on digital education platform overnight. Subsequently, we have summarized some of the readily available online solutions that could be adopted as such to deliver online education to the students followed by the recommendation on practices that must be followed once the educational institutions may resume their working after COVID-19.

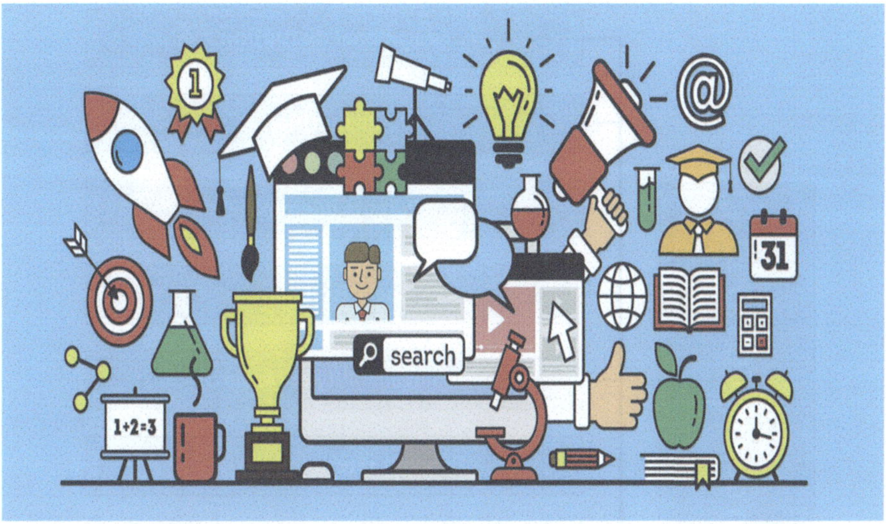

Fig. 10.1 Universities adopted ways to fight COVID-19 situation [6]

10.2 Challenges Faced by Education System Across the World

The coronavirus outbreak will have a deep and long-lasting impact on global education system. At this tough time, there are many questions that need to be addressed before jumping to the specific solution for the betterment of students. In this section, various challenges have been discussed in detail that need open discussion. The pictorial representation of challenges faced by the whole education system worldwide due to COVID-19 is shown in Fig. 10.2.

10.2.1 Educational Disruption

The educational institution provides its students with basic learning and prepares them for a better future. When institution closes, students get deprived of opportunities for growth and development. Figure 10.3 shows the statistics of disruption of studies faced by students due to school closures worldwide in February and March 2020. This educational disruption impacts adversely the underprivileged students who in general have less educational opportunities beyond schools/colleges [5].

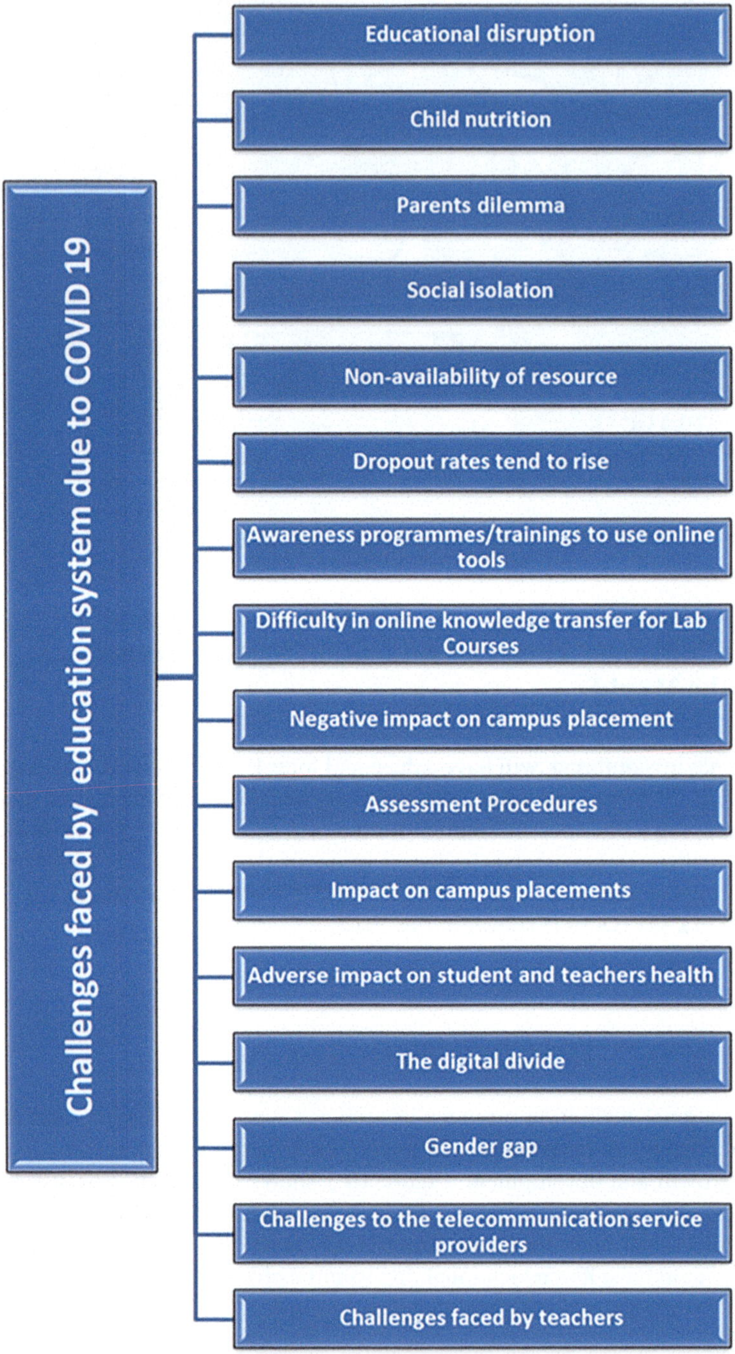

Fig. 10.2 Challenges faced by world education system due to COVID

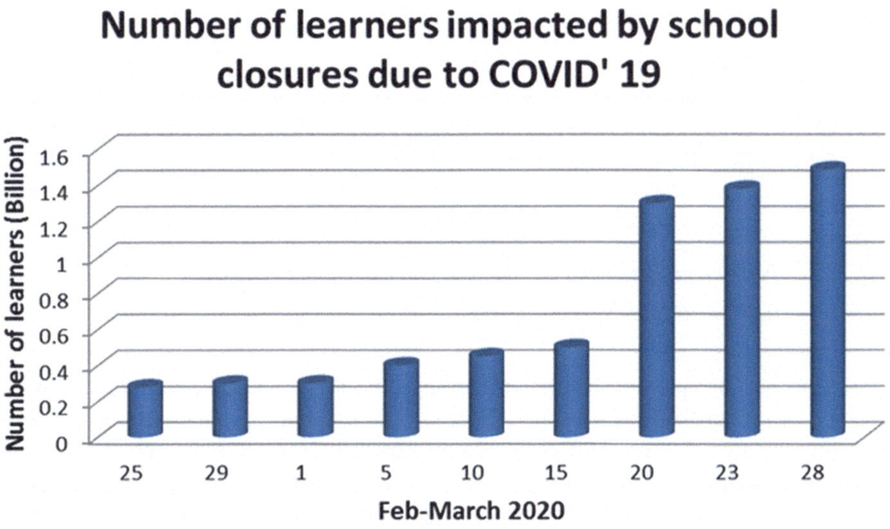

Fig. 10.3 The number of learners impacted due to school closure [7]

10.2.2 Child Nutrition

Countries around the world offer a variety of school meal programs for students. School meals are a source of nutritious foods in developed countries. But, in developing countries like India, mid day meal is the reason for many parents to send their children to school and continuing their education. For such countries, students depend on free or reduced price meals provided in institutions for food and nutrition. With existing COVID-19 situation, these students will not be able to continue their education and will also be malnourished [8].

10.2.3 Parent Dilemma of Home Schooling

The kids are sent to schools to elevate their skills. The time spent in schools promotes social competencies and mindfulness in them. The basic notion of sending a child to the school is to enhance the child's ability. When the school is closed, parents are requested to facilitate their kids in learning at home. In a country like India, it is very challenging for parents with limited education and constrained resources to face the scenario [9]. By and large, the working parents are more likely to take leaves from their places of work in order to take care of their kids in the course of lockdown, which in many instances leads to loss of pay and negatively influences their productivity. The scenario is worst when both mother and father are in the clinical profession.

10.2.4 Social Isolation

During school time, kids participate in social activities and interact with their peers and teachers. Due to the school closure, many children lose this social connection vital for gaining knowledge and overall personality development.

10.2.5 Non-availability of Resources to the Students and Teachers

UNESCO has also pointed out that disrupting schooling can cause hardship to families and other hardships, including a decrease in economic productivity, as parents are obliged to work with their childcare responsibilities [10]. Currently, half of all students outside the classroom, or 830 million learners worldwide, do not have access to a computer. In a recent survey, it has been observed that 40% of the population do not have Internet connectivity. As shown in Figure 10.4, at many geographical locations, lack of Internet access or improper Internet connectivity is a major obstacle in online learning, particularly for students coming from deprived communities.

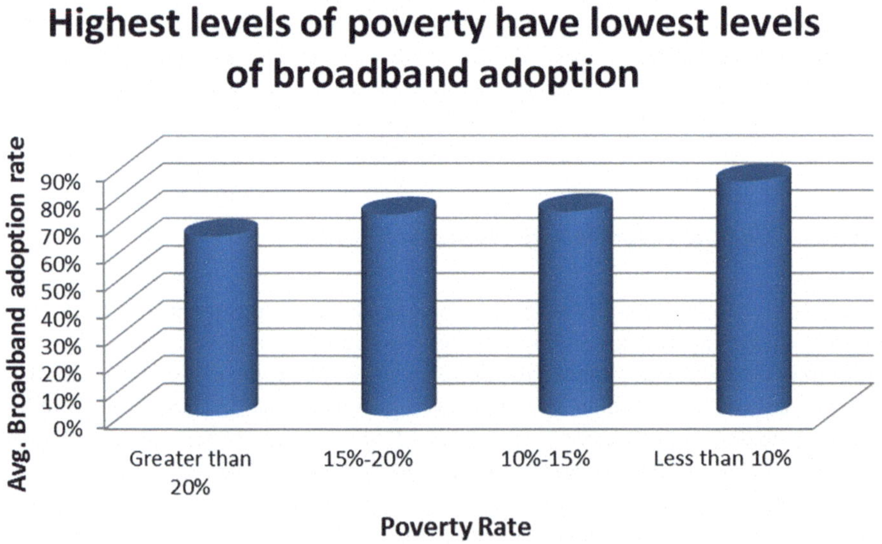

Fig. 10.4 Represents poverty rate vs. average broadband adoption rate [11]

10.2.6 Dropout Rates Tend to Rise

With the existing COVID-19 situation, it is very difficult to predict when exactly the schools/universities will open. And it is even more difficult to anticipate that people will send their kids back to school, especially in case of extended closures. In this scenario, the chance of increase in dropout rate is very high and is a matter of great concern to most of the educational institutions.

10.2.7 Awareness Programs/Trainings to Use Online Tools

In many developing countries, schools and universities teach students according to traditional blackboard and chalk practices. With the outbreak of COVID-19, such schools and teachers have no choice but to take on online teaching learning pedagogies. However, many teachers are unfamiliar or indifferent to online education using technology-led materials. A typical online course requires content preparation and state-of-the-art audio visual techniques to connect the content with students. Converting an offline course may require additional work to bring it online. Thus, online trainings/short-term courses/FDPs are also required to train the faculty for effective online teaching [12].

10.2.8 Difficulties in Transferring Knowledge Online for Laboratory Courses

The basic notion behind a successful online course is student engagement. Knowledge components can be effectively communicated in online mode. However, the practical aspects where hands-on practices are required cannot be transferred in online mode. For example, to do design-based experiments in online mode can be a foremost challenge and sometimes may not be feasible. This issue is a major concern of the education sector that needs immediate attention and resolution.

10.2.9 Negative Impact on Campus Placement

The university graduate placements may be severely affected due to COVID-19 epidemic this year. The final year graduates this year have experienced major teaching and assessments interruptions, and eventually they are graduating in the beginning of global recession. Thus, many of them would have to accept less paid jobs and this could be the everlasting implications for them [13].

10.2.10 Assessment Procedures

The sudden closure of institutions/universities has not only adversely impacted the learning of the students worldwide; unfortunately, the school closure situation has coincided with the key assessment period of the students, and their exams are either postponed or have been cancelled this year. As a result, parents and teachers fail to assess a student's learning capabilities which can have long-term negative consequences for him or her [14]. One potential alternative for the cancelled assessments is to use "predicted grades" [15], but generally such measurements are often inaccurate [16–20].

10.2.11 Adverse Effects on Student Health

Recent reports have indicated that people who spend more time on a computer or mobile phones have difficulty in concentrating and Internet obsession that can seriously affect their lives. It can lead to social isolation which may decrease their academic performance and sometimes depression also. Procrastination problem affects most of the students who do online courses. This sleep deprivation affects them negatively resulting in poor memory retention and academic performance. With COVID-9 outbreak, the online learning option led new E-learners to spend long study hours to take courses and complete assignments. Sometimes, it may also affect students' health like weak muscle, joint pain, weak eyesight, etc.

10.2.12 The Digital Divide

The biggest challenge in continuing online education is unequal access to the electronic devices, such as computers and smartphones, and irregular power supply in countries like India and Internet connections. Access to electricity is important for digital education, both to power devices and to connect to the Internet. In developed countries, electricity may not be an issue, but in developing countries like India, electricity quality and the number of hours available each day are issues. Computers/laptops with good Internet courses are mandatory for online courses. Smartphones could also serve this purpose. However, smartphones are good for apps, but not for time-consuming assignments or research. Thus, the digital divide is evident across class, gender, region, or place of residence. It has been reported that in India, among 20% of people below poverty line, only 2.7% people have computer in their house and 8.9% have Internet facilities [21]. The situation is exacerbated in remote areas.

10.2.13 Gender Gap

The Internet and Mobile Association of India has reported that in 2019, 67% of the Internet users were men and only 33% of Internet users were women. The inequality is more pronounced in rural areas, with men and women accounting for 72% and 28%, respectively. General inequalities in the virtual world can lead to increased educational inequality in learners if governments continue to provide online education without the necessary support [22, 23].

10.2.14 Challenges Faced by the Telecommunication Service Providers

To continue online learning by the students, regular and predictable Internet connectivity is a must. During this lockdown period, many telecom service providers like BSNL, Vodafone, and Reliance Jio must offer additional data package and free Internet hours to the students and educational institutions. Without good Internet access, it is difficult to arrange online classes to students sporadically due to poor Internet connectivity and signal fading issues. In some cases as in J&K, due to restricted 2G network services instead of 4G, students could not access online classes [24]. To continue online learning on a regular basis has also a cost implication, and many students are not able to bear Internet services cost. So far, no communication has been made by the governments on the reimbursement of Internet bills to the students or on providing free or subsidized data packs to the students. With this prevailing situation, many students may not be able to afford these data packages as their families have lost their source of income.

10.2.15 Challenges Faced by Teachers

Bringing the classroom online does not mean effective distance learning. Interaction among students and teachers is a very crucial part in learning. The online learning requires strict discipline by the student. Teachers are also facing challenges as many of them are not digitally adept. The exposure to the online teaching is very little to most of them. Teaching courses online requires training on developing lesson plans and preparing lecture materials in the form of audio and video [25–28]. Figure 10.5 lists some of the available tools that one can use to create digital educational content.

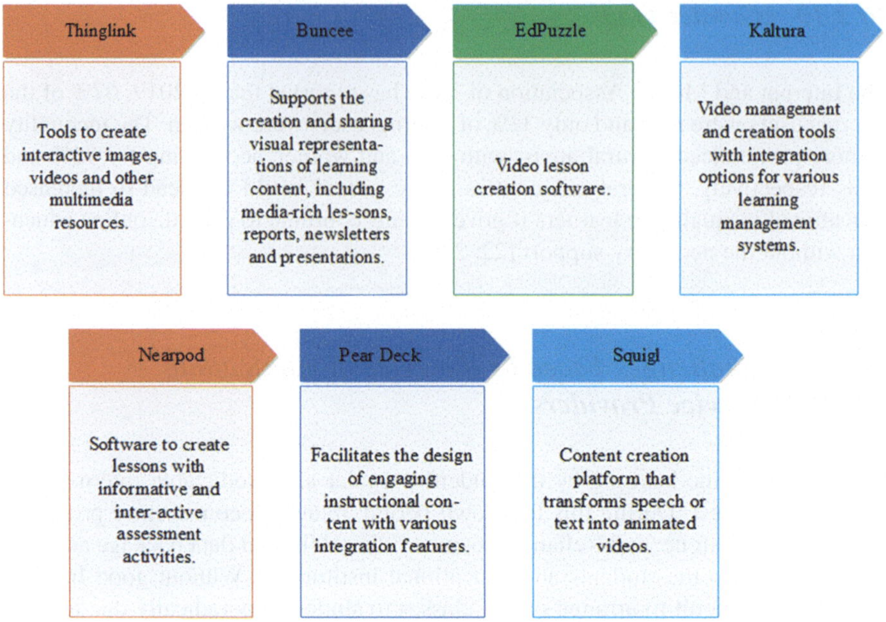

Fig. 10.5 Tools for teachers to create digital learning content

10.3 Transition Phase of Indian Education System

The nationwide lockdown due to the coronavirus has led to the adoption of digital tools in various fields, including education. Universities, schools, and colleges have switched to e-learning to continue the uninterrupted flow of knowledge. Despite the current restriction, universities, schools, and colleges have switched to e-learning in order to keep up with the continuous flow of knowledge, which is expected to expand in line with the growing number of coronavirus cases in different parts of the country. The discussions about the adoption of digital technologies for educational purposes have been going on for some time. But what used to be a discussion has now become a reality due to corona breakdown throughout the world. It has now become a hierarchy of strategic actions, and the wave of digital transformation has positively affected the education sector of the industry. At times like these, it is more important than ever that education not be discontinued; otherwise, it can have serious consequences for the mental well-being and development of our students [29]. A unique educational model is anticipated to emerge from COVID-19. The pandemic has forced the educational policy makers around the world to understand the shortcomings of the current education system. To apprehend the shortcomings of the contemporary training system, the need of digital literacy is strongly felt worldwide that could draw big difference between traditional and non-traditional teaching. In this section, a number of probable solutions related to continuing the

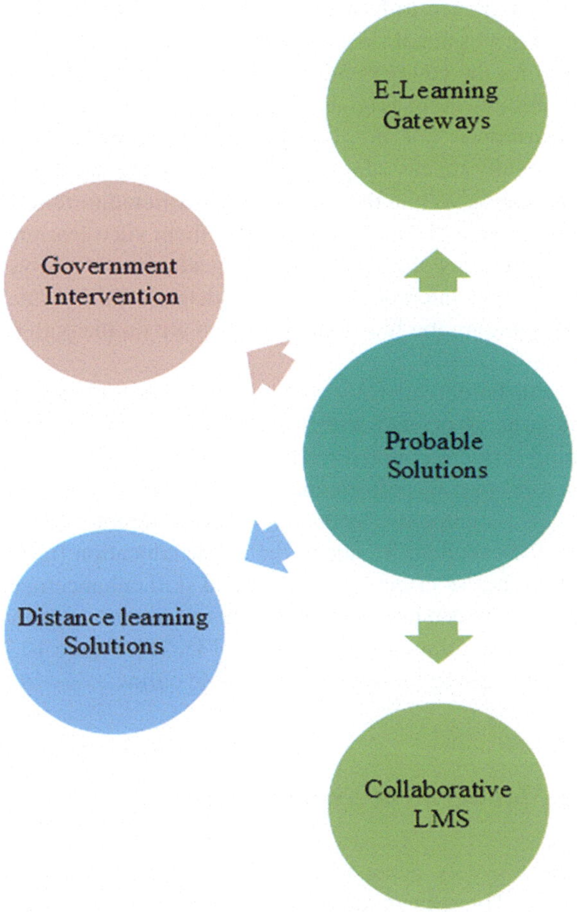

Fig. 10.6 Represents the probable solutions during COVID-19 pandemic

education during COVID-19 are highlighted in Fig. 10.6 with their respective details as follows.

10.3.1 E-Learning Gateways

The lockdown has accelerated adoption of digital technology by educational institutes to work in tandem. It is considered to be an ideal time to experiment with and to deploy new technologies to make online education delivery possible and meaningful. Without hampering students' learning, digital transformation has become a new means to the educational institutions across the country. Many educationists consider the existing situation as a chance to be more productive and efficient by adopting modern and accelerated professional skills via online learning.

E-learning provides a gateway for the young minds to indulge in learning regardless of the lockdown which continues them productive and helps them not loose connect with the subjects. E-learning is not simply a platform for training from distance these days; but it additionally means adapting new and fascinating digital tools to make learning more interesting. While the students are restricted to remain indoors and cannot go to school, the school can always come to them via e-learning platforms like illumnus itself which uses collaborative learning administration systems to make schooling seamless and interactive. In the hindsight of this brutal pandemic, the education sector is among the few domains which are on the path of being positively transformed.

By the time this pandemic will be defeated, we additionally have a chance of overcoming all the issues and cons associated with the typical and unorganized structure of schooling. E-learning services coupled with collaborative LMS providing Auto-Quiz creation, instructors' overall performance reviews, expertly curated content material library, one-tap assignments, instant messaging, doubt-clearing sessions, etc. will turn out to be the excellent friends of the whole education fraternity [30–34]. Realizing the importance of effective teaching and skill enhancement of the instructors, the partnerships between universities, online education organizations, and tech providers may also be continued after pandemic [35, 36]. Figure 10.7 provides some of the self-directed learning tools readily available online.

10.3.2 Digital Learning Management Systems

The success of any online course largely depends upon the content and content delivery to keep students engaged. The subject knowledge can be delivered effectively in online mode. However, the skills cannot be transferred through online mode. For example, conducting an analog design laboratory in an online mode could be very challenging. Figure 10.8 shows some of the trendy digital learning management system tools for lab courses.

10.3.3 Teacher's Knowledge Diversification

The COVID-19 situation has emerged as an opportunity to the students to learn things online from subject experts and for teachers to diversify their knowledge. The time flexibility allows students to study the course as per their convenience. For a typical online course, instructor has to prepare the contents carefully, and using audio and video facilities, delivery of these contents is made to the students. For example, in India, IITs are following this practice of use of the technology

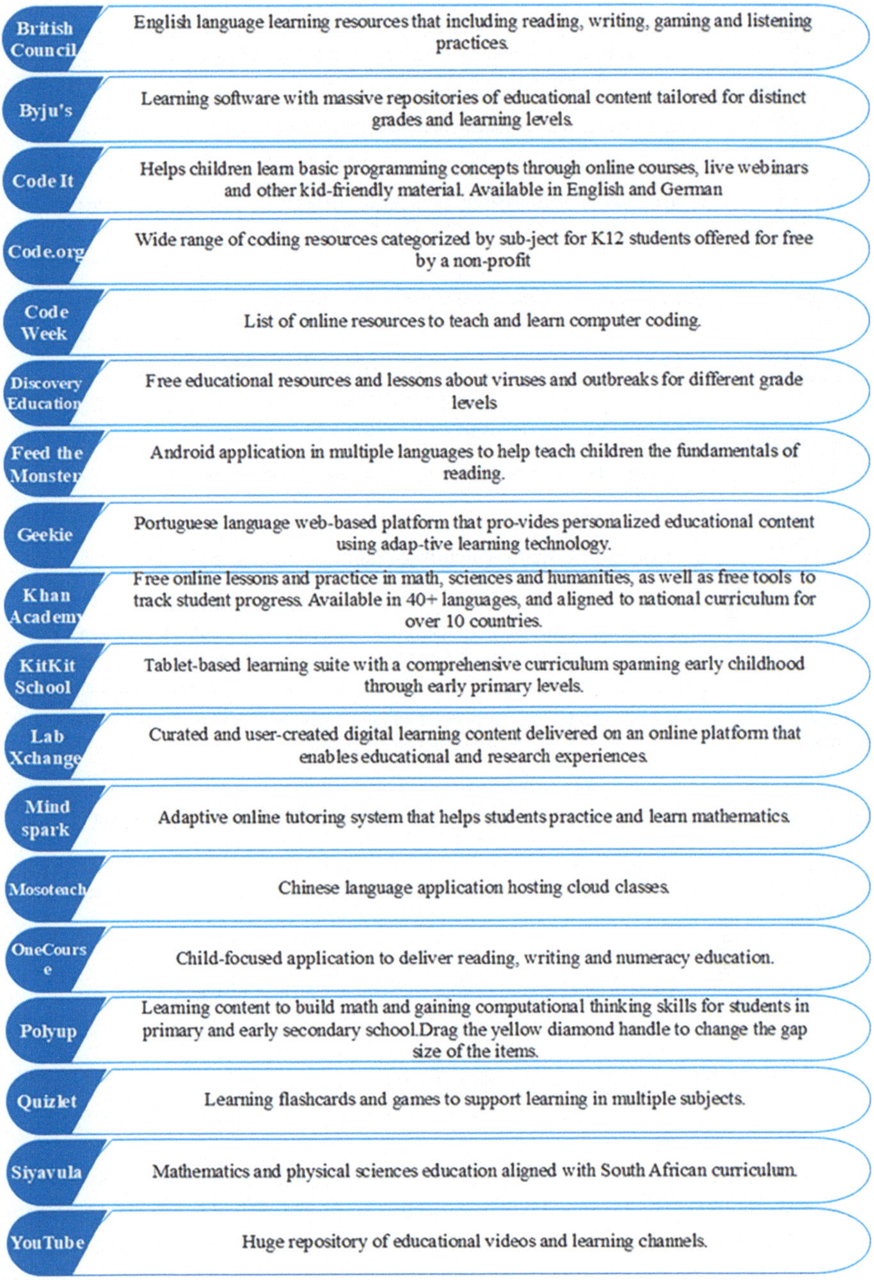
British Council
English language learning resources that including reading, writing, gaming and listening practices.
Byju's
Learning software with massive repositories of educational content tailored for distinct grades and learning levels.
Code It
Helps children learn basic programming concepts through online courses, live webinars and other kid-friendly material. Available in English and German
Code.org
Wide range of coding resources categorized by sub-ject for K12 students offered for free by a non-profit
Code Week
List of online resources to teach and learn computer coding.
Discovery Education
Free educational resources and lessons about viruses and outbreaks for different grade levels
Feed the Monster
Android application in multiple languages to help teach children the fundamentals of reading.
Geekie
Portuguese language web-based platform that pro-vides personalized educational content using adap-tive learning technology.
Khan Academy
Free online lessons and practice in math, sciences and humanities, as well as free tools to track student progress. Available in 40+ languages, and aligned to national curriculum for over 10 countries.
KitKit School
Tablet-based learning suite with a comprehensive curriculum spanning early childhood through early primary levels.
Lab Xchange
Curated and user-created digital learning content delivered on an online platform that enables educational and research experiences.
Mind spark
Adaptive online tutoring system that helps students practice and learn mathematics.
Mosoteach
Chinese language application hosting cloud classes.
OneCours e
Child-focused application to deliver reading, writing and numeracy education.
Polyup
Learning content to build math and gaining computational thinking skills for students in primary and early secondary school.Drag the yellow diamond handle to change the gap size of the items.
Quizlet
Learning flashcards and games to support learning in multiple subjects.
Siyavula
Mathematics and physical sciences education aligned with South African curriculum.
YouTube
Huge repository of educational videos and learning channels.

Fig. 10.7 Self-directed learning content

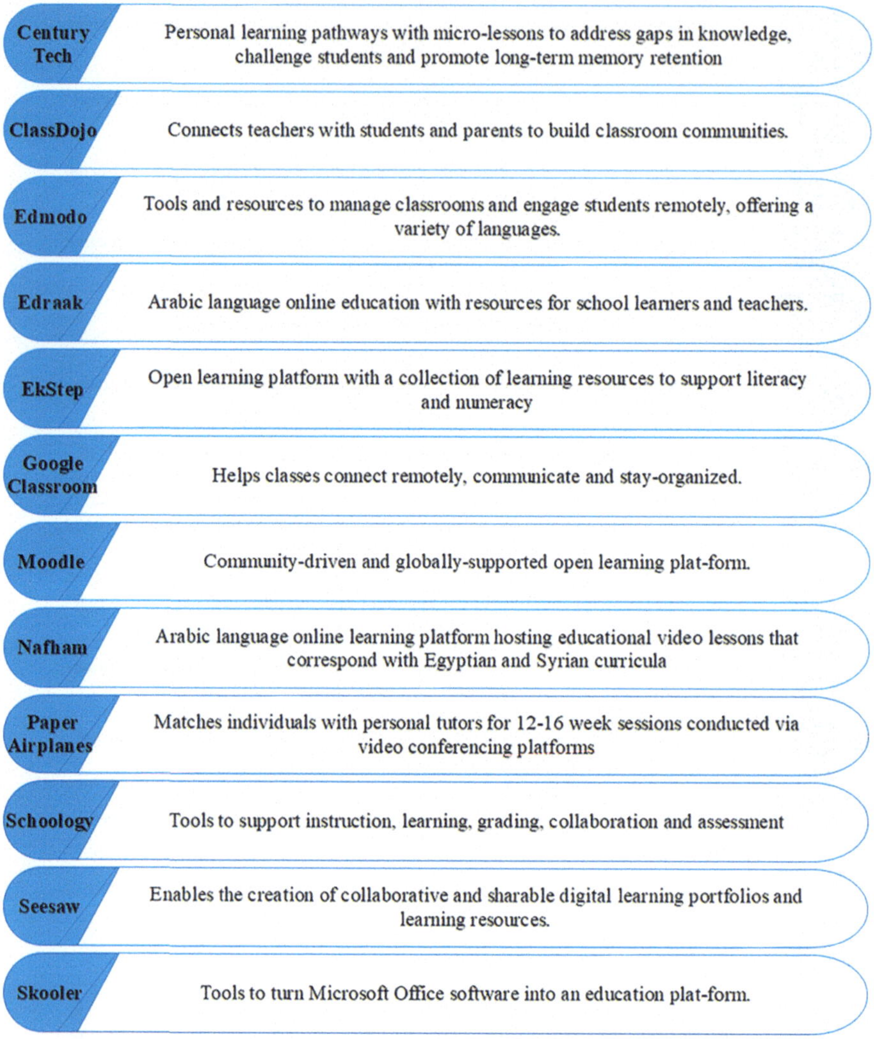

Fig. 10.8 Digital learning management system (DLMS) [10]

infrastructure to run online courses on platforms like NPTEL. Many other similar platforms are listed in Figure 10.9. No doubt, it requires great efforts to change offline courses contents to make it online. Thus, teachers are required great efforts to convert these contents online as the trend of online education is gaining momentum with the existing pandemic situation.

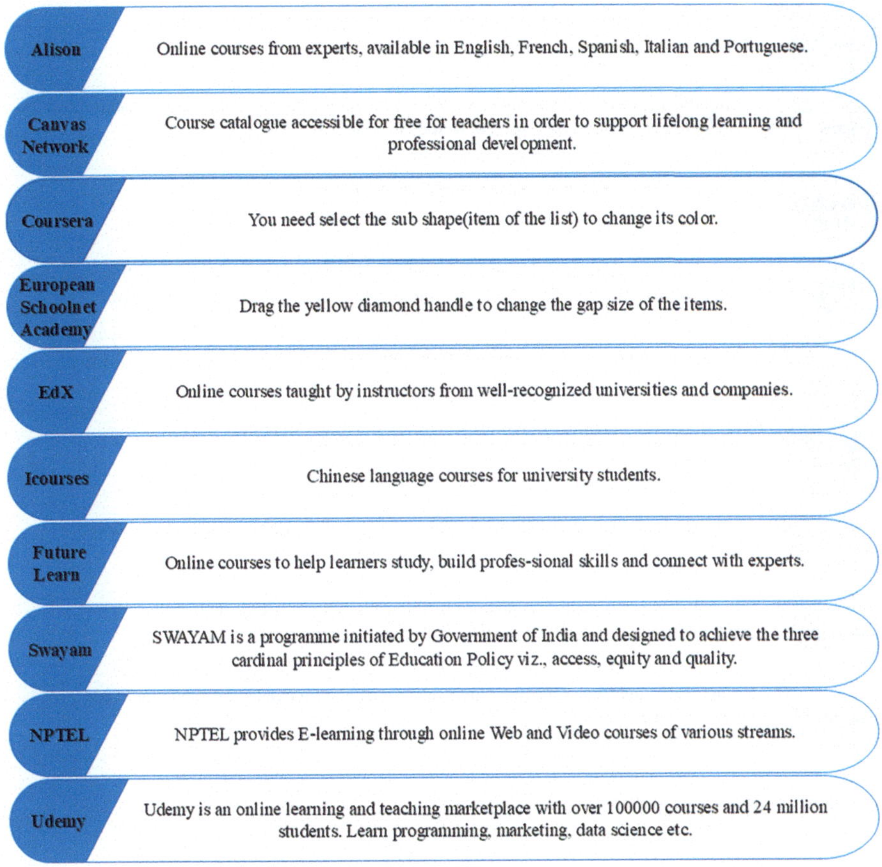
Alison
Online courses from experts, available in English, French, Spanish, Italian and Portuguese.
Canvas Network
Course catalogue accessible for free for teachers in order to support lifelong learning and professional development.
Coursera
You need select the sub shape(item of the list) to change its color.
European Schoolnet Academy
Drag the yellow diamond handle to change the gap size of the items.
EdX
Online courses taught by instructors from well-recognized universities and companies.
Icourses
Chinese language courses for university students.
Future Learn
Online courses to help learners study, build profes-sional skills and connect with experts.
Swayam
SWAYAM is a programme initiated by Government of India and designed to achieve the three cardinal principles of Education Policy viz., access, equity and quality.
NPTEL
NPTEL provides E-learning through online Web and Video courses of various streams.
Udemy
Udemy is an online learning and teaching marketplace with over 100000 courses and 24 million students. Learn programming, marketing, data science etc.

Fig. 10.9 Massive Open Online Course (MOOC) platforms [10]

10.3.4 Collaborative LMS

Digital India campaign launched by the Government of India will now serve as the foundation for bridging the learning gap that exists at the moment. Collaborative LMS makes the offline to digital transition simpler for the administrations as they can easily manage their institutes simply like they do on regular schooling days. The customers can set up yearly direction structures, conduct virtual classes, send notices and timetables at the click of a button, and certainly can get a bird's-eye view of the overall institute's performance. Virtual lecture rooms and online tools used on these e-learning platforms allow the academicians/school staff to engage students the same as in a classroom environment. These tools can also aid in organizing teachers and parent meetings and staff/management meetings and can save both time and money while offering the quintessential interactivity. This is an era of transformation no matter the harsh times and although the training industry is on the

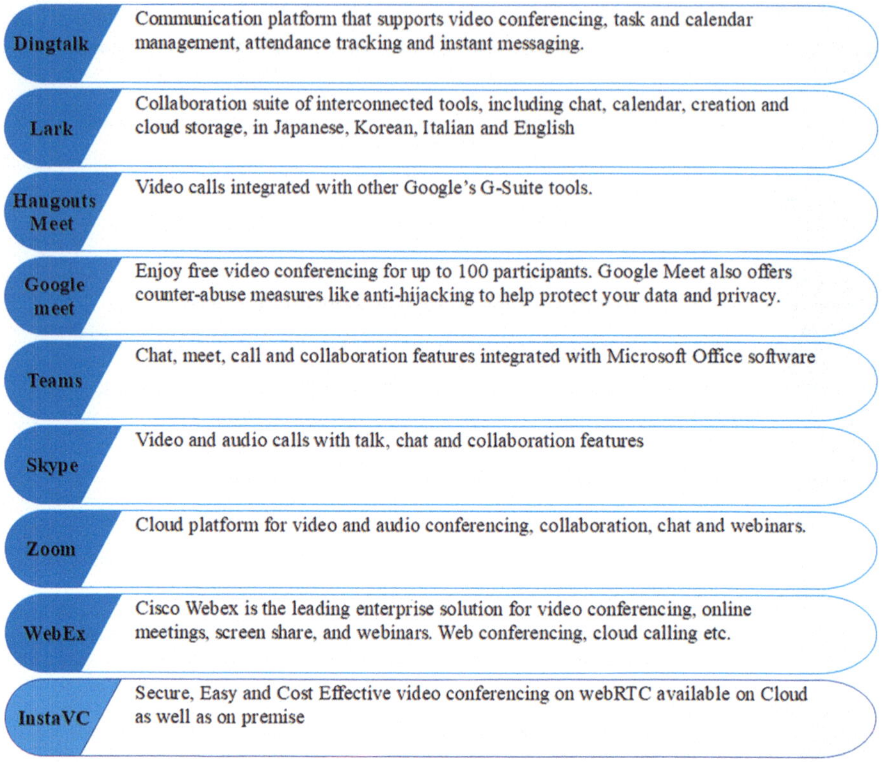
Dingtalk
Communication platform that supports video conferencing, task and calendar management, attendance tracking and instant messaging.
Lark
Collaboration suite of interconnected tools, including chat, calendar, creation and cloud storage, in Japanese, Korean, Italian and English
Hangouts Meet
Video calls integrated with other Google's G-Suite tools.
Google meet
Enjoy free video conferencing for up to 100 participants. Google Meet also offers counter-abuse measures like anti-hijacking to help protect your data and privacy.
Teams
Chat, meet, call and collaboration features integrated with Microsoft Office software
Skype
Video and audio calls with talk, chat and collaboration features
Zoom
Cloud platform for video and audio conferencing, collaboration, chat and webinars.
WebEx
Cisco Webex is the leading enterprise solution for video conferencing, online meetings, screen share, and webinars. Web conferencing, cloud calling etc.
InstaVC
Secure, Easy and Cost Effective video conferencing on webRTC available on Cloud as well as on premise

Fig. 10.10 Collaborative platforms supporting live video conference [10, 36–41]

verge of being absolutely altered for good. There is no looking back from here. The advantages of adopting e-learning services today will have a very tremendous and powerful influence on our future. Some of the collaborative platforms that support video conference are listed in Fig. 10.10.

10.3.5 Distance Learning Solutions

Some of the educational platforms and applications that are listed in Figure 10.11 aim to aid teachers, parents, and school administrators to help student in his studies and to provide him social care and interaction during school closure. Most of these solutions are free and available in multiple languages.

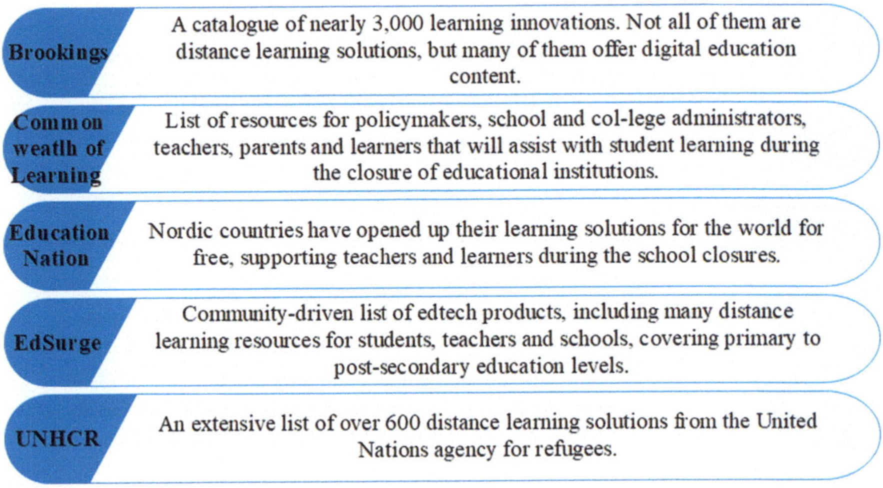

Fig. 10.11 External repositories of distance learning solutions [10]

10.3.6 Government Initiatives

In response to educational institutions' closure, governments and private companies have come forward with numerous initiatives for the benefits of the students. Ever since the lockdown started, the government has taken all necessary measures to avoid any kind of disruption in the studies of students. To facilitate them, a variety of e-learning portals and apps have been launched by the Indian government and educational authorities such as ePathshala, DIKSHA portal, STEM-based games, Swayam, etc. Some of the worldwide available mobile apps for reading and learning are tabulated in Fig. 10.12.

10.4 Recommendations

A key aspect of coping with COVID-19 situation is to guarantee that services are being delivered in every possible manner. The IT professionals can adapt themselves to this transition phase as most of them are already working on their laptops and smart devices even in office and they can simply plug in at homes now. But students have had to make far bigger adjustments as learning has always been in classrooms which they can't go to now. Moreover, many of them are not well equipped with technology required for remote learning. Here, the Digital India vision of the legislature is developing as an imperative instrument for settling the current emergency due to COVID-19. The lockdown has speed up adoption of computerized innovation. Business houses, educational spots, exploration, PC, information management strategies, and online education arrangements have been compelled

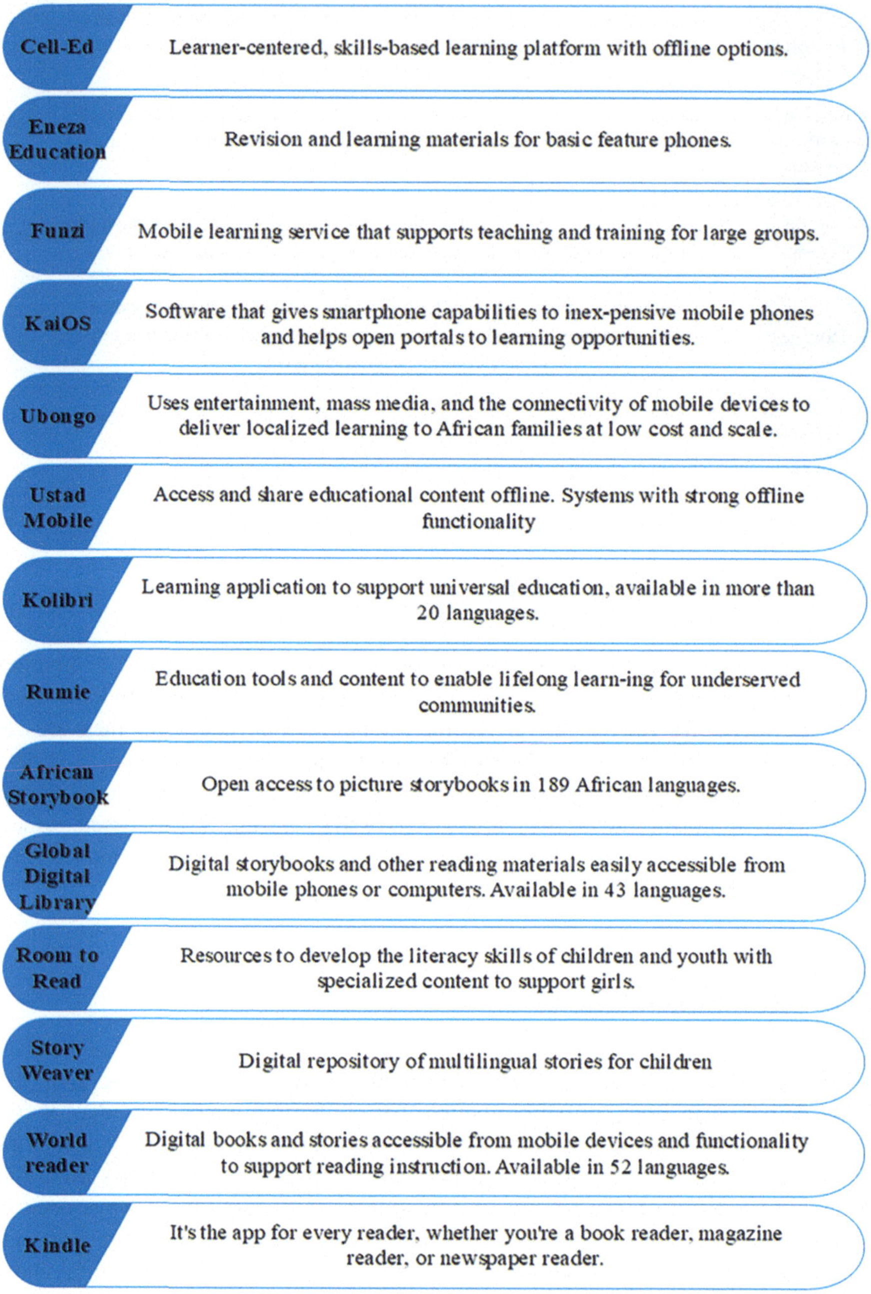

Fig. 10.12 Mobile platforms for online learning [42, 43]

to work fast and improve in quality and delivery time to deal with such circumstances [44–48]. This is a perfect opportunity to analyze and send new gadgets to make training delivery important to students who can't go to institutes. It's an opportunity to be increasingly effective and gainful while growing as good as ever proficient abilities/information through web-based learning and appraisal.

It is additionally a reality that utilization of innovation in teaching is resulting in various ideas in the system, for example, the move from educator-driven teaching to student-driven education. An extreme change in point of view is required in the mentality of policy makers, specialists, students, and extraordinarily educationists. Teacher selection ought to continuously be connected to innovation amicability and intelligence for innovation adoption. Correspondingly, accreditation parameters and models need reexamination. COVID-19 has just quickened selection of innovations to convey teaching. To beat the current bottlenecks in adoption of web-based learning, following recommendations are made to adapt to existing circumstance [49]. The pictorial view of recommendations is presented in Fig. 10.13.

10.4.1 Educational TV Programs

While a greater part of the youngsters can get access to online talks by means of Internet on advanced cells or on work areas/workstations, there is as yet a group of children forsaken, particularly the individuals who study in government schools. The administration should begin with certain TV slots through which poor kids can approach education as now the greater part of the families have TVs at home. The TV channels ought to have bifurcation as per various classes, and talks/projects can be broadcast during school timings.

10.4.2 Overcome Language/Infrastructure and Technology Barrier

In the current situation, many students don't have smart phones or workstations to use applications like Zoom, Skype, and so forth. Moreover, many of them can't comprehend the lectures in English. For such students, sound recordings of the lectures in Hindi can be sent to them. Those who are unable to access this facility can be taught later on when the schools reopen after the lockdown. For future e-learning, the government should also come forward with schemes to provide smart mobile phones to the students at easy installments. The government should also make e-learning mandatory for specific topics to ensure teachers and students are familiarized with this digital learning process.

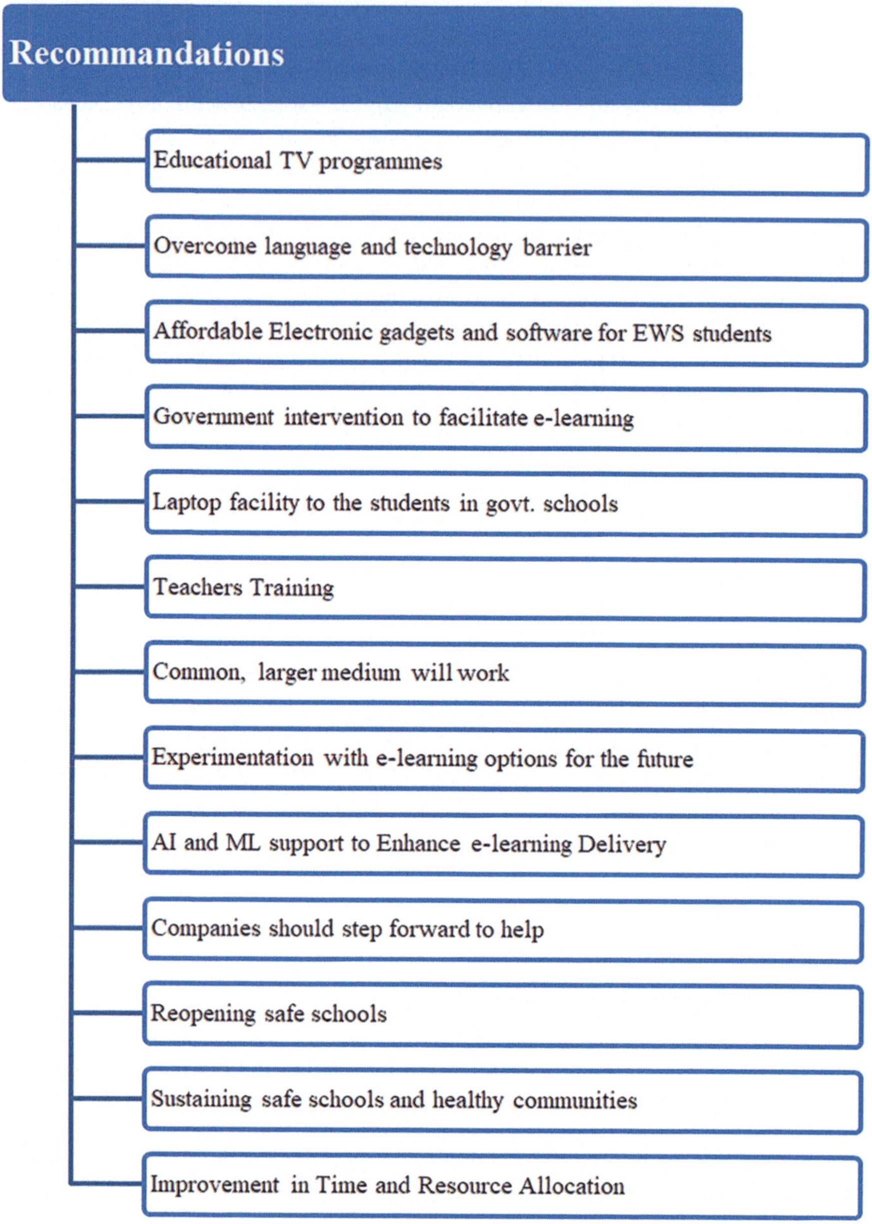

Fig. 10.13 Recommendations to improve Indian education system after COVID-19

10.4.3 Affordable Electronic Gadgets and Software for EWS Students

Digital distance learning is in trend these days and many Indian universities, for example, IGNOU, have started many such programmes for higher classes. With the existing pandemic situation, the focus is now shifting towards the online delivery of the digital contents at the primary level. It requires the availability of cheap handheld devices with multimedia facilities and excellent storages capacity to retain the study material within it for every class. Such devices must be distributed to EWS-kids free of cost to facilitate students further, the contact numbers of the course instructors must also be embedded in these smart devices.

10.4.4 Government Intervention to Facilitate E-Learning

In India, economically weak students join government institutions as they comparatively have less tuition fees and free food facility. Some of these schools or colleges lack in basic facilities such as boards and chalks for writing. And therefore, it is unreasonable to imagine their participation at digital learning platform. Thus, a strong government intervention is required so that government students may also be private exposed to learning that matches with the quality of education in other top institutions.

10.4.5 Laptop Facility to the Students in Govt. Schools

Keeping in view the poor infrastructure facilities in government school and colleges, the government, NGOs and private firms should come forward to arrange laptop or smart phones for the students. Laptop and smart phone manufacturing companies should design these laptops with embedded softwares for online learning. Government intervention is also required to arrange such gadgets at subsidized rates for the students.

10.4.6 Teachers' Trainings and Other Infrastructure Requirements

To make online education equally effective as the classroom teaching, the teachers must be trained in delivering course contents efficiently and effectively. Secondly, the students as well as teachers must have PC with good configuration and smartphones. Thirdly, all villages and remote areas must have good internet facility.

10.4.7 Common, Larger Medium Will Work

Children from all strata of society can get online education if they are educated through a much common and larger medium. Schools authorities can do this by broadcasting video lectures for the students on All India Radio or Doordarshan and other similar platforms. The time table of different classes must be announced on different radio stations. In addition to this, the curriculum books like NCERT must be translated into audio and video form for primary school students.

10.4.8 Experimentation with E-Learning Options for the Future

The existing corona situation must be considered as an opportunity to experiment with available digital technologies such as, WhatsApp, Facebook, and YouTube on PDAs to access educational videos. The schools authorities must approach smart phone manufacturing companies those who are ready to provide free or cheap handsets to the needy students. The telecommunication service providers should also offer cheap data plans to the students and school authorities should help EWS students to avail these plan rather than investing in school buildings, infrastructures and equipments.

10.4.9 Artificial Intelligence (AI) and Machine Learning (ML) Support to Enhance E-Learning Delivery

Face-to-face learning allows students to interact with the instructor in the classroom. It also helps the teacher to understand the perception of the learner. The E-learning platforms and LMS systems embedded with AI and ML models can predict both teaching and learning patterns to facilitate both teacher and students to adapt the learning programs on the basis of behaviors, assessments, and understanding. The ML plays a very important role in online learning through effective data analysis and automation. It enables administrators and trainers to identify the weak areas of the learner on analytical patterns and algorithms and add new information to predict learning outcomes. On the basis of the automation and decision-making models, the AI tools can constantly monitor the alignment of the newly developed program with the learning objective. Moreover, ML also allows administrators to automate personalized training paths for individual students. It analyses patterns and trends to adjust the learners' coursework automatically to meet training needs. In addition to this, ML can also help the faculty to understand students' need to learn. The ML programs apply predictive algorithms to assessment of current and past performance of the student(s) and enable the faculty to identify targeted online training recommendations.

10.4.10 Companies Should Step Forward to Help

The taxes paid by the conscious occupants of India must be spent in this social motive and for the strengthening of substantially less special understudies and instructors. To deal with the existing Covid-19 situations, both, government and private institutes would have to play a significant role in the digital empowerment of less privileged students and teachers. The handset manufacturing companies should design cheap smart phones or laptops for them. NGOs and civil societies too should also come forward to facilitate them to access digital online classes. The government must start digital classrooms for the economically weak students so they do not lack in knowledge.

10.4.11 Reopening Safe Schools

School systems need proper planning for reopening schools as quickly and responsibly as possible. The teachers must be provided with accurate information and training on the public health crisis, using schools as an opportunity to quickly monitor and trace any re-emergence, and providing any additional physical or mental health support that students may need, especially in high-incident areas.

10.4.12 Sustaining Safe Schools and Healthy Communities

Access to schools is important for implementing wider public health programs. Equally important is having a contingency plan for future emergencies. We hope that children and students in the most affected areas will be able to return to school sooner and other schools will not be affected. But don't forget global education during or after the crisis [51]. Investment in education not only provides the normality and ways for youth to fully participate in the economy and society but also promotes the innovation and skills and talents needed to fight the next pandemic or crisis.

In the coming weeks and months, many governments will have to make tough preferences about their funding in education. The crisis will simply entice resources. Faced with this choice, it needs to be remembered that cutting-edge kids are tomorrow's nurses, epidemiologists, doctors, researchers, and professionals in the subject of public health. We need to proceed to make investments in training these days so that the world can be higher organized for tomorrow's epidemics and crises.

10.4.13 Improvement in Time and Resource Allocation

ML programs automate many processes in learning modules and enable instructors and administrators to spend time on other aspects of the learning process, e.g., be with the development of online modules for the creation of other subject areas or laboratory simulations and practical courses.

10.5 Conclusion and Future Scope

With the immediate closure of schools in March 2020 to stop the spread of coronavirus, many countries have opted for online distance learning platforms to continue educational services. The studies of the students must not suffer; therefore, many countries started putting their educational resources on their websites. In some of the nations, teachers are asked to prepare online digital content and to give online classes to the students. The success of running online classes depends largely on availability of the digital infrastructure and familiarity with the tools. In developed countries with robust connectivity, online distance learning is not a big challenge, whereas in developing countries like India, digital divide is more pronounced and the penetration of Internet, smartphone, or television access and reachability is not equal for all the students.

In this chapter, we have addressed various challenges that Indian education system has faced recently due to the immediate closure of the institutions. To deal with this situation, there are many online learning applications and tools available for immediate adoption by the educational institutions as an open source. However, the key challenge is to prepare the course contents in a structured way to engage students in online learning. The partnership with private corporations active in education sector can be fruitful to get already developed contents/course materials. At the same time, telecom service providers should also come forward with zero-charge data plans for downloading the contents from the Ministry of Education. Other than the infrastructure and connectivity issues, the teachers and administrators should have hands-on experience on digital tools and technologies for effective online teaching. Thus, online short-term courses and faculty development programs must be organized for them so that they have apt knowledge about the usage of tools required to make their online classes interactive and interesting to keep students engaged in learning.

References

1. Chahrour, M., Assi, S., Bejjani, M., Nasrallah, A.A., Salhab, H., Fares, M.Y., Khachfe, H.H.: A bibliometric analysis of COVID-19 research activity: a call for increased output. Cureus. **12**, e7357 (2020). https://doi.org/10.7759/cureus.7357

2. Xiang, Y.T., Yang, Y., Li, W., Zhang, L., Zhang, Q., Cheung, T., Ng, C.H.: Timely mental health care for the 2019 novel coronavirus outbreak is urgently needed. Lancet Psychiatry. **7**, 28–29 (2020). https://doi.org/10.1016/S2215-0366(20)30046-8
3. Spina, S., Marrazzo, F., Migliari, M., Stucchi, R., Sforza, A., Fumagalli, R.: The response of Milan's emergency medical system to the COVID-19 outbreak in Italy. Lancet. **395**, 49–50 (2020). https://doi.org/10.1016/s0140-6736(20)30493-1
4. As coronavirus spreads, the decision to move classes online is the first step. What comes next? (2020). https://www.chronicle.com/article/As-Coronavirus-Spreads-the/248200. Accessed 6 Mar 2020
5. UNESCO. COVID-19 educational disruption and response (2020). https://en.unesco.org/themes/education-emergencies/coronavirus-school-closures. Accessed 25 Mar 2020
6. https://www.npr.org/2020/03/06/812462913/6-ways-universities-are-responding-to-coronavirus
7. https://www.weforum.org/agenda/2020/03/infographic-covid19-coronavirus-impact-global-education-health-schools/
8. Wheeler, C.C., Erhart, L.M., Jehn, M.L.: Effect of school closure on the incidence of influenza among school-age children in Arizona. Public Health Rep. **125**, 851–859 (2010). https://doi.org/10.1177/003335491012500612
9. Luca, G.D., Kerckhove, K.V., Coletti, P., Poletto, C., Bossuyt, N., Hens, N., Colizza, V.: The impact of regular school closure on seasonal influenza epidemics: a data-driven spatial transmission model for Belgium. BMC Infect. Dis. **18**, 29 (2018). https://doi.org/10.1186/s12879-017-2934-3
10. https://en.unesco.org/covid19/educationresponse/solutions
11. https://www.brookings.edu/blog/the-avenue/2020/03/20/as-classes-move-online-during-covid-19-what-are-disconnected-students-to-do/
12. Coronavirus: universities are shifting classes online—but it's not as easy as it sounds (2020). http://theconversation.com/coronavirus-universities-are-shifting-classes-online-but-its-not-as-easy-as-it-sounds-133030. Accessed 9 Mar 2020
13. Oreopoulos, P., von Wachter, T., Heisz, A.: The short- and long-term career effects of graduating in a recession. Am. Econ. J. Appl. Econ. **4**(1), 1–29 (2012)
14. Andersen, S.C., Nielsen, H.S.: Learning from performance information. J. Public Admin. Res. Theory. **30**(3), 415–431 (2020)
15. Murphy, R., Wyness, G.: Minority report: the impact of predicted grades on university admissions of disadvantaged groups. CEPEO Working Paper Series No 20-07 Centre for Education Policy and Equalising Opportunities, UCL Institute of Education (2020)
16. Burgess, S., Greaves, E.: Test scores, subjective assessment, and stereotyping of ethnic minorities. J. Labor Econ. **31**(3), 535–576 (2013)
17. Rangvid, B.S.: Systematic differences across evaluation schemes and educational choice. Econ. Educ. Rev. **48**, 41–55 (2015)
18. Maurin, E., McNally, S.: Vive la revolution! Long-term educational returns of 1968 to the angry students. J. Labor Econ. **26**(1), 1–33 (2008)
19. Piopiunik, M., Schwerdt, G., Simon, L., Woessman, L.: Skills, signals, and employability: an experimental investigation. Eur. Econ. Rev. **123**, 103374 (2020)
20. Fredriksson, P., Hensvik, L., Nordström Skans, O.: Mismatch of talent: evidence on match quality, entry wages, and job mobility. Am. Econ. Rev. **108**(11), 3303–3338 (2018)
21. https://www.thehindubusinessline.com/opinion/columns/the-cheat-sheet/digital-divide-in-times-of-covid-19/article31349014.ece
22. WHO. Coronavirus disease (COVID-2019) situation reports (2020). https://www.who.int/docs/default-source/coronaviruse/situation-reports/20200314-sitrep-54-covid-19.pdf. Accessed 25 Mar 2020
23. WHO. Coronavirus disease (COVID-19) pandemic (2020). https://www.who.int/emergencies/diseases/novel-coronavirus-2019. Accessed 20 Mar 2020

24. https://corporate.cyrilamarchandblogs.com/2020/05/covid-19-its-impact-on-the-telecommunications-sector-in-india/
25. Gewin, V.: Five tips for moving teaching online as COVID-19 takes hold. Nature. **580**(7802), 295–296 (2020). https://doi.org/10.1038/d41586-020-00896-7
26. THE. Will the coronavirus make online education go viral? (2020). https://www.timeshighereducation.com/features/will-coronavirus-make-online-education-go-viral. Accessed 24 May 2020
27. THE. Educating despite the COVID-19 outbreak: lessons from Singapore (2020). https://www.timeshighereducation.com/blog/educating-despite-covid-19-outbreak-lessons-singapore. Accessed 20 May 2020
28. https://www.weareteachers.com/free-online-learning-resources/
29. Shock, fear, and fatalism: as coronavirus prompts colleges to close, students grapple with uncertainty (2020). https://www.chronicle.com/article/Shock-FearFatalism-As/248240. Accessed 12 Mar 2020
30. Timmis, S., Broadfoot, P., Sutherland, R., Oldfield, A.: Rethinking assessment in a digital age: opportunities, challenges and risks. Br. Educ. Res. J. **42**, 454–476 (2016). https://doi.org/10.1002/berj.3215
31. Raaheim, A., Mathiassen, K., Moen, V., Lona, I., Gynnild, V., Bunæs, B.R., Hasle, E.T.: Digital assessment–how does it challenge local practices and national law? A Norwegian case study. Eur. J. High. Educ. **9**, 219–231 (2019). https://doi.org/10.1080/21568235.2018.1541420
32. Kearns, L.R.: Student assessment in online learning: challenges and effective practices. MERLOT J. Online Learn. Teach. **8**(3), 198–208 (2012) https://jolt.merlot.org/vol8no3/kearns_0912.pdf. Accessed 9 Mar 2020
33. Cheating in the digital age: do students cheat more in online courses? (2010). https://www.westga.edu/~distance/ojdla/spring131/watson131.html. Accessed 9 Mar 2020
34. Alruwais, N., Wills, G., Wald, M.: Advantages and challenges of using eAssessment. Int. J. Inf. Educ. Technol. **8**, 34–37 (2018). https://doi.org/10.18178/ijiet.2018.8.1.1008
35. https://www.khanacademy.org/
36. https://youtu.be/aaY9IkHHay8
37. https://www.microsoft.com/en-in/microsoft-365/microsoft-teams/group-chat-software
38. https://support.zoom.us/hc/en-us/articles/360029527911
39. https://support.skype.com/en/faq/FA10613/how-do-i-make-a-call-in-skype
40. https://www.youtube.com/watch?v=GbcrnI_TLy8
41. https://www.youtube.com/watch?v=M6L-nZGIUTE&feature=emb_rel_end
42. https://elearningindustry.com/mobile-based-education-apps-transforming-industry
43. Harvard University. Coronavirus (COVID-19) (2020). https://www.harvard.edu/coronavirus. Accessed 28 May 2020
44. Kawano, S., Kakehashi, M.: Substantial impact of school closure on the transmission dynamics during the pandemic flu H1N1-2009 in Oita, Japan. PLoS One. **10**, e0144839 (2015). https://doi.org/10.1371/journal.pone.0144839
45. Coronavirus COVID-19 global cases by the Center for Systems Science and Engineering (CSSE) at Johns Hopkins University (JHU) (2020). https://coronavirus.jhu.edu/map.html. Accessed 20 Mar 2020
46. Khachfe, H.H., Chahrour, M.A., Sammouri, J., Salhab, H.A., Eldeen Makki, B., Fares, M.Y.: An epidemiological study on COVID-19: a rapidly spreading disease. Cureus. **12**, e7313 (2020). https://doi.org/10.7759/cureus.7313
47. Remuzzi, A., & Remuzzi, G., "COVID-19 and Italy: what next?," The Lancet (2020)
48. Coronavirus COVID-19—latest update on Kingston University's response (2020). https://www.kingston.ac.uk/news/article/2306/27-mar-2020-coronavirus-covid19-latest-update-on-kingston-universitys-re. Accessed 27 Mar 2020

49. Bedford, J., Enria, D., Giesecke, J., Heymann, D.L., Ihekweazu, C., Kobinger, G., Lane, H.C., Memish, Z., Oh, M.D., Schuchat, A., Ungchusak, K.: COVID-19: towards controlling of a pandemic. The Lancet. **395**(10229), 1015–1018 (2020)
50. https://analyticsindiamag.com/adoption-of-e-learning-during-crises-lockdowns/
51. Al-Rabiaahab, A., Temsahabc, M.H., Al-Eyadhy, A.A., et al.: Middle East Respiratory Syndrome-Corona Virus (MERS-CoV) associated stress among medical students at a university teaching hospital in Saudi Arabia. J. Infect. Public Health. **13**(5), 687–691 (2020). https://doi.org/10.1016/j.jiph.2020.01.005

Chapter 11
Perspectives on the Definition of Data Visualization: A Mapping Study and Discussion on Coronavirus (COVID-19) Dataset

Ajantha Devi and Anand Nayyar

Abstract Data visualization is an arrangement that presents data in manners that enable the utilization of human subjective and visual capacities. It is the method used to convert crude information into some visual structure. It uses designs and visuals to help with the psychological burden of comprehending big data. The burden put on general well-being because of the coronavirus is exacerbated by the ceaseless rise of new strains and unanswered inquiries concerning viral spread inside the host. Observations regarding the course of coronaviruses in people have been step by step expanded and extended to numerous regions worldwide. These observation programs have created an enormous amount of genomic information regarding coronaviruses, which encourages the investigation of the infection by computational strategies that are proficient and cost effective.

The main focus of this chapter is the development of visualization techniques to comprehend the advancement of coronaviruses. The strategies depend on unaided dimensional decrease methods, which can be applied to every individual genome fragment or to the total genome succession of the infection. These strategies are a takeoff from the customary phylogenetic tree development worldview in light of the fact that an exceptionally enormous number of high-dimensional info arrangements can be prepared and results are seen legitimately in an a few-dimensional Euclidean space.

Keywords Data visualization · Coronavirus · Public health · Disease surveillance · Social network analysis

A. Devi (✉)
Research Head, AP3 Solutions, Chennai, Tamil Nadu, India
e-mail: ap3solutionsresearch@gmail.com

A. Nayyar (✉)
Graduate School, Faculty of Information Technology, Duy Tan University, Da Nang, Viet Nam
e-mail: anandnayyar@duytan.edu.vn

© The Author(s), under exclusive license to Springer Nature Switzerland AG 2021

F. Al-Turjman et al. (eds.), *Emerging Technologies for Battling Covid-19*, Studies in Systems, Decision and Control 324,
https://doi.org/10.1007/978-3-030-60039-6_11

11.1 Introduction

With the broad utilization of computers, huge amounts of data are generated every day in many different disciplines, including scientific and engineering fields, economics, and social sciences. The need to understand and develop insights from big data is urgent. However, the data are large, complex, and often unstructured, which makes it difficult for us to discover the underlying patterns and reveal the hidden relationships.

Dissimilar to the conventional investigation method, which combines the information into a few numbers, visualization approaches [1] couple human and machine analysis by utilizing the human visual framework to aid information revelation. Visualization permits more parts of the information to be watched and enables collaborations for increasingly deliberate investigation. The utilization of graphical diagrams gives a general way to change the information and its connections into a theoretical view for investigating complex connections and improving information understanding.

Producing graph-based portrayals for various types of data is challenging due to the following reasons. As a matter of first importance, users are keen on particular connections derived from different types of data. For multivariate data collections, they might be keen on considering the connections among factors. For instance, when the auto showcase is considered, they might need to know the correlation between price and brand.

11.2 Visualization of Scientific Data

Wang and Tao classified the methods utilizing graph-based portrayals in logical perception depending on their applications into four categories: partition-wise, relationship-wise, structure-wise, and provenance-wise. Works identified within this chapter fall into the categories of partition-wise and relationship-wise. In particular, the four connections reviewed here are as follows: hierarchical relationships, data evolution, variable relationships, and relationships among field lines.

11.2.1 Exploring Hierarchical Relationships

A tree is a unique sort of graph that does not contain cycles. It is often used to represent hierarchical relationships. In this subsection, we focus on two sorts of chains of important developments: data partitioning and data clustering.

Data Partitioning Data partitioning progressively parcels the spatiotemporal data into smaller pieces, which enables clients to analyze the data in a versatile way. Octree is a broadly utilized structure to segment a solitary volume. During preprocessing, they originally divided the data set into space-time squares utilizing an octree for singular compression. At that point, they pressed information checks into the illustration's memory, then remade and rendered the data in the GPU. In addition to being the inward structures for parcels, trees act as interfaces that guide clients in their investigation. Wang and Shen presented the hierarchical navigation interface, an interface with numerous planned perspectives for level-of-detail (LOD) choice and rendering. There are three perspectives: the volume rendering view, the tree view that displays the chain of command cut, and a tree map that assists clients with pinpointing the objective districts for exploration.

Data Clustering Other than dividing the area, different methodologies apply clustering techniques to group data pieces and structure chains of command that could be normally spoken to by trees. Gu and Wang applied three hierarchal clustering algorithms to gather the example focuses dependent on their connections and eliminate the pecking order when utilizing trees. Equal directions are used to visualize the connections between example focuses for each degree of the tree.

11.2.2 Understanding Data Evolution

Contemplating the advancement in a time-varying volumetric data is significant in numerous scientific and engineering fields. It enables researchers to watch the progressions and check their hypotheses. Graph-based perception aims at helping researchers to realize the development in the information through disentangling the fundamental advancement connections and picturing them as charts. A significant test is to distinguish highlights and concentrate the connections. One commonly utilized arrangement is distinguishing client-characterized highlights and matching them in neighboring time steps. Another arrangement is to examine the likelihood of changes starting with one component then onto the next, which permits emotional element changes.

Feature Matching For the component coordinating methodologies in 3D volume tracking, features are coordinated through their qualities or areas, under the assumption that the progressions in neighboring time steps are small. A commonly embraced technique extricates old limited features from each time step and afterward relates them over time.

11.3 Data Visualization Regarding the COVID-19 Pandemic

Data visualization [1–3] in its most fundamental structure is essentially mapping data to geometry and shading. In addition, a significant part of visuals is to have the option to guide to the information, ensuring that its substance is unblemished, and in any case, the visualizations will show up as only shapes. Having the option to pick a specific viewable signal is essential. These signs by and large change dependent on the job needing to be done, which relies upon how different shapes, sizes, and shades are seen. Figure 11.1 presents the ten most common prompts.

The main obvious sign is position, which helps in spotting clusters, patterns, and outliers by plotting all the information immediately. One model type is a scatterplot, where data centers, addressed as spots, are settled on a choice reliant on their *X* and *Y* arrangements and where they are comparative with others. Scatterplots can be valuable when the information is huge in size, because it draws all the information inside the *X*- and *Y*-plane, therefore requiring less space.

COVID-19 [4–6] is a fatal pandemic that the world is currently facing. The principle reason for coronavirus infection data-visualization [1–3] is to convey data unmistakably and viably utilize distinctive graphical presentations. Visualization is a helpful medium for examining, comprehending, and transmitting data because it has a few potential uses in the domain.

Python is viewed as one of the top programming languages for handling data visualization because it is recognized for its huge and dynamic logical figuring network and has numerous libraries that take into consideration more prominent adaptability. It can likewise control the particular components of the charts that are made and make those particulars repeatable through code. In addition, python is extraordinary at taking care of information and can handle a lot of information without crashing; it is particularly valuable for analyses and heavy computation. Finally, Python has a spotless and simple to-peruse sentence structure that software programmers like, and it can work off of a lot of modules to make information illustrations (Fig. 11.2).

1. Data acquisition: is the place where you read information from different wellsprings of unstructured information, semi structured information, or fully organized information that may be put in a spreadsheet, comma-isolated document, website page, database, and so forth.
2. Data cleaning: is the place where you expel uproarious information and set tasks expected to keep just the significant information.
3. Exploratory analysis: is the place where you inspect your cleaned information and make factual preparing fits for explicit examination purposes.
4. An analysis model should be made. Progressed apparatuses, for example, AI calculations, can be utilized in this progression.
5. Data visualization is the place the outcomes are plotted utilizing different frameworks provided by Python to help in the dynamic procedure.

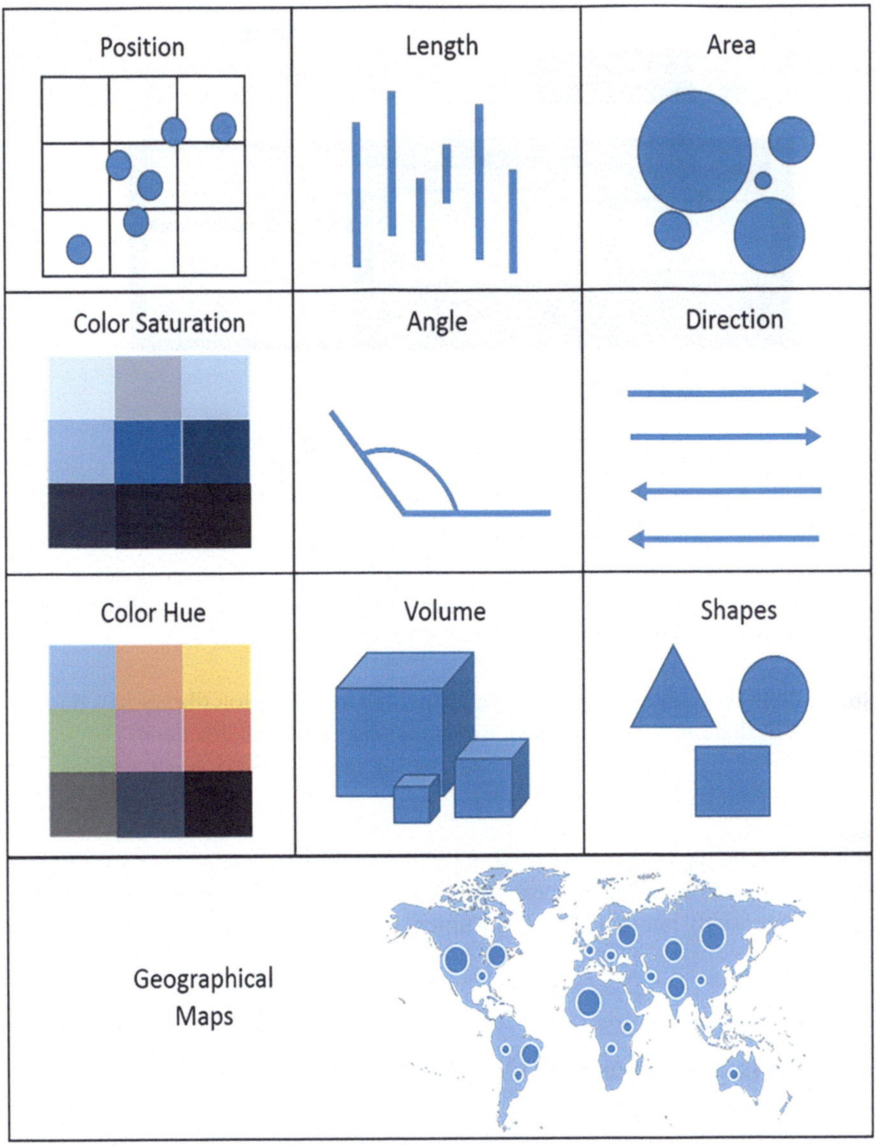

Fig. 11.1 Type of plots on visualization

11.3.1 Data Visualization Libraries

Matplotlib Matplotlib is one of the most famous Python bundles utilized for data visualization. It is a cross-platform library for making 2D plots from data in arrays. It gives an object-oriented API that helps in installing plots in applications utilizing Python GUI.

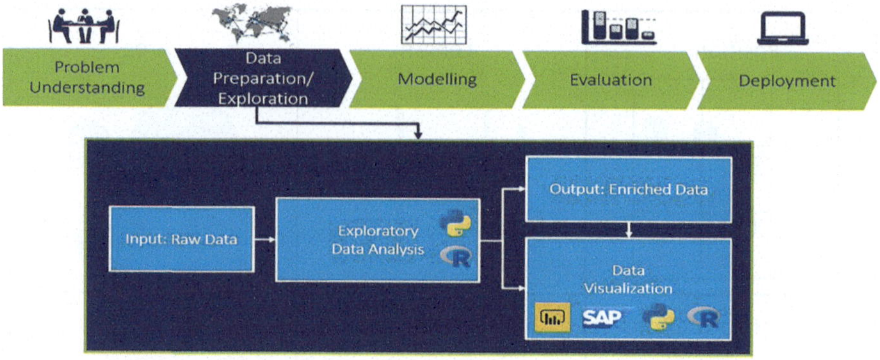

Fig. 11.2 Process of data visualization

Tool boxes, for example, PyQt and WxPythonotTkinter. It tends to be utilized in Python and IPython shells, Jupyter note pad and web application servers as well.

Seaborn It is a library based on Matplotlib. It enables one to make their representations prettier, and furnishes us with a portion of the basic data visualization needs (such as mapping a shading to a variable or utilizing faceting). Seaborn is increasingly incorporated for working with Pandas Data Frames.

Plotly Plotly.js is an explanatory JavaScript data visualization library based on D3 and WebGL that bolsters a wide scope of statistical, scientific, financial, geographic, and three-dimensional perceptions. Backing for making Plotly.js perceptions from Python is given by the plotly.py library.

Folium It tells the best way to make a Leaflet web map from scratch with Python and the Folium library. The process should create a map.html document. Afterward, you can essentially put that HTML document on a live server and have the guide on the web.

11.4 Data Visualization: Case Study on COVID-19

COVID-19 has affected more than 11 million individuals worldwide and in excess of 500,000 lives in Europe and the United States, overwhelming the numbers in China [7–10] where the pandemic began last December. The World Health Organization (WHO) announced the coronavirus a pandemic because of the across the board size of the episode and has cautioned that the most extreme period of COVID-19 [4–6] is yet to come. The United Nations said the coronavirus pandemic is the most noticeably awful worldwide emergency since World War II.

In this examination, we perform a time-intermittent observation of COVID-19 in the adjoining United States [11] utilizing an imminent space-time check measurement. We recognize developing groups of COVID-19 [4, 5] in the United States at the province level, and give day-by-day results [12] during the investigation time of January 22, 2020–June 25, 2020.

11.4.1 COVID-19 Confirmed Cases Using Plotly with Scattergeo

See Figs. 11.3 and 11.4.

```
In [11]: df['text'] = df['Country'] + " " + df["4/13/20"].astype(str)
         fig = go.Figure(data = go.Scattergeo(
             lon = df["Long"],
             lat = df["Lat"],
             text = df["text"],
             mode = "markers",
             marker = dict(
                 size = 12,
                 opacity = 0.8,
                 reversescale = True,
                 autocolorscale = True,
                 symbol = 'square',
                 line = dict(
                     width = 1,
                     color = 'rgba(102, 102, 102)'
                 ),
                 cmin = 0,
                 color = df['4/13/20'],
                 cmax = df['4/13/20'].max(),
                 colorbar_title = "COVID 19 Reported Cases "
             )
         ))

         fig.update_layout(
             title = "COVID19 Confirmed Cases Around the World as on 13th April 2020",
             geo = dict(
                 scope = "world",
                 showland = True,
             )
         )
         fig.write_html('first_figure.html', auto_open=True)
```

Fig. 11.3 COVID-19 confirmed cases: code using Plotly

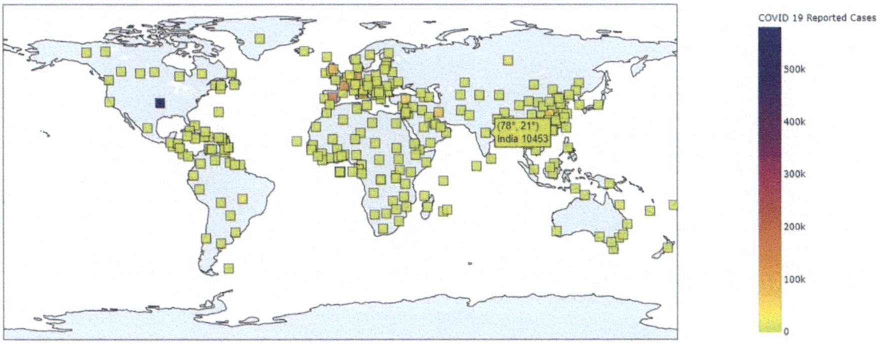

Fig. 11.4 COVID-19 confirmed cases worldwide as of April 13, 2020

11.4.2 COVID-19 Confirmed Cases Using Plotly with Express

Plotly with Express is a high-level API that wraps a graph object, where a multi-bar plot can be implemented in a single line (Figs. 11.5 and 11.6).

- All the nations began to recognize COVID-19 cases from the end of January with the exception of China [7–10], which revealed to the world that the focal point of the infection was in China.
- China showed a development in number of cases from January till mid-February, and after that, the quantity of cases has been consistent in China.
- The United States [11] has been the most noticeably affected nation in the world, and as of April 19 the quantity of cases that had been contracted was 700,000 and it had expanded to in excess of 800,000 on April 22, 2020.
- Italy, Spain, and France [11, 13–17] nearly follow a similar example and the quantity of cases contracted there was approximately 200,000 as of April 22, 2020.
- In India, the condition was better contrasted with different nations [18, 19] as the quantity of cases contracted was just 22,000, which is extremely few when contrasted with different nations as of April 22, 2020.

```
In [6]: fig = px.line(df_filtered, x="Date", y = "Confirmed_Plus", color="Country/Region",
                      title="Daily Confirmed Cases In Five Asian Countries")
        fig.write_html('first_figure.html', auto_open=True)
```

Fig. 11.5 COVID-19 confirmed cases: code using Plotly with Express

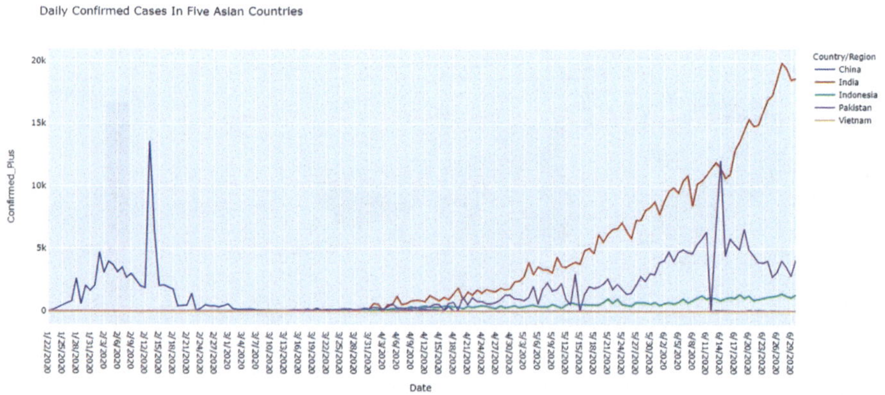

Fig. 11.6 COVID-19 confirmed cases worldwide as of June 29, 2020

11.4.3 Reported COVID-19 Cases Using Plotly with Choropleth

- A geometry as a geojson object. This is the place where things are somewhat befuddling and not obviously referenced in its documentation. You might give a geojson object. On the off chance that you give a geojson object, at that point, that item will be utilized to plot the earth highlights, yet in the event that you do not give a geojson object, at that point, the capacity will, as a matter of course, utilize one of the inherent geometries.
- A pandas DataFrame object for the characteristic data_frame. Here we label our DataFrame, new_df, as we did before.
- We will utilize the information of the confirmed section to choose the shade of every nation polygon.
- Further, we will utilize the date segment to make the animation_frame. In this way, as we slide over the dates, the shades of the nations will change according to the qualities in the confirmed segment (Figs. 11.7 and 11.8).

Instances of coronavirus disease 2019 (COVID-19) are expanding exponentially in Europe and North America, as shown in Fig. 11.9. These settings have among the most vigorous readiness plans; in any case, most have been not able to satisfy the requirements placed on their well-being frameworks by this pandemic. In total, 33% of nations have abilities to react to a well-being crisis in accordance with the International Health Guidelines. Struggling nations are lopsidedly influenced

```
In [4]: colors = ["#F9F9F5", "#FAFAE6", "#FCFCCB", "#FCFCAE",  "#FCF1AE", "#FCEA7D", "#FCD97D",
                  "#FCCE7D", "#FCC07D", "#FEB562", "#F9A648",  "#F98E48", "#FD8739", "#FE7519",
                  "#FE5E19", "#FA520A", "#FA2B0A", "#9B1803",  "#861604", "#651104", "#570303",]


        fig = go.Figure(data=go.Choropleth(
            locationmode = "country names",
            locations = new_df['Country'],
            z = new_df['Total_Cases'],
            text = new_df['Total_Cases'],
            colorscale = colors,
            autocolorscale=False,
            reversescale=False,
            colorbar_title = 'Reported Covid-19 Cases',
        ))

        fig.update_layout(
            title_text='Reported Covid-19 Cases as on 13th April 2020',
            geo=dict(
                showcoastlines=True,
            ),
        )

        fig.write_html('first_figure.html', auto_open=True)
```

Fig. 11.7 Reported COVID-19 cases: code using Plotly

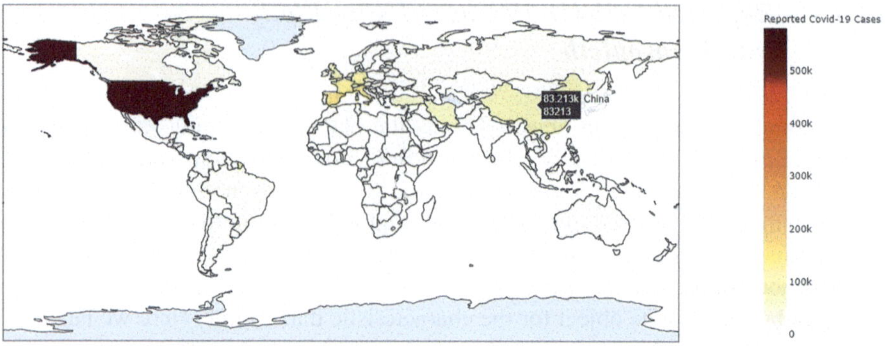

Fig. 11.8 Reported COVID-19 cases worldwide as of April 13, 2020—China

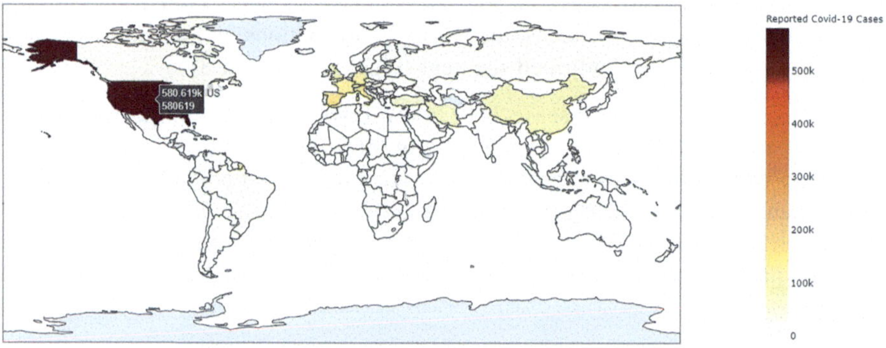

Fig. 11.9 Reported COVID-19 cases worldwide as of April 13, 2020—US

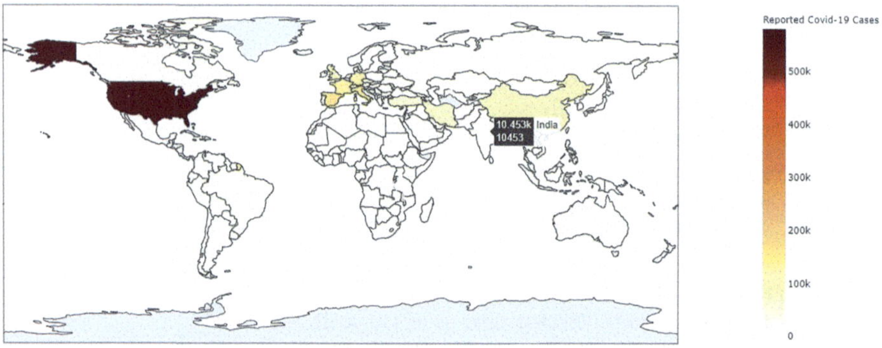

Fig. 11.10 Reported COVID-19 cases worldwide as of April 13, 2020—India

because of the results of contention on their well-being frameworks, foundations, establishments, economies, and general public well-being, leaving them badly arranged to oversee pandemics, for example, COVID-19 (Fig. 11.10).

11.4.4 COVID-19 Daily Confirmed and Recovery Cases in India: Bar Chart

See Figs. 11.11, 11.12, 11.13, and 11.14.

11.4.5 Recovery Rate in Italy: Using Plotly with Indicator and Gauge Mode

The reason for "indicator" is to picture a solitary worth determined by the "value" property. Three unmistakable visual components are accessible to speak to that value: number, delta, and check. Any mix of them can be determined through the "mode" attribute. High level attributes are:

```
In [7]: filterIn = df_filtered["Country/Region"] == "India"
        df_In = df_filtered[filterIn]

        fig = px.bar(df_In, title= "COVID-19 Daily Confirmed and Recovery Cases in India", x="Date", y="Confirmed_Plus",
                     color="Recovered_Plus",
                     labels={"Confirmed_Plus": "New Confirmed Cases"},
                     hover_data=["Confirmed_Plus", "Recovered_Plus", "Deaths_Plus"])
        fig.write_html('first_figure.html', auto_open=True)
```

Fig. 11.11 COVID-19 daily confirmed and recovery: code for Bar chart—India

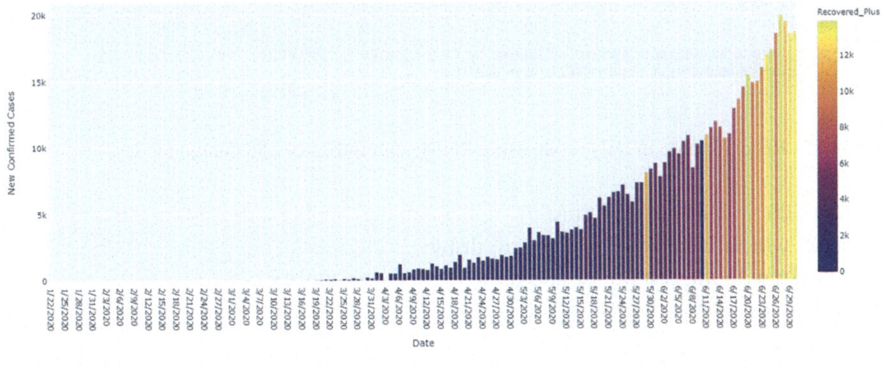

Fig. 11.12 COVID-19 daily confirmed and recovery cases in India—Bar chart—India

```
In [11]: filterIt = df_filtered["Country/Region"] == "Italy"
         df_It = df_filtered[filterIt]

         fig = px.bar(df_It, title= "COVID-19 Daily Confirmed and Recovery Cases in Italy", x="Date", y="Confirmed_Plus",
                      color="Recovered_Plus",
                      labels={"Confirmed_Plus": "New Confirmed Cases"},
                      hover_data=["Confirmed_Plus", "Recovered_Plus", "Deaths_Plus"])
         fig.write_html('first_figure.html', auto_open=True)
```

Fig. 11.13 COVID-19 daily confirmed and recovery: code for Bar chart—Italy

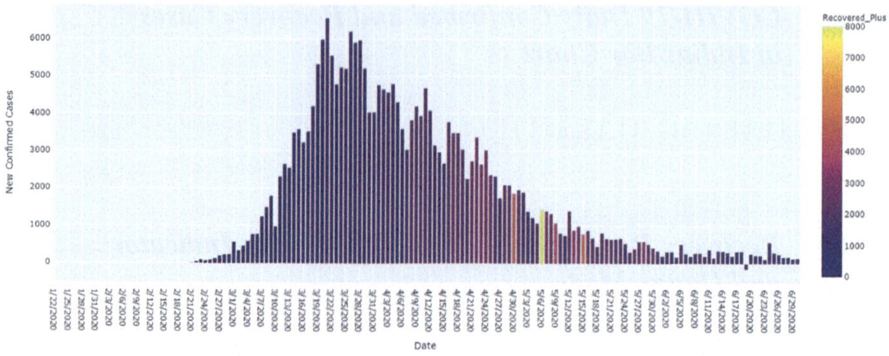

Fig. 11.14 COVID-19 daily confirmed and recovery: cases in India—Bar chart—Italy

```
In [26]: import plotly.graph_objects as go

         fig = go.Figure(go.Indicator(
             mode = "gauge+number",
             value = 48877,
             domain = {'x': [0, 1], 'y': [0, 1]},
             title = {'text': "Recovery in Italy"},
             gauge = {
                         'axis': {'range': [None, 160000], 'tickwidth': 1, 'tickcolor': "darkblue"},
                         'bar': {'color': "darkblue"},
                         'steps' : [
                             {'range': [0, 40000], 'color': "lightcoral"},
                             {'range': [40001, 80000], 'color': "orange"},
                             {'range': [80001, 120000], 'color': "yellow"},
                             {'range': [120001, 160000], 'color': "green"}
                         ],

                         'threshold' : {'line': {'color': "red", 'width': 4}, 'thickness': 0.75, 'value': 157114}
                     }
         ))

         fig.update_layout(paper_bgcolor = "lavender", font = {'color': "darkblue", 'family': "Arial"})
         fig.write_html('first_figure.html', auto_open=True)
```

Fig. 11.15 Recovery rate in Italy: code using Plotly with Indicator and Gauge mode

- value: the incentive to picture
- mode: which visual components to draw
- align: how to align number and delta (left, focus, right)
- domain: the degree of the figure (Figs. 11.15, 11.16, 11.17 and 11.18)

11.4.6 COVID-19 Confirmed Cases Using Seaborn

Seaborn gives profoundly appealing and useful charts/plots. It is anything but difficult to utilize and is blazingly quick. It tends to be utilized to manufacture practically every statistical chart. It is based on matplotlib, which is likewise a visualization library. Seaborn is a dataset [12] with arranged plotting capacity that can be utilized regarding the two information types: casings and exhibits. It improves the representation intensity of matplotlib, which is only utilized for fundamental plotting such as visual diagrams, line graphs, and pie charts (Figs. 11.19 and 11.20).

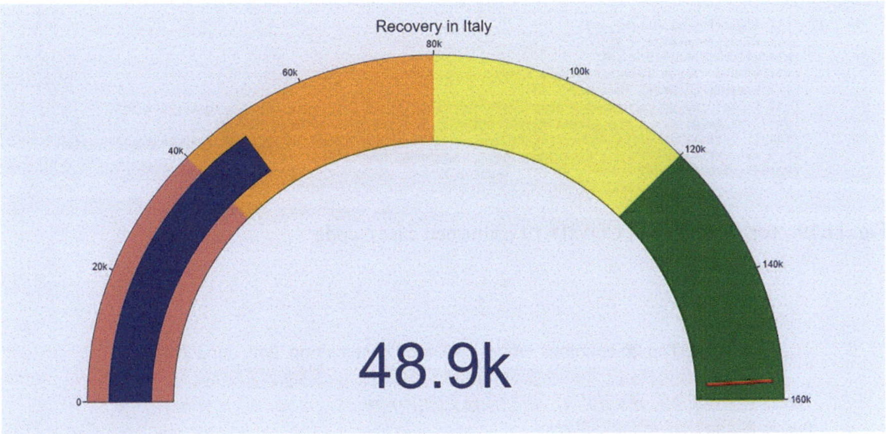

Fig. 11.16 Recovery rate in Italy: using Plotly with Indicator and Gaüge mode

```
In [15]: fig = go.Figure(go.Indicator(
             mode = "gauge+number",
             value = 80587,
             domain = {'x': [0, 1], 'y': [0, 1]},
             title = {'text': "Recovery rate in Spain"},
             gauge = {
                         'axis': {'range': [None, 180000], 'tickwidth': 1, 'tickcolor': "darkblue"},
                         'bar': {'color': "darkblue"},
                         'steps' : [
                             {'range': [0, 50000], 'color': "lightcoral"},
                             {'range': [50001, 100000], 'color': "orange"},
                             {'range': [100001, 150000], 'color': "yellow"},
                             {'range': [150001, 180000], 'color': "green"}
                         ],

                         'threshold' : {'line': {'color': "red", 'width': 4}, 'thickness': 0.75, 'value': 179358}
                     }
         ))

         fig.update_layout(paper_bgcolor = "lavender", font = {'color': "darkblue", 'family': "Arial"})
         fig.write_html('first_figure.html', auto_open=True)
```

Fig. 11.17 Recovery rate in Spain: code using Plotly with Indicator and Gauge mode

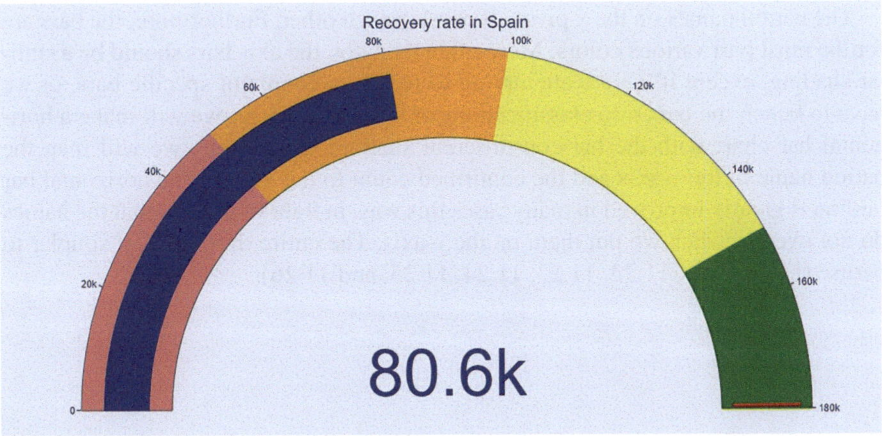

Fig. 11.18 Recovery rate in Spain: using Plotly with Indicator and Gauge mode

```
In [51]: plt.figure(figsize= (15,10))
         plt.xticks(fontsize = 15)
         plt.yticks(fontsize = 15)
         plt.xlabel("Total cases",fontsize = 30)
         plt.ylabel('Country',fontsize = 30)
         plt.title("Top 20 countries - most confirmed cases as on 24th June 2020" , fontsize = 25)
         ax = sns.barplot(x = top_casualities.confirmed, y = top_casualities.country)
         for i, (value, name) in enumerate(zip(top_casualities.confirmed,top_casualities.country)):
             ax.text(value, i-.05, f'{value:,.0f}',  size=10, ha='left',  va='center')
         ax.set(xlabel='Total cases', ylabel='Country')
```

Fig. 11.19 Top 20 countries COVID-19 confirmed cases: code

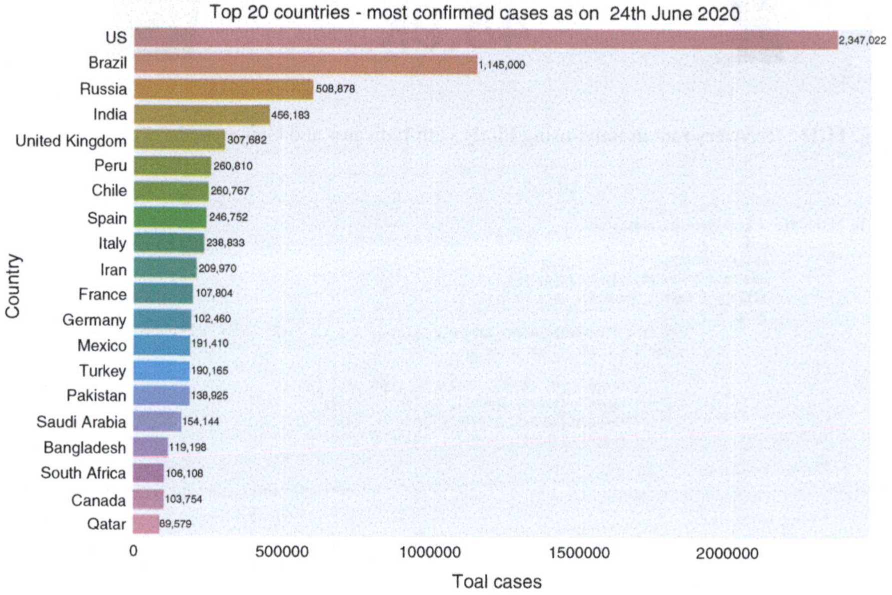

Fig. 11.20 Top 20 countries COVID-19 confirmed cases worldwide as of June 24, 2020

The nation names on the x pivot all overlap each other. Furthermore, the bars are for the most part various colors. More often than not, the axis bars should be a similar shading, except if we are attempting to feature a couple of specific bars, or we have to bunch the bars into classifications of some sort. Here, we will make a horizontal bar chart with the bars on different shading. To do this, we will map the nation name to the *y*-axis and the confirmed count to the *x*-axis. The horizontal bar outline is greatly improved in many cases this way, in light of the fact that the names do not overlap when we put them on the *y*-axis. The entire thing is a lot simpler to peruse (Figs. 11.21, 11.22, 11.23, 11.24, 11.25, and 11.26).

```
In [53]: plt.figure(figsize= (15,10))
         plt.xticks(fontsize = 15)
         plt.yticks(fontsize = 15)
         plt.xlabel("Total cases",fontsize = 30)
         plt.ylabel('Country',fontsize = 30)
         plt.title("Top 20 countries - most active cases as on 24th June 2020" , fontsize = 25)
         ax = sns.barplot(x = top_actives.active, y = top_actives.country)
         for i, (value, name) in enumerate(zip(top_actives.active, top_actives.country)):
             ax.text(value, i-.05, f'{value:,.0f}',  size=10, ha='left',  va='center')
         ax.set(xlabel='Total cases', ylabel='Country')
```

Fig. 11.21 Top 20 countries COVID-19 active cases: code

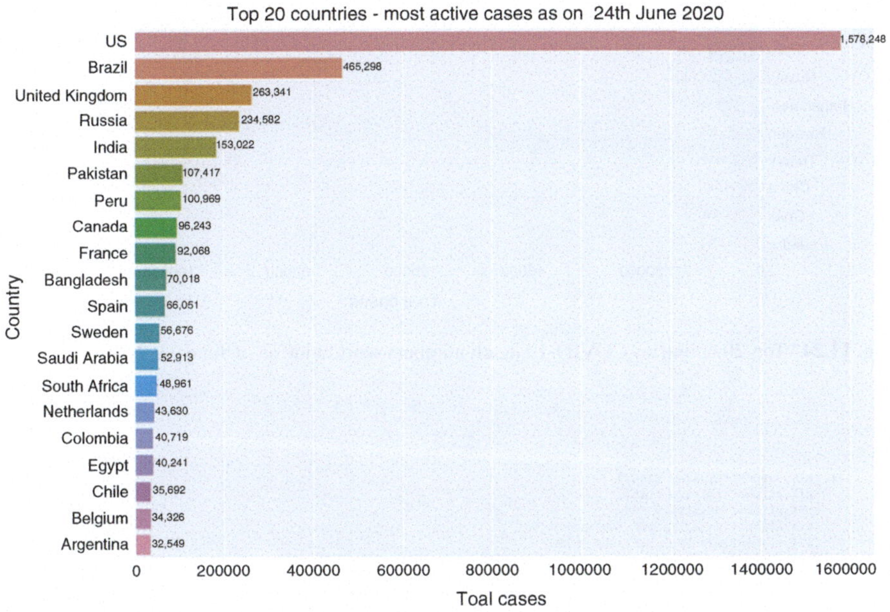

Fig. 11.22 Top 20 countries COVID-19 active cases worldwide as of June 24, 2020

```
In [55]: plt.figure(figsize= (15,10))
         plt.xticks(fontsize = 15)
         plt.yticks(fontsize = 15)
         plt.xlabel("Total cases",fontsize = 30)
         plt.ylabel('Country',fontsize = 30)
         plt.title("Top 20 countries - most deaths as on 24th June 2020" , fontsize = 25)
         ax = sns.barplot(x = top_deaths.deaths, y = top_deaths.country)
         for i, (value, name) in enumerate(zip(top_deaths.deaths,top_deaths.country)):
             ax.text(value, i-.05, f'{value:,.0f}',  size=10, ha='left',  va='center')
         ax.set(xlabel='Total cases', ylabel='Country')
```

Fig. 11.23 Top 20 countries COVID-19 death numbers: code

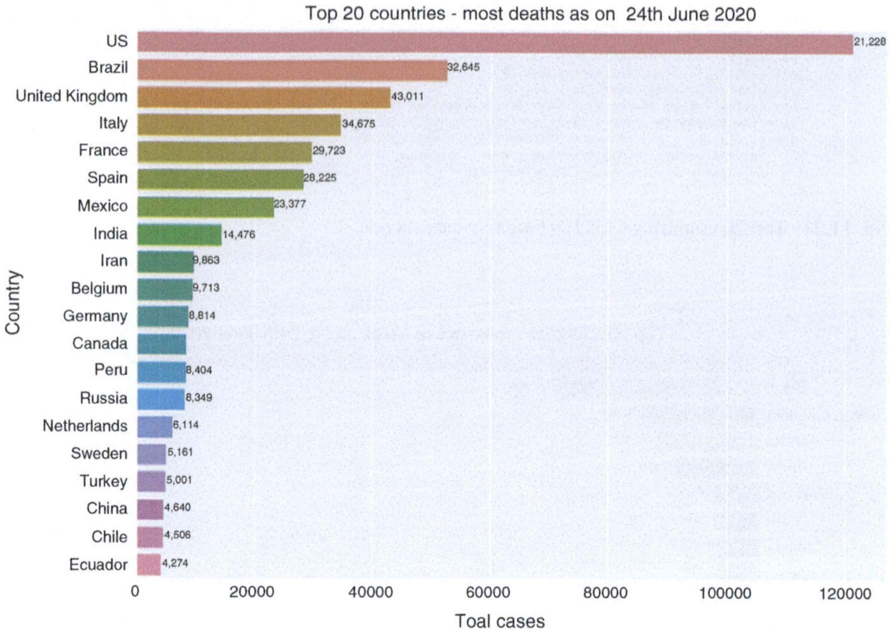

Fig. 11.24 Top 20 countries COVID-19 death numbers worldwide as of June 24, 2020

```
In [57]: plt.figure(figsize= (15,10))
         plt.xticks(fontsize = 15)
         plt.yticks(fontsize = 15)
         plt.xlabel("Total cases",fontsize = 30)
         plt.ylabel('Country',fontsize = 30)
         plt.title("Top 20 countries - most recovered cases as on 24th June 2020" , fontsize = 25)
         ax = sns.barplot(x = top_recovered.recovered, y = top_recovered.country)
         for i, (value, name) in enumerate(zip(top_recovered.recovered,top_recovered.country)):
             ax.text(value, i-.05, f'{value:,.0f}',  size=10, ha='left',  va='center')
         ax.set(xlabel='Total cases', ylabel='Country')
```

Fig. 11.25 Top 20 countries COVID-19 recovered cases: code

11.5 Conclusion

In this chapter, initially we showed the complete number of instances of COVID-19 alongside the absolute recovered and losses over the continents with the assistance of plots and outlines. From the data introduced and cases assessed above, we infer that among various countries, the USA has been seriously affected by COVID-19 as contrasted with different nations [18, 19]. Various elements have driven a few nations to endure a higher infection rate than others. Subsequent to contemplating, we have arrived at the resolution that lockdown and travel limitations have assumed a significant role in containing COVID-19.

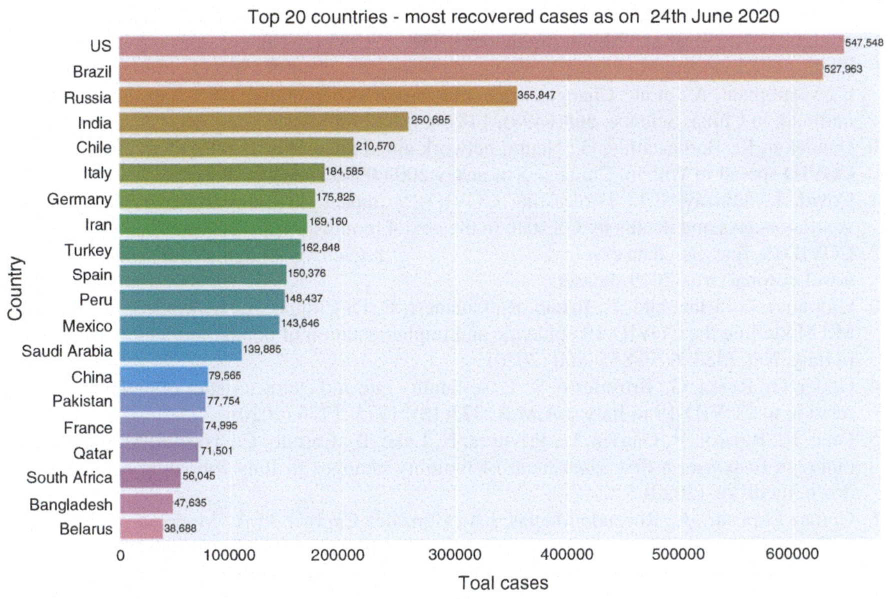

Fig. 11.26 Top 20 countries COVID-19 recovered cases worldwide as of June 24, 2020

We have likewise presumed that because COVID-19 has an elevated number of cases that this implies it has a noteworthy infectiousness as compared with other plagues and has a lower death rate.

References

1. Mohammed, T.T., Al-ameen, S.: SSCSMCS 2019 data visualization with real world data using Python. ResearchGate, April (2019). https://www.researchgate.net/publication/333671090_Data_Visualization_with_Real_World_Data_Using_Python
2. Oberoi, A., Chauhan, R.: Visualizing data using Matplotlib and Seaborn libraries in Python for data science. Int. J. Sci. Res. Publ. **9**(3), p8733 (2019). https://doi.org/10.29322/ijsrp.9.03.2019.p8733
3. Weihs, C., Ickstadt, K.: Data science: the impact of statistics. Int. J. Data Sci. Anal. **6**(3), 189–194 (2018). https://doi.org/10.1007/s41060-018-0102-5
4. Sajadi, M.M., Habibzadeh, P., Vintzileos, A., Shokouhi, S., Miralles-Wilhelm, F., Amoroso, A.: Temperature and latitude analysis to predict potential spread and seasonality for COVID-19. [ISSRN 3550308] (2020)
5. Bukhari, Q., Jameel, Y.: Will coronavirus pandemic diminish by summer? [ISSRN 3556998] (2020)
6. Wang, J., Tang, K., Feng, K., Lv, W.: High temperature and high humidity reduce the transmission of COVID-19. [ISSRN 3551767] (2020)
7. Zhou, F., Yu, T., Du, R., Fan, G., Liu, Y., Liu, Z., Xiang, J., Wang, Y., Song, B., Gu, X., et al.: Clinical course and risk factors for mortality of adult inpatients with COVID-19 in Wuhan, China: a retrospective cohort study. Lancet. **395**, 1054–1062 (2020)

8. Leung, C.: Risk factors for predicting mortality in elderly patients with COVID-19: a review of clinical data in China. Mech. Ageing Dev. **188**, 111255 (2020)
9. Zhang, J., Litvinova, M., Liang, Y., Wang, Y., Wang, W., Zhao, S., Wu, Q., Merler, S., Viboud, C., Vespignani, A., et al.: Changes in contact patterns shape the dynamics of the COVID-19 outbreak in China. Science. **368**(6498), 1481–1486 (2020)
10. Dandekar, R., Barbastathis, G.: Neural network aided quarantine control model estimation of COVID spread in Wuhan, China. arXiv, arXiv:2003.09403 (2020)
11. Covid, I., Murray, C.J.: Forecasting COVID-19 impact on hospital bed-days, ICU-days, ventilator-days and deaths by US state in the next 4 months. medRxiv (2020)
12. COVID19_line_list_data.csv. https://www.kaggle.com/sudalairajkumar/novel-corona-virus-2019-dataset
13. Giordano, G., Blanchini, F., Bruno, R., Colaneri, P., Di Filippo, A., Di Matteo, A., Colaneri, M.: Modelling the COVID-19 epidemic and implementation of population-wide interventions in Italy. Nat. Med. **6**(6), 855–860 (2020)
14. Onder, G., Rezza, G., Brusaferro, S.: Case-fatality rate and characteristics of patients dying in relation to COVID-19 in Italy. J.A.M.A. **323**(18), 1775–1776 (2020)
15. Pepe, E., Bajardi, P., Gauvin, L., Privitera, F., Lake, B., Cattuto, C., Tizzoni, M.: COVID-19 outbreak response: a first assessment of mobility changes in Italy following national lockdown. medRxiv (2020)
16. Gómez Expósito, A., Rosendo Macías, J.A., González Cagigal, M.Á.: Modelado y Análisis de la Evolución de una Epidemia Vírica Mediante Filtros de Kalman: El Caso del COVID-19 en España; Technical report; Universidad de Sevilla: Sevilla, Spain (2020)
17. Oliver, N., Barber, X., Roomp, K., Roomp, K.: The covid19 impact survey: assessing the pulse of the COVID-19 pandemic in Spain via 24 questions. arXiv, arXiv:2004.01014 (2020)
18. Sayre, R., Karagulle, D., Frye, C., Boucher, T., Wolff, N.H., Breyer, S., Touval, J.: An assessment of the representation of ecosystems in global protected areas using new maps of world climate regions and world ecosystems. Global Ecol. Conserv. **21**, e00860 (2020). https://doi.org/10.1016/j.gecco.2019.e00860
19. Average yearly temperature by country, Lebanese Economy Forum. https://web.archive.org/web/20150905135247/http://lebanese-economyforum.com/wdi-gdf-advanced-datadisplay/show/EN-CLC-AVRT-C/. Last Accessed 13 Apr 2020

Chapter 12
Disaster Management Using Recent Technologies During COVID-19

Ruby Jain, Manimala Puri, and Bhuvan Jain

Abstract As we came across in earlier chapters, during the time of worldwide lockdown, various sectors like industry, healthcare, and agriculture are facing a lot of difficulty in meeting the basic needs of the people due to issues identified in supply chain management. Apart from addressing the discussed problems, governments have various other issues to address, such as enforcing the proper lockdown among the people; providing the citizens with basic necessities like food, groceries, and vegetables, from the retailers; enforcing and monitoring law and order during the lockdown period pertaining to areas like transportation, markets, shops, public gatherings, and medical facilities; and identification and treatment of people suffering from coronavirus attack. Apart from these general issues, there were some other challenges faced that attracted attention such as blocking of false messages generated, related to COVID-19, etc. The chapter aims at addressing these issues using various technologies like drones for monitoring activity, AI technology for planning and prediction in order to curtail the growth rate of coronavirus infections using algorithms, etc.

Keywords Spoofing of malicious messages · Drones · AI algorithm · Economic slowdown · COVID-19 · Technological era

---

R. Jain (✉) · M. Puri
Symbiosis Skills and Professional University, Pune, India
e-mail: ruby.jain@ssou.ac.in

B. Jain
DPU IDL Pune, Pune, India

© The Author(s), under exclusive license to Springer Nature Switzerland AG 2021

F. Al-Turjman et al. (eds.), *Emerging Technologies for Battling Covid-19*, Studies in Systems, Decision and Control 324,
https://doi.org/10.1007/978-3-030-60039-6_12

12.1 Introduction

The lesson taught by COVID-19 disaster calls for a huge measure of attentiveness toward health organization. It is crucial in the country to tackle such disasters, which appeared all of a sudden and affected a huge number of people irrespective of geographic boundaries with tremendous pace and virulence. Acceptable readiness in health-related infrastructure is never wasteful, and same infrastructure can come handy in the future as well—whether natural or human-influenced pandemic [1]. Since COVID-19 is a contiguous infection, relevant reframing of health organizations may be required to tackle such disasters [2].

While deliberating natural disasters, apart from earthquakes, the other common natural disasters include cyclone, flood, drought, and Tsunami; early warning systems are already in place in India [3]. Issuance and dissemination of such early warnings in India are well institutionalized by the respective nodal agencies and National/State Disaster Management Agencies, For all kind of disasters its not possible to have preparations already available and on the same way all distasters can't always be attentive [4].

For landslides, due to non-availability of credible statistics, forecast of its time of manifestation is challenging, and India is still not prepared with any efficient operational chronological forecast model for initial warning. For 60% of landslide-prone areas (2.55 lakh km^2), India is now conscious about the spatial positions where forthcoming landslides are likely to occur due to the attendance of a trigger, which in utmost cases is the sophisticated volume of torrential rainfall [5]. GSI, being the nodal agency for landslides, has already prepared and uploaded such geo-information on landslide susceptibility maps on its Bhukosh web portal to be used in 17 landslide-prone states [6].

Tehsil/district-level shelter homes are required to save human lives. One of the major consequences of COVID-19 is the possible protraction or hesitation, and preserving social distance (a basic requirement in case of COVID-19) would be an issue in such shelter homes [7].

This may result in an obvious space crisis in such shelter homes and may lead to additional expenses in obtaining and dealing with more number of provisional shelters. For arrangement, such parameters should continuously be taken into account [8].

It is always useful to accept the fact that the annual recurrence of such natural disasters due to heavy rainfall will remain; therefore, extra caution and satisfactory readiness must be ascertained in case of such natural disasters by all the concerned agencies.

Basically, this chapter is further divided in six sections including introduction, and Sect. 12.2 includes measures undertaken by the government to control COVID-19 like restriction of mass gathering, maintaining social distancing, and lockdown. Section 12.3 addresses issues faced due to lockdown like economic slowdown, country-based statistics about unemployment, and social impact of lockdown. Section 12.4 focuses on new technologies to help handle the pandemic. The impact of COVID-19 on financial sector, supply chain industry, transportation, warehousing, inventory management, healthcare, and safety in offices is discussed. Section 12.5 addresses technologies that can be used to address issues like drones as surveillance camera, drones as broadcasting machine, and AI-based technologies like ML- and NLP-based solutions. Section 12.6 addresses the impact of research in dealing with the epidemic by call for papers and designing specify search engines and so.

12.2 Measures Undertaken by the Government to Control COVID-19

The new policies introduced by the government to control the pandemic are as follows [9, 10]:

1. Restriction of mass gathering: Various countries have implemented lockdown as a measure to control the wide spread of coronavirus. The measures undertaken have resulted in closing of malls, market places, universities, and factories as well as travel restrictions and freeze on transport facilities, giving rise to various losses incurred upon sectors such as industry, retail markets, education, and tourism.
2. Social distancing: Post lockdown, social distancing has restricted the productivity of major sectors that are currently operating with 30% of operating staff; such companies are struggling in order to maintain their financial margins [11].
3. Lockdown: The complete lockdown called upon by the government has almost put a halt to the operation of various sectors apart from those operating over virtual or online platforms. This measure has said to have brought a major setback to the sectors operating in physical spaces but has favored those companies operating on virtual platforms due to the sudden shift of various sectors such as education, delivery, and purchase markets into online mode.

12.3 Issues Faced Due to Lockdown

The lockdown and various other policies implemented by the government have resulted in the following issues [12].

12.3.1 Economic Slowdown

Taking an example of the 2008 Financial Crisis, COVID-19 put the same yet severe strain on the economy all over the world. Since the beginning of COVID-19, the fear of the contagion has taken the operational capability of the market to a downtrend, eventually leading many countries to implement lockdown measures, which also affect the financial markets as well. Upcoming reports from WTO and other government and nongovernment agencies suggest and forecast the financial downturn of their respective economy [13].

Due to the economic crisis, the expected losses have touched one trillion USD all over the world, which has also impacted the investor psychology due to the spread of the virus. Loss of wealth has put the pressure on major investors to direct the investment from equity to safe products, i.e., bonds and government securities, due to which the heavy pull over equities has taken the market down to negative return [14]. The impact does not only affect the equities but also the commodity market. Since the COVID-19 spread, oil price has been heavily affected. On April 27, 2020, West Texas Intermediate (WTI) oil price benchmark index turns index closing at −37.63 a barrel. Brent Crude reaches 18-year low to 20$ a barrel, making a new high in US oil inventories [15].

The recession has been affecting the third-world countries, which is apparently due to heavy pressure on meeting the fiscal target and barely be able to run the economic cycle. To increase the debt and put more pressure on the balance sheet and to raise funds and broaden the fiscal deficit, major economies such as USA which was severely affected during the 2008 crisis has pumped $2.3 trillion into the economy to keep the liquidity in check. Unfortunately, this event is inevitable in nature and has been testing each and every government's decision-making with respect to running the economy. However, it is yet to be ascertained the extent to which this crisis is going to test the world economy [16].

12.3.2 *Unemployment*

Another major factor that has been impacted due to COVID-19 is the unemployment rate and the value addition that has been created by it. Due to heavy lockdown, a large number of workforce have been out of job, and a large number of small-scale businesses have been affected for not being able to meet the working capital requirement, therefore leading them to shut down [17].

The unemployment rate in India has touched a record high of 27.11%. Considering the population in India, due to the unavailability of proper data with respect to the unorganized sector, the given number might be much higher, affecting the large part of small-scale businesses in the environment. Although not all businesses have been affected, the essential service sectors are still active, i.e., hospital and FMCG, pharmacies and electricity, water supply, etc. Although these sectors are facing pressure from both demand and supply side, operation capability is under control [14, 16].

At the moment, India is on the verge of crossing two million mark of COVID-19 cases, unfolding the large-scale movement of people from their work city to their home town and facing issues such as the unavailability of transport, food, and shelter. As part of fiscal measure, the Government has started providing the minimum wage of Rs. 500 to the citizens below the poverty line to meet their essential needs [18].

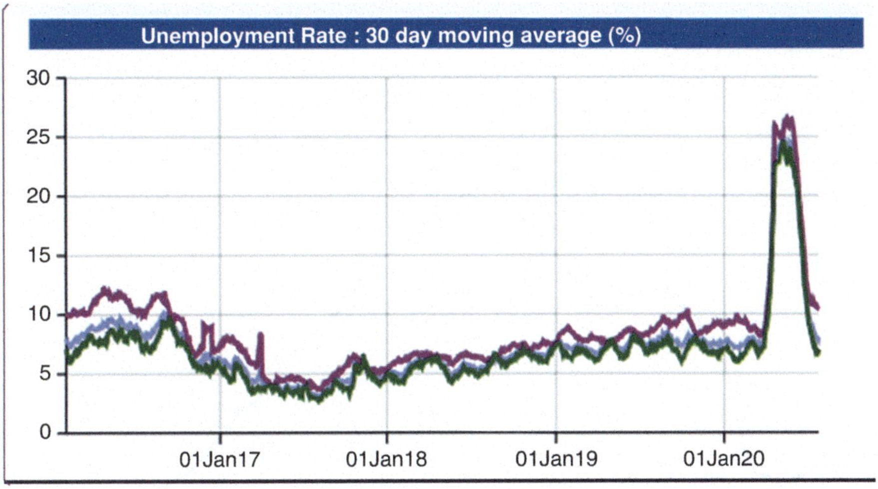

Fig. 12.1 Unemployment comparison for 2017–2020

By considering the state of employment in developed countries, which has be facing/faced extreme rise in the COVID-19 cases, had to face the major push back in the employment sector. Figure 12.1 shows the rate of employment projected for 2019–2020 in comparison to 2018–2019.

Various countries facing the issue of unemployment due to COVID-19 are discussed as follows [18, 19]:

12.3.2.1 Italy

In Italy, the unemployment rate has dropped to 8.4% in March, touching the lowest of 9 years. Due to heavy lockdown and fear among the people for not going out, the job market has dropped sharply. Economists suggest that the situation could be worse and the unemployment rate could even drop to 10.5%. Eventually, it leads to become a contouring factor for unemployment in European Union.

12.3.2.2 European Countries

From years market recovery has been on a recovery mode since 2008 financial crisis, Has be curtailed by the economic disruption. The unemployment rate in the EU rose to 6.6% in April, subsequently biggest for several years, touching nearly 240,000. The Eurozone jobless rate rose to 7.3%. Approximately, 40 m of Europeans have enrolled for the furlough schemes, in which a part of their wages is paid by government (Fig. 12.2).

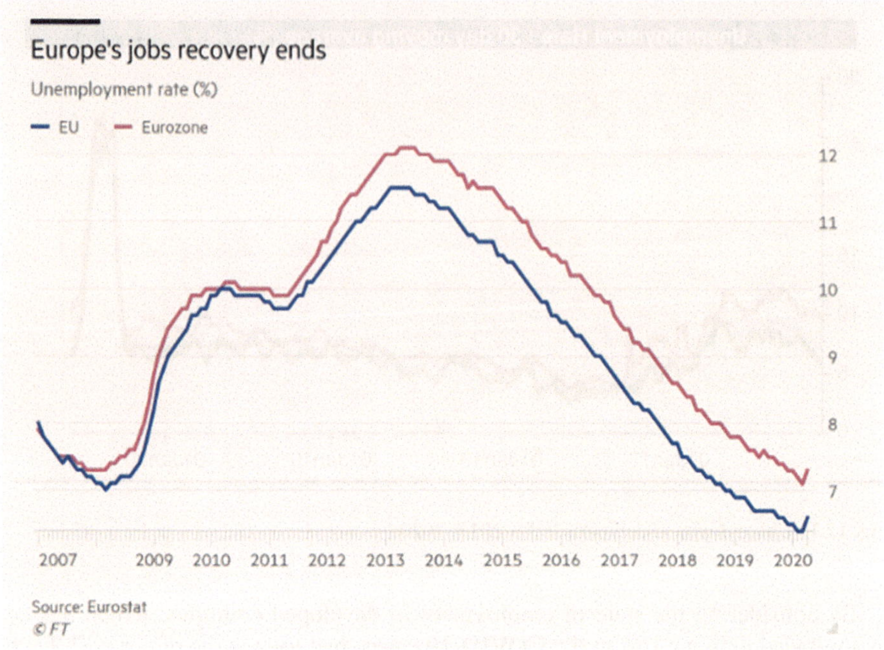

Fig. 12.2 Increase of unemployment for Europe

In the past 6 weeks, due to heavy layoffs by major small- and large-scale private industries, more than 30 m people have filed for unemployment benefits [20].

12.3.2.3 United States of America

The United States of America is one of the hardest hit countries due to the pandemic, with the COVID-19 cases touching nearly 25 million. Due to heavy restriction in the economic capital states such as New York and California, a large number of workforce have lost their job, with April and May being the toughest months. In the history of the country, unemployment rate crosses 14% and 13% mark in the month of April and May, respectively.

Being a major global player, countries that rely on them as their market have been severely affected. Figure 12.3 shows the unemployment report in the USA provided by the article [18, 19].

12.3.2.4 United Nations

The United Nations projected a worldwide loss of 25 million of job due to COVID-19 crisis. The International Labor Organization, which is a United Nations Institution, assesses the employment outlook of countries worldwide and puts forth urgent measures on a large scale based on three pillars.

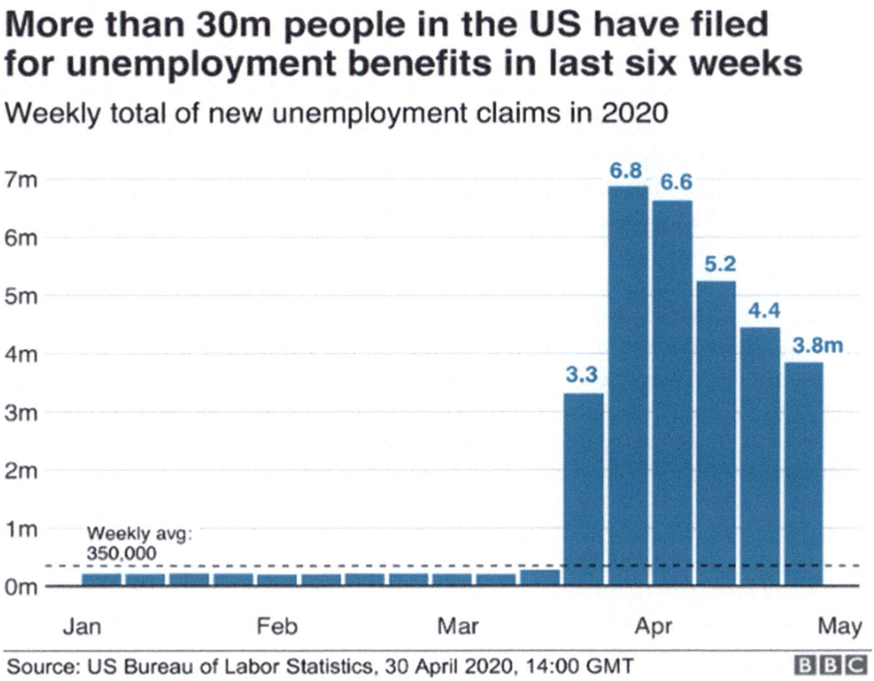

Fig. 12.3 Unemployment rate in the USA

- Protecting worker in the workplace
- Stimulating the economy and employment
- Supporting jobs and income

Apart from these, fiscal and monetary measures have also been suggested for specific sectors. ILO reports provide different scenarios of how unemployment will be impacted due to coronavirus.

12.3.3 Social Issues

Living in the globalization era allows humans to connect with others in another part of the world, eventually helping to grow the various economic and noneconomic ecosystems. Alas, the COVID-19 effect has affected the chain of globalization on various levels, such as political, cultural, and social levels.

Issues such as social distancing with friends and family and closure of various entertainment outlets, parks, schools, colleges, and malls affected not only the social activity but also the academic aspect as well as put pressure on parents to guide their children in the period of crisis. The vulnerable section of the society even faces issues such as depression and anxiety [14, 21].

12.4 The New Technological Era

Financial repercussions have started to surface due to these turbulent times, and many economists forecast a profound downturn of unknown span. While some supply chains are spinning extremely firm to keep up, others such as "VW in automotive" are being forced to ramp down.

For supply chain planners, one downside to overcome to move forward is the dynamic called the "inventory bounce." When demand reaches a new stable state which is lower than the earlier stable state, there must be a cut in manufacturing to tolerate the pipeline of stock to a lower new stable state level. At that point, manufacturing essentially *increases* a bit to match the new demand [10, 12].

In the previous major economic downturn 10 years ago, the inventory bounce fooled some upstream supply chains into assuming that demand was rebounding. The bullwhip effect started to have an effect and the bounce became more powerful and created enormous chaos and anguish among people.

12.4.1 Transportation

Apart from allowing the truck drivers and warehouse employees back to their job, logistics operators had to struggle in order to meet the working capital requirements and supply chain inefficiencies.

Fear of crowd infection has not only stopped the public gathering but also the public transport. Major cities such as Delhi and Mumbai have seen reduction in public transport usage of 20–30%. Despite the limited frequencies, due to no alternative there are instances of crowded vehicles which have been frequently observed. One of the major challenges with respect to transport, with relevance to the whole of the world, is the lack of enough research on building understanding about modality model by change [22].

There have been studies that put emphasis on the use of non-AC buses, which is being justified by the inference that viruses could be spread easily in indoor air conditioned areas.

A recent research conducted by the International Association of Public Transport (UITP) and the World Bank have found that over 67% of bus operators are in the task of providing essential services.

If considering the whole supply chain value system, there are many barriers which can have a greater influence on the supply chain network which consists of variables such as lack of labor, lack of availability of local transport, local law enforcement agencies, and slow movement [23].

12.4.2 *Warehousing*

According to Logistics Managers Index Report, both the transport and inventory level have taken a negative turn, and this pattern can go down as we move forward, since there have been disruption on the supply chain side. Hence, there is a need to evaluate and assess the situation of current warehouse and fulfillment center and make changes accordingly.

12.4.3 *Inventory Management*

The impact of COVID-19 has been felt throughout the supply chain, and there have been a lot of concerns for retailers on managing the inventory. Taking variables such as season and time decay, retailers and wholesalers need to build a short-term and a long-term strategy to meet the demand post-COVID.

Inventory management is not only limited to the supply that comes from China itself but also the disruption at the local level, and the supplier who buys their inputs from other's parts of the country have also been heavily affected. During the lockdown, a lot of inventories have been closed, apart from mandates by a few state governments to keep the supply of essential goods and products unrestricted. These measures have allowed industries such as FMCG and Pharma to keep working without any disruption from the administrative side [24].

12.4.4 *Officer Health and Safety*

The local administration based upon the rural and urban municipality contributes heavily, providing major preventive measures despite the diversity prevailing in our country, where no single form of preventive model applicable in one region can fit over all divergent regions in India [22, 24].

Due to unpreparedness, initially COVID-19 has posed major challenges for different departments to make a robust policy with respect to implementing preventive measures. Hence, a coordinated effort by different public health institutions, such as ICMR and local state bodies, is essentially required.

12.5 Technologies to Address Various Issues

The COVID-19 epidemic that led to more than 661,000 deaths and infected more than 16.7 million people worldwide has forced us to rethink how governments, organizations, and societies around the world can work with minimum or without any physical contact. Currently, the frontline warriors and heroes of the nation are typically the medical professionals, local police, private security guards, and few government officials exposing themselves to risk of infection caused due to COVID-19. In such cases technologies such as Artificial Intelligence, Big Data, GIS and Mapping, Location Technology, and autonomous machines currently play a major role as a weapon responding to the COVID-19 pandemic.

Few of such technologies are discussed in the following sections [25, 26].

12.5.1 Drones

In this battle against the imperceptible opponent, drones have been put to optimal use by authorities and people in numerous ways to prevent the spread of the coronavirus outbreak through maintaining and ensuring social distancing.

Below are few effective uses of drones to combat COVID-19.

12.5.1.1 Surveillance

A major policy adopted by authorities across the globe to prevent the spread of the virus is to implement and ensure that they are taking appropriate measures to avoid human contact. Most countries took measures such as:

- Closure of nonessential public places
- Ban on mass gatherings
- Ensuring social distancing to limit physical contact

However, there are various places where individuals are not mandated with the requirement to comply with the restrictions. Either knowingly or unknowingly or lack of awareness regarding what latest restrictions are, law enforcement authorities such as the local police or municipal authorities are currently using drones as shown in Fig. 12.4 in order to monitor human movement as well as unauthorized social gatherings, if any, that could cause threat to the society with infection spread. The introduction of drones at this time of major crisis has reduced the probability of risk caused due to infection to police officials and other staff, since it enables them to monitor the areas remotely [22, 26].

However, the use of drones for surveillance involves privacy and individual rights with respect to mainstream media as well as social media platforms.

12.5.1.2 Broadcast

- In addition to street surveillance, authorities are also using drones in order to broadcast various messages as well as important information regarding lockdown measures, especially in rural areas which lack open communication chan-

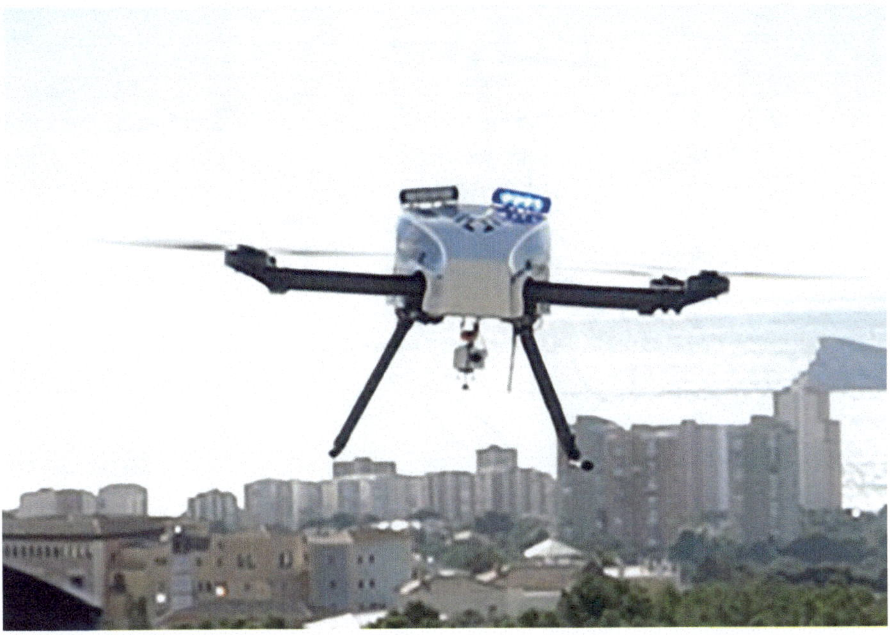

Fig. 12.4 Drones as surveillance camera

nels as shown in Fig. 12.5. Drones equipped with loudspeakers are currently serving as broadcast machines by making public announcements pertaining to various protocols to be followed during lockdown and post-lockdown such as keeping people indoors, taking necessary precautions, mandating social distancing, and enforcing the use of masks while stepping out [28]. China and many European countries are currently using drones for broadcasting messages to the public [22, 25].

12.5.2 AI-Based Technologies

The COVID-19 literature has at this time exposed an investigative evolution in much the same way as the disease's diffusion. The NIH's COVID-19 Portfolio, a website built as a repository of articles relating to coronavirus, can also track papers related to the SARS-CoV-2 coronavirus and the disease it causes, currently lists more than 28,000 articles, much beyond any researcher can read. The rapid growth of artificial intelligence (AI) tools may help researchers and clinicians in order to quickly work out through the literatures available by characteristically emphasizing the article most associated with their concentration area present within the literature [2, 26].

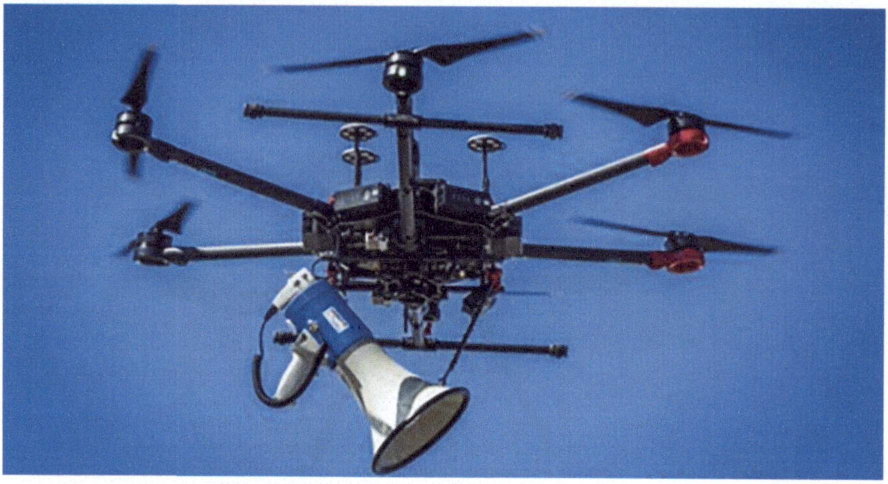

Fig. 12.5 Drones as a broadcasting machine. (Image courtesy: Getty Images/AFP [27])

With the result of the amalgamation of influences, i.e., accessibility of a huge collection of significant articles, with explicitly the urgency of the epidemic itself, progressive research technology based on Natural-Language Processing (NLP) and Machine-Learning (ML) tools have used AI in order to find the studies that are most relevant to the user, including extra findings and analysis done over the result based on certain specific cases [29].

> "Thinking beyond the current emergency situation caused due to the pandemic, these tools can help to bridge fields by making it easier to identify solutions from other disciplines" (quoted by Amalie Trewartha) [4, 19].

12.6 Various Other Uses of AI Technology During COVID-19

Currently, various tools are still under the improvement phase, where their effectiveness is mostly unverified. Hence they cannot be used to make medical or research pronouncements. Oren Etzioni, in Seattle, stated "Even using AI, a vaccine is not going to emerge full-blown." But researchers and various AI developers hope that the new expertise would assist researchers to emphasize their efforts. Few of such tools discussed by the developers are as follows [30].

12.6.1 Call to Action

The White House Office of Science and Technology Policy invited the AI community in order to develop tools for mining the COVID-19 literature on 16 March. To get them started, the White House worked with numerous administrations to announce the COVID-19 Open Research Dataset (CORD-19), stipulating a pool of 13,000 full-text papers on SARS-CoV-2 and other coronaviruses as shown in Fig. 12.6. AI-2 formatted all such relevant files for easier parsing by algorithms and adds new papers regularly. The collection now has roughly 68,000 papers and 67,000 abstracts. Dozens of such tools have emerged thereafter [2, 14].

- To focus AI researchers' efforts, the White House generated a set of questions to answer. Kaggle presents these questions there to dozens to its users and awards weekly a prize of US$1000 to the team that comes up with the best answers. Medical-student volunteers sort through the results and compile the best answers into a set of tables on a central page, which is currently acting as a continuously updated reference. Currently, it has a record of more than 1000 accounts having submitted the algorithms.
- José Morey, the chief medical-innovation officer currently working in Liberty Biosecurity, a research firm in Arlington, Virginia, used the resulting reference lists in order to draft, within a short span of a few days, a summarized risk factors for COVID-19 severity.
- "The CORD-19 data set is inadvertently proving to be a super-interesting pragmatic test" for AI-based literature analysis, as suggested by Anthony Goldbloom, chief executive of the website Kaggle, a Google subsidiary in San Francisco, California, which hosts machine-learning competitions.
- Goldbloom have further stated that competitors generally show the trait of using one of two AI methods. The first is an "old-school information retrieval method" that requires explicit rules that look for specific keywords in papers and analyze the text around them. The second uses deep neural networks, which is a type of machine-learning method, trained on large data sets in order to recognize text related to a question or topic.

12.6.2 Search Engines

A huge collection of tools exists in and outside the Kaggle competitions. For example, Google's COVID-19 Research Explorer allows users to raise various related queries such as naming rapid molecular diagnostics for COVID-19. The tool thereafter puts forth a list of papers, with key passages highlighted.

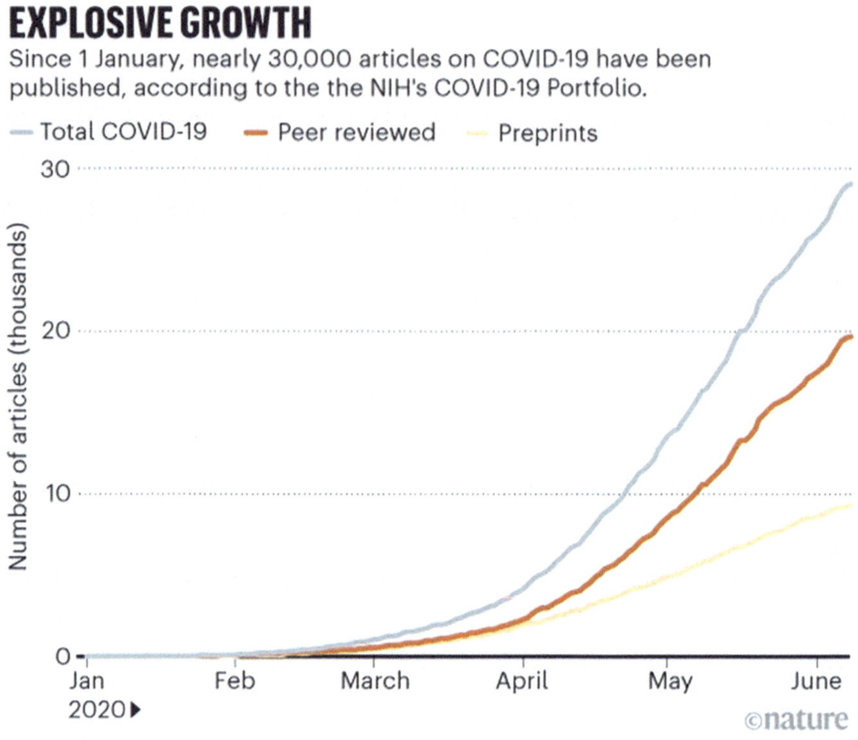

Fig. 12.6 Explosive growth of publication pertaining to COVID-19

Keith Hall, a computer scientist leading the project from New York City regarding the development of COVID-19 Research Explorer, was already working over a biomedical-research tool before the pandemic. When COVID-19 appeared, he went ahead to comment that the pandemic made it a little more obvious that he could work over providing a tool that may prove to be helpful for researchers to work with though it was not fully integrated with other Google products [30].

12.7 Conclusion

The chapter addressed the monetary impact of COVID-19 on various countries. It roughly discussed the issues like unemployment problem that is increasing in many developing countries and also its impact on other countries dependent on them for their economic upliftment. The chapter also highlighted various other issues faced by different sectors and the reason they need to change their mode of operation in order to meet their financial objectives. The chapter finally discussed the various AI-based technologies and how they can be used to regulate the day-to-day life while implementing the newly laid policies to fight the spread of COVID-19.

References

1. Vyas, M.: Unemployment rate touches 26%. Centre for Monitoring Indian Economy (CMIE) (2020). Accessed 24 Apr 2020
2. Sharma, Y.S.: Unemployment rate falls to pre-lockdown level: CMIE. The Economic Times (2020). Accessed 24 June 2020
3. Goyal, M.: Covid-19: how the deadly virus hints at a looming financial crisis. The Economic Times (2020). Accessed 23 Mar 2020
4. Research, Centre for Policy. Podcast: how has India's lockdown impacted unemployment rates and income levels? Scroll.in. Accessed 24 Apr 2020
5. Covid-19 lockdown estimated to cost India $4.5 billion a day: Acuité Ratings. Business Line (2020). Accessed 11 Apr 2020
6. PTI. Experts peg India's cost of coronavirus lockdown at USD 120 bn. The Hindu @businessline (2020). Accessed 25 Mar 2020
7. Lockdown relaxation—more than half of India's economy may reopen from Monday, says Nomura. Business Insider. Accessed 18 Apr 2020
8. Mukherji, B.: Coronavirus impact: Indian industry seeks relief measures to aid economy. Livemint (2020). Accessed 23 Mar 2020
9. Chaudhry, S.A.: Covid-19 puts India's food supply chain to a stress-test. The Hindu @businessline (2020). Accessed 26 Mar 2020
10. Das, G.: 136 million jobs at risk in post-corona India. Livemint (2020). Accessed 2 Apr 2020
11. Young Indian startups hit as investors get cautious. Outlook India. IANS (2020). Accessed 1 Apr 2020
12. Rajat, P.: CDS Bipin Rawat: forces must shun imports, go for 'Make In India', says Gen Bipin Rawat | India News—Times of India. The Times of India (2020). Accessed 10 May 2020
13. Goswami, S., Singh, S.: 'We've to learn to live with Covid-19', says Delhi deputy CM Manish Sisodia. Hindustan Times (2020). Accessed 5 May 2020
14. Covid-19: Maharashtra freezes all spending on development projects until March, say reports. Scroll.in. Accessed 5 May 2020
15. Yadav, S.: Coronavirus | Madhya Pradesh caught between pandemic and penury. The Hindu. ISSN 0971-751X (May 2020). Accessed 31 May 2020
16. Brown, G.W.: Iterative solutions of games by fictitious play. In: Koopmans, T.C. (ed.) Activity Analysis of Production and Allocation. Wiley, New York (1951)
17. Brueggemann, T., Kern, W.: An improved deterministic local search algorithm for 3-SAT. Theor. Comput. Sci. **329**, 303–313 (2004)
18. Bryn, S., Page, L.: Bringing Order to the Web: A Hypertext Search Engine. Stanford University, Mimeo (1998)
19. Davis, J.P., Eisenhardt, K.M., Bingham, C.P.: Complexity Theory, Market Dynamism and the Strategy of Simple Rules. DRUID Working Paper (2008)
20. Denrell, J., Fang, C., Levinthal, D.A.: From T mazes to labyrinths: learning from model-based feedback. Manag. Sci. **50**(10), 1366–1378 (2004)
21. PTI. Covid-19 pandemic won't affect S-400 deliveries: Indian Ambassador in Russia. The Print (2020). Accessed 24 Apr 2020
22. Denrell, J.: Adaptive learning and risk taking. Psychol. Rev. **114**(1), 177–187 (2007)
23. https://www.focusedmomentum.com/strategic-planning. Accessed 20 June 2020
24. Moldoveanu, M.: Algorithmic foundations for business strategy (2007). Accessed 20 June 2020
25. Eisenhardt, K., Martin, J.A.: Dynamic capabilities: what are they? Strateg. Manag. J. **21**, 1105–1121 (2000)
26. Fogel, D.B.: Evolutionary Computation: Toward a New Philosophy of Machine Intelligence. IEEE Press, Piscataway (1995)
27. Van Hoorn, M.: Opshot-Netherlands-health-virus (2020). https://www.gettyimages.in/detail/news-photo/this-picture-taken-on-april-4-shows-a-drone-used-by-police-news-photo/1209132628?adppopup=true. Accessed 20 Jul 2020

28. Nayyar, A., Nguyen, B.L., Nguyen, N.G.: The Internet of Drone Things (IoDT): Future Envision of Smart Drones. In: First International Conference on Sustainable Technologies for Computational Intelligence, pp. 563–580. Springer, Singapore (2020)
29. Tambe, P., Cappelli, P., Yakubovich, V.: Artificial intelligence in human resources management: challenges and a path forward Sage Journal. **61**(4) (2019)
30. Bylander, T., Allemang, D., Tanner, M.C., Josephson, J.: The computational complexity of abduction. Artif. Intell. **49**, 25–60 (1991)

Chapter 13
COVID-19 Impact on Educational System Globally

Muhammad Ibrahim Khalil, Mamoona Humayun, and N. Z. Jhanjhi

Abstract Education plays a very important role in the development of the society. A good educational system produces good citizens. The nations which compromise their education live far behind in the race of development. The advancement of ICT has brought drastic positive changes in the educational system and made the knowledge available and accessible from everywhere. The E-Learning system is also prevailing in most modern societies, and a lot of people who are not able to attend regular classes are getting benefit from it. However, it cannot be the supplement of traditional face-to-face learning mechanisms. The blend of the traditional educational system with E-Learning is very fruitful, and a lot of developed societies are getting its benefit. Recently, the rapid growth of COVID-19 all over the world has put the traditional education system to halt. The policy of lockdown and isolation has put billions of children away from school. Most governments have officially declared school closure to prevent the widespread of COVID-19. In such a situation, online learning is the only solution to run the vehicle of the educational system. However, the current E-Learning infrastructure was not expecting this rapid paradigm shift from the traditional educational system toward E-Learning. Therefore, a lot of issues are reported daily such as Internet connectivity, security breaches, conducting the assessment, etc. In this paper, we will provide the impact of COVID-19 on the educational system worldwide and the strategies that might be useful to fill the gap created by school closure during COVID-19.

Keywords COVID-19 · E-Learning · Online learning · ICT · Digital learning

---

M. I. Khalil (✉)
Department of Computer Science, Bahria University, Islamabad, Pakistan
e-mail: 01-243191-008@student.bahria.edu.pk

M. Humayun
Department of Information systems, College of Computer and Information Sciences, Jouf University, Sakakah, Kingdom of Saudi Arabia

N. Z. Jhanjhi
School of Computer Science and Engineering (SCE), Taylor's University, Subang Jaya, Malaysia

© The Author(s), under exclusive license to Springer Nature Switzerland AG 2021

F. Al-Turjman et al. (eds.), *Emerging Technologies for Battling Covid-19*, Studies in Systems, Decision and Control 324,
https://doi.org/10.1007/978-3-030-60039-6_13

13.1 Introduction

Education is a collective mechanism in which essential intellectual awareness, life skills, and cultural expectations are taught to children throughout the society. Every nation in the world has some kind of academic system, but such systems differ widely. Before the situation in COVID-19, the traditional education system was running smoothly; learning in the classroom is very beneficial because of the direct interaction between students and teachers. Working at the school allows students and instructors to get to know each other more. This helps teachers to get to know students, assess their strengths and shortcomings, serve as mentors, and direct students into their future potential. In the conventional classroom, students will express their opinions directly with the instructor and explain their own concerns while receiving definitive responses to their queries (Fig. 13.1).

The daily leisure events revive the students, and they get some relaxation from the tension of the studies they love and are having fun because of these recreational activities. Throughout the classroom, the students know easily. This is mainstream education's most popular aspect, and it's the productive learning style. Before COVID-19 the research institutes were providing valuable knowledge of research subjects, enhancing logical thinking skills, increasing awareness of the scope and difficulty of analytical study, building realistic skills, increasing comprehension of the essence of research, promoting curiosity in science and learning literacy, and strengthening collaboration skills. The realistic knowledge was provided by educational institutes; research laboratory equipment teaches students how to create a compelling case and perform experiments for the new developments.

Before COVID-19 starts, the total students enrolled in different departments were around 1.5 billion. Currently students have less opportunities for learning at home because almost all the science students don't have access to laboratories. They are unable to perform their practical exams. Every country is trying to

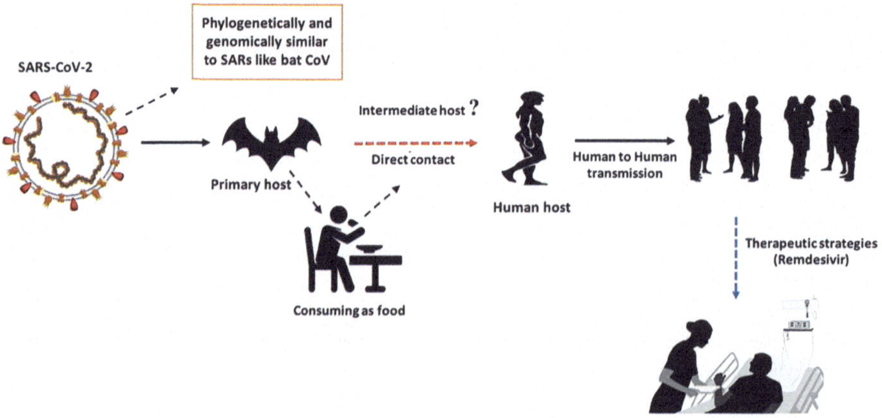

Fig. 13.1 Coronavirus disease (COVID-19) [1]

facilitate students by providing them remote options. Most of the universities have taken corporate account from different companies in order to schedule different remote sessions. It's impossible for every country to provide learning environment to all the 1.5 billion students across the globe. Around 6.3 billion teachers have been affected due to this pandemic.

The COVID-19 has changed, in a matter of a night, how the future can educate the students. The reforms provide us with a quick look at how schooling has progressed over a night. One aspect that comes to mind in such an environment is remote education by webinars, virtual learning management systems, and online courses. For the first time, E-Learning serves an ability to create a useful stand. Theoretically we have several resources at hand, as remote learning is not a new subject. In comparison to the roots that go back many hundred years, the Internet has given us many useful alternatives. In this situation, it's impossible to override teacher's interaction with students. So, we begin testing webinar sites first. Overall, they allow for collaboration on training materials, real-time contact through audio and video, and other activities, such as quizzes and assignments that can be used as evaluation techniques. Institutions performed Web wonders. In very short span, the sector has done what others thought due to the efforts of IT specialists.

Before COVID-19 the educational system was not facing many challenges, and students were attending their classes conveniently and were directly interacting with their teachers and class fellows; besides study students were also engaging themselves in extra cocurricular activities, as they facilitate the development of various domains of mind and personalities such as intellectual, emotional, moral, social, and aesthetic development. Everyday new inventions were taking place in the field of science and technology. As COVID-19 has terribly affected the world, it was not feasible to open the educational institutes, but on the other hand, it was not possible to take the education of students for granted. Educational institutes have adopted the online education system as it is one of the best solutions in the prevailing situation and continuing the learning process.

We have tried to cover the impact of COVID-19 along with its suspected origin. Education system situation before COVID-19. How colleges and universities are dealing with this pandemic along with their strengths. How remote and online learning opportunities are helping students and the issue associated with the connectivity of different collaboration tools. In this document, we have also tried to cover the learner and students impacted due to this virus and how education system changed over the nights. This document also has details on the challenges and problem that education system was facing before COVID-19. How existing tools are helping students to connect and attend the class session along with pros and cons of the software. We have learned the following lessons from COVID-19:

- It's time to reform the current school framework.
- Online classes must be conducted using collaboration tools.
- The role of the teacher needs to be refined.
- Partnership between the public-private sectors is mandatory for the development of education software.

- Strategies to educate students in the interconnected world should be defined.
- Technology should be unlocked to minimize social interaction.

This chapter attempts to identify the COVID-19 impacts on the education system globally that caters the challenges to sustain the education. Education needs to be addressed with the challenge of a short time around the world. Includes the existing distance learning tools and techniques with their pros and cons. Detailed discussion on the role of technology for helping to continue education and the future planning to address any emergency situation. Lastly summarizing the main findings and suggest some future directions.

13.2 Literature Review

At the end of December 2019, a new coronavirus (called SARS-CoV-2) triggered an infectious disease outbreak (COVID-19) that emerged in Wuhan, China, and spread rapidly in China and abroad. In this market, animal species are being sold. The coronavirus disease (COVID-19) is likely to originate from animal species and then is transferred to humans. Transmission is verified from humans to humans. The time of incubation varies from 5 days, which can go up to 14 days. On March 12, 2020 [2], the WHO has called the disease COVID-19 a pandemic. According to a recent Chinese survey, nearly 80% of patients has moderate disease, and the overall occurrence of case fatality rate is about 2.3% but reaches 8.0% in patients aged 70–79 years and 14.8% in those aged 80. Effective care is required urgently to stabilize symptomatic individuals but also to reduce the transmission time of the virus to minimize public dissemination [3]. The repositioning of old medicines for use as antiviral therapy is an essential strategy among candidate drugs to treat COVID-19, and knowledge regarding safety profile, side effects, and medication interactions are well established [4].

Coronaviruses are a class of viruses that cause mammal and bird diseases, including human respiratory tract infections. These infections are usually moderate, but rarer types like Middle East respiratory syndrome (MERS) and severe acute respiratory syndrome (SARS) can be lethal. The COVID-19 disease spread quite rapidly and took just 30 days to travel from Hubei to the rest of Mainland China. With many people coming back from long vacations, the virus spread to other countries as well [5]. The Chinese National Health Commission released more details on the epidemic on January 12, 2020 reporting viral pneumonia [6]. In a sequencing study of patients' isolates, the virus was described as a novel coronavirus. In addition, a genetic code for the diagnosis of viral infection has been developed [7]. Further tests have showed that some people had acquired illness and had no record of visiting the seafood shop. These studies have also shown the ability of the human being to transmit this infection and have consequently been reported in more than 100 countries around the world. Owing to near communication with an infectious individual, prone to coughing, sneezing, nasal droplets or aerosols, the human to the infection spreads [8].

Countries also collectively closed colleges and training facilities, impacting more than 80% of the world's student population. Several countries have adopted municipal school cuts, and such reductions are likely to be frequent. There is a large body of literature on the closing of educational facilities to reduce the dissemination of infectious diseases in the community by cutting off substantial transmission chains. Given the warning over the latest COVID-19 pandemic, the majority of universities worldwide have either postponed or cancelled all campus events, such as lectures, conferences, sports [9].

The Nation, through the Ministry of Health, declared in a press conference that all classrooms, colleges, and universities will be suspended because of fears about the spread of coronavirus (COVID-19), which allegedly ravaged several regions of China [10], the United States, Italy, Spain, and other sections of Europe and Africa. This suggested that high school students completed term 1 of the academic year 2020 in both public and private schools without sitting for their end-of-term exams so at the conclusion of any of the three academic year periods, both public and private schools must hold appraisal assessments. The early closing of educational facilities was a successful move by the government to secure students by future COVID-19 threats because educational atmospheres are areas where hundreds of students gather, rendering those unsafe sites where disease would propagate rapidly (Fig. 13.2) [11].

The condition rapidly escalated with the closing of schools from 29 countries based on the COVID-19 epidemic evidence and expectations that it decreases social contact among students and hence the transmission intersection. School closures may have a beneficial impact on casualties during an epidemic, either by reducing infection and the amount of incidents or by growing the health-care staff eligible for patient care [12]. According to UNESCO during COVID-19 pandemic, over 90% of the world's students are not attending school. Some schools started the online class using webinars because this was the only way to continue education in this

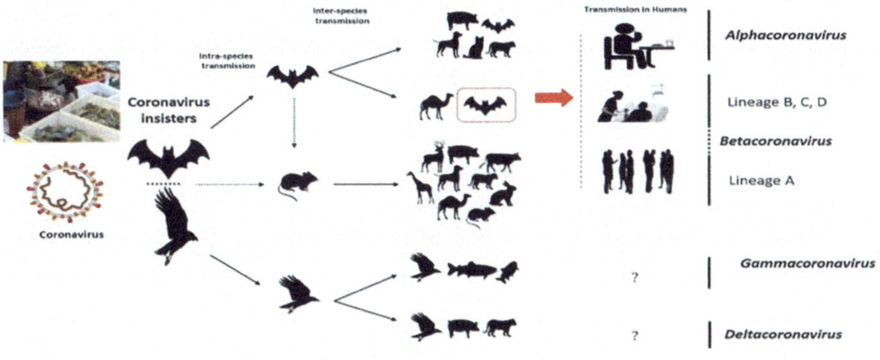

Fig. 13.2 COVID-19 transmission cycle [1]

pandemic. Many schools announce the summer/winter vacations because they don't have E-Learning environment. Colleges and universities also started online learning education in order to continue the learning process.

Current obstacles for delivering services and educating people in the context of insecurity, the allocation of wealth and the loss of traditional learning opportunities. Our evolutionary strategy is meant to be a universally applicable technique for enhancing our current landscape [13]. Effective contact between learners, clinical teachers, and administrative staff was recorded to strengthen mutual confidence and promote adequate cooperation [14]. The anticipated difficulties could be changing electronic classrooms face-to-face education that is essential for students with hearing problem; it may be more perplexing because most of the students may not have Internet access and wireless-enabled laptops.

Education is the most important step toward the progress of any country. All the education institutes needs to hire motivational speaker to conduct motivational speeches during this pandemic so that all the students remain motivated for attending the online classes and remain positive about their learning. Low-bandwidth consuming software tools should be used for online learning so that the students living in the village and small towns with limited access to Internet can get benefits of online learning opportunities. Education institutes need to publish their books on their official website, because students will not be having access to the library books. One the most important things is that all the lectures should be recorded and need to be available on the official institution website that will help the student to attend missing lectures.

Distance education has traditionally provided via phone, but thanks to expanded usage of the Web and technical advancements, it is now accessible on the device or smartphone screen through different resources such as telephone, multimedia networking apps, and social connectivity such as networks, student clubs, student bundles, and video conference platforms such as ezTalks Cloud Meetings [15]. Personal cloud storage resources are becoming increasingly common. With a flood of companies joining the sector and an increasing promise of inexpensive storage space, cloud storage is projected to produce a large volume of Internet traffic early. There is relatively little information regarding the design and efficiency of these structures and the workload they face [16]. One of the best cloud storage software tools is Dropbox, and some E-Learning software tools are Microsoft Teams, Zoom, and Webex.

- Pros
  - Usually, you can set your own study pace too.
  - It's your decision, when and where you're learning.
  - Wherever you reside, it doesn't matter—you can get a degree from everywhere in the country.

- Cons
  - You need an Internet connection.
  - You should have knowledge about how to operate the tools.
  - If you lose a connection, you will be disconnected from the online session.
  - Student should have microphone and camera for interaction.

In 2001, an initial evaluation of the technical capacities of four Internet-based online video conferencing devices (CUseeMe, ICUII, Virtual VoxPhone Black, and NetMeeting) was performed with language teachers and device specialists, and NetMeeting was established as the most effective oral and visual connectivity support platform in DLE [17, 18].

Currently there are a lot of tools available for video conferencing. A detailed comparison is given below (Table 13.1):

Main challenges are arranging online classes in an effective manner. Fully functional LMS (learning management system) is required for uploading assignment and conducting online quizzes and exams. There are concerns to be worried as extended school closing and home detention during the spread of the disease may have adverse impacts on the physical and mental fitness of children. Data shows that children who are out of school (e.g., weekends and summer holidays) have less active activity, a slightly longer turnaround period, erratic sleeping habits, and fewer healthy diets. The psychological effect on children and adolescents is a more serious but easily overlooked problem. Stressors such as excessive duration of time; sickness issues; anger and loneliness; lack of paperwork; lack of regular contact with parents, friends, and instructors; lack of personal rooms at home; and loss of family income may have much more detrimental and irreversible consequences on adolescents [18].

Table 13.1 Video conferencing tools' feature comparison

Features	zoom	Google Hangouts	skype	Cisco webex	Microsoft Teams	slack
Video	Yes	Yes	Yes	Yes	Yes	Yes
Screen Sharing	Yes	Yes	Yes	Yes	Yes	Yes
Meeting recording	Yes	Yes	Yes	Yes	Yes	Yes
Max users	Up to 500 depends on plan	Up to 250 depends on plan	50	Up to 1000 depends on plan	Up to 250	Unlimited
Mobile-friendly	Yes	Yes	Yes	Yes	Yes	Yes
Join via link	Yes	Yes	No	Yes	Yes	Yes
Drawing tools	Yes	Yes	No	Yes	Yes	Yes
No student sign-up	Yes	No	No	Yes	No	No

The IT-based methodologies include webinars, virtual learning management systems, and video conferencing tools to help education system to fight against COVID-19. Teachers worldwide appear to be capable of managing virtual classroom, communicating with students on social media platforms, and teaching students affected by the COVID-19 pandemic through distance learning. In numerous educational establishments, learning management systems (LMSs) were adopted to improve pedagogy through their features and applications. Educational institutes were encouraged to use LMSs to enhance the working atmosphere of students and their instructors working together.

The role of technology in education, in its Web creation relationship. Stating that, the value of conventional learning methods and educational strategies cannot be ignored, because one should still teach algebra, for example, in a discursive manner and it gives students and instructors the ability to feel the pleasure of participating, or active involvement [19]. Technologies obviously can touch a far larger student population, irrespective of spatial and/or social restrictions [20]. Technology shifts the position of teachers from instruction to help and encouragement, which shifts reliance on some times and locations we want students, particularly young students, to "do" school. Let's assume that while COVID-19 is reflections in our rear view, the inventions and technologies that enabled our students and educational institutions get through it are normal and frequently used resources in the great challenge of educating children (Fig. 13.3).

Continued adoption of structured and informal education across classrooms, linked to community-based risk management, promises the creation of a "health culture" of communities less fragile and more responsive to future catastrophe impacts [21]. Institutions should be trained in a manner that provides them with adapted information and strengthens their capacity to handle and plan for disasters and maintain preparation for future emergencies. Future preparation would include the efficient distribution of capital. By enhancing their understanding of the partnership between preparedness and catastrophe risk management, schooling will enable individuals to take preparatory steps. In fact, trained citizens will have a stronger idea about what preparedness steps can be taken.

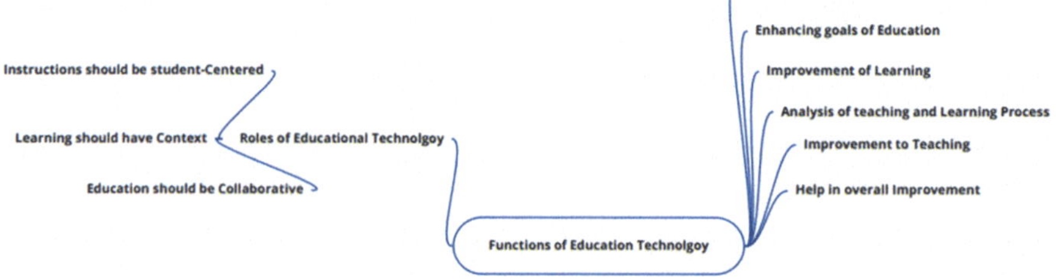

Fig. 13.3 Education technology in the twenty-first century

13.3 Discussion

The COVID-19 pandemic is a health problem in the first place. Most nations (rightly) have agreed to shut down schools, colleges, and universities. Online teaching evolves at an untested, unparalleled rate [22]. A number of experiments were essentially cancelled. Obviously, such challenges may only pose a short-term problem but may also have long-term consequences for the students who have been impacted. It is predicted that inequalities between students would increase. Closing schools, colleges, and universities is crippling student schooling across the globe. Significant assessments of professional qualifications for the whole class are cancelled. We're likely to see these actions globally depending on the duration of the lockdown. But it is also likely that certain student occupations will profit from interruptions [23]. In higher education, several universities and colleges are replacing standardized tests with electronic evaluation instruments; this is a different environment for both teachers and students, so evaluations are expected to contain a larger measuring error than average. In higher education, many universities and colleges are replacing traditional exams with online assessment tools; this is a new area for both teachers and students, and assessments are likely to have greater measurement errors than usual. Public-private education collaborations may rise in value as a remedy [24]. In developed countries such as Pakistan, a positive development in future education can be rendered to account for student loses, and school changes may gain in the future. The benefit of that would be that the joint approach of government and private educational establishments will prove to be in the benefit of the students in the future. In fact, there is a need to reduce the expense of obtaining online schooling in places where online education is delivered utilizing digital platforms such as Microsoft Team, Zoom, Google Classroom, WhatsApp, etc. To receive information, the Education Commission will keep in good contact with the educational establishments. The responsible authority will also have a forum for students to lodge concerns regarding online schooling so that they can be further implemented [25]. Colleges and colleges have provided for the budget limitations by growing the proportion of their paid teaching personnel. Although it poses its obstacles, it is also a huge opportunity to break out of old habits and develop fresh, strong, meaningful learning models that take advantage of technology. In the longer run, this year's college application process will be more complicated owing to standardized assessments, online education, and improvements to criteria. New applications in the home are likely to drop because many students and their parents will no longer be in a position to pay tuition fees when they are laid off. In a very short time, the faculty and staff have transitioned all learning to online and virtual, and this will undoubtedly have an impact on student success and retention.

The adoption of project-based learning and collective preparation to full credit hours will facilitate that. In fact, simplifying criteria for degrees will often go a long way toward not just encouraging applicants but also training colleges for potential cohorts. Similarly, professionals require ways to participate successfully. Instead of conventional coursework, colleges should opt into mentored learning opportunities and online professional growth services [26]. Decision-makers will therefore utilize and distribute capital wisely in a manner that enables smaller institutes to leverage information from larger universities. This may involve capturing video or audio presentations and shared usage of electronic conference sites.

In a case study of Peking University, the educational institutes have initiated initiatives to create an accessible education network focused on knowledge and network technology digitally since the beginning of the twenty-first century. The number, complexity, and length of the teaching material are suitable for the training of students and the properties of online learning activities. Due to the low concentration of students in online learning, it is necessary to change the pace of the teaching so that the teacher's information is presented effectively. Teaching assistants and professors must give their students timely input, such as online video tutoring and e-mail guidance. Certain measures must be adopted to enhance the degree and depth of student attendance. Principle of contingency plan preparation. Due to the huge amount of online education [27].

For most colleges, particularly those campuses which emphasize an intimate college experience, the necessary transition to online learning has been challenging. Particularly if foreign students are eligible to enroll online in fall courses, there would be questions of electronic connectivity as well as freedom of expression and considerations of thinking for certain people with more austere regimes [28]. Additionally, owing to different time zone variations, many foreign students will not be willing to take part in real-time classes conducted remotely, and in the case that foreign students cannot be given a transitional solution, higher education organizations would suffer fewer diverse student demographics and greater financial pressure. In short now the future is online education and online learning. All the institutions are refining their process in order to conduct online classes and exams.

13.4 Conclusion

Educational institutes need to respond skillfully and creatively to stay ahead of the events. As well as key project management and marketing positions, exposure to epidemiological experience is crucial for senior leadership. Moreover, as no two universities work in nature or design similar, a one-size-fits-all solution would go out of the window. The higher education sector in the world has a tremendous potential to build on when a growing amount of employers seek educational programs that closely match the requirements of modern global industry. Universities will need to incorporate equity-based measures as many students may not have the tools or access needed to complete the online coursework. Steps to address future instability and risks to plan execution need to be assessed and enforced. Finally, in comparison to their own budgetary issues, higher education organizations ought to consider fair workplace choices from teachers to janitors and third-party suppliers. When Earth marches forward from the darkest day of the novel coronavirus pandemic, the higher education industry has a great chance to turn a fresh leaf and use that ability to push further into a better future. It would take a desire to step outside of conventional frames and to introduce creative, flexible, and constructive initiatives around the board. I hope that a day will arrive where educators will express their experiences and help each other in a way that creates trust like we've never seen before. And I hope the planet is more respected for how challenging it is to educate a student but also for how valuable and vital educational initiatives are to our future.

13.5 Future Directions

Our work shows that online learning has been shown to improve knowledge processing and take less time, suggesting that the coronavirus improvements could have induced remaining here. We believe that schools that rely on electronic program management services to administer online programs have had a more challenging time in making this move. We need confidence in investing in such a competitive market, however, does not continue as it used to in the short to mid-term. Private sector roles for development of innovative online learning solution now become very important. Collaboration tools need to be tested in the future. Reviews of tools need to be published of the official website so that institutions can share their feedback with each other. The COVID-19 crisis could well transform our environment, and our global perspective can also tell us how schooling must evolve to help educate our young learners for what the future can bring. Educating peoples in an interconnected world is the future, redesign of educator's position, providing life skills for the future and technology enabling to provide knowledge.

References

1. Shereen, M.A., Khan, S., Kazmi, A., Bashir, N., Siddique, R.: COVID-19 infection: origin, transmission, and characteristics of human coronaviruses. J. Adv. Res. **24**, 91 (2020). https://www.sciencedirect.com/science/article/pii/S2090123220300540
2. World Health Organization: WHO Director-General's Opening Remarks at the Media Briefing on COVID-19-11 March 2020. WHO, Geneva (2020). https://www.who.int/dg/speeches/detail/who-director-general-s-opening-remarks-at-the-media-briefing-on-covid-19%2D%2D-11-march-2020
3. Wang, M., Cao, R., Zhang, L., Yang, X., Liu, J., Xu, M., Shi, Z., Hu, Z., Zhong, W., Xiao, G.: Remdesivir and chloroquine effectively inhibit the recently emerged novel coronavirus (2019-nCoV) in vitro. Cell Res. **30**(3), 269–271 (2020)
4. https://www.nature.com/articles/s41422-020-0282-0?fbclid=IwAR3c5iy9h65X1cnkrL6i6fJcWwi0ygN1LtI67SkcgREM4DyxxAcPauRuf5w
5. Colson, P., Rolain, J.M., Lagier, J.C., Brouqui, P., Raoult, D.: Chloroquine and hydroxychloroquine as available weapons to fight COVID-19. Int. J. Antimicrob. Agents. **55**, 105932 (2020). http://119.18.194.205:100/filesdown/xg/xgwk035.pdf

6. Surveillances, V.: The epidemiological characteristics of an outbreak of 2019 novel coronavirus diseases (COVID-19)—China, 2020. China CDC Week. **2**(8), 113–122 (2020). https://slma.lk/wp-content/uploads/2020/02/TheEpidemiologicalCharacteristicsofanOutbreakof2019NovelCoronavirusDiseases28COVID-1929E28094China2C20201.pdf
7. Wang, C., Horby, P.W., Hayden, F.G., Gao, G.F.: A novel coronavirus outbreak of global health concern. Lancet. **395**(10223), 470–473 (2020). https://www.thelancet.com/journals/lancet/article/PIIS0140-6736(20)30185-9/fulltext?fbclid=IwAR0_jlY1L9TutpZ-CO4PoKJsC8vNEnu5Vq_x582iyULg-9ML2UHF67Kw3_kE
8. Phan, L.T., Nguyen, T.V., Luong, Q.C., Nguyen, T.V., Nguyen, H.T., Le, H.Q., Nguyen, T.T., Cao, T.M., Pham, Q.D.: Importation and human-to-human transmission of a novel coronavirus in Vietnam. N. Engl. J. Med. **382**(9), 872–874 (2020). https://doi.org/10.1056/NEJMc2001272
9. Torani, S., et al.: The importance of education on disasters and emergencies: a review article. J. Educ. Health Promot. **8**, 85 (2019). https://doi.org/10.4103/jehp.jehp_262_18. https://www.ncbi.nlm.nih.gov/pmc/articles/PMC6512217/
10. Sahu, P.: Closure of universities due to coronavirus disease 2019 (COVID-19): impact on education and mental health of students and academic staff. Cureus. **12**(4), e7541 (2020). https://doi.org/10.7759/cureus.7541. https://www.ncbi.nlm.nih.gov/pmc/articles/PMC7198094/
11. Riou, J., Althaus, C.L.: Pattern of early human-to-human transmission of Wuhan 2019 novel coronavirus (2019-nCoV), December 2019 to January 2020. Eur. Secur. **25**(4), 2000058 (2020). https://www.eurosurveillance.org/content/10.2807/1560-7917.ES.2020.25.4.2000058;jsessionid=nxJbp_ICxsCTbSUjj0hFsqt0.i-0b3d9850f4681504f-ecdclive
12. Sintema, E.J.: Effect of COVID-19 on the performance of grade 12 students: implications for STEM education. Eur. J. Math. Sci. Technol. Educ. **16**(7), em1851 (2020). https://www.ejmste.com/article/effect-of-covid-19-on-the-performance-of-grade-12-students-implications-for-stem-education-7893
13. Viner, R.M., Russell, S.J., Croker, H., Packer, J., Ward, J., Stansfield, C., Mytton, O., Bonell, C., Booy, R.: School closure and management practices during coronavirus outbreaks including COVID-19: a rapid systematic review. Lancet Child Adolesc. Health. **4**, 97 (2020). https://www.sciencedirect.com/science/article/pii/S235246422030095X
14. Schwartz, A.M., Wilson, J.M., Boden, S.D., Moore Jr., T.J., Bradbury Jr., T.L., Fletcher, N.D.: Managing resident workforce and education during the COVID-19 pandemic: evolving strategies and lessons learned. JBJS Open Access. **5**(2), e0045 (2020). https://journals.lww.com/jbjsoa/Fulltext/2020/06000/Managing_Resident_Workforce_and_Education_During.4.aspx?context=LatestArticles
15. Meng, L., Hua, F., Bian, Z.: Coronavirus disease 2019 (COVID-19): emerging and future challenges for dental and oral medicine. J. Dent. Res. **99**(5), 481–487 (2020). https://doi.org/10.1177/0022034520914246
16. Mohamed, A.A.H.: Effectiveness of distance education using mobile applications on performance level some sports activities in PE lesson. AJSSA. **1**, 39 (2018). https://ajssa.journals.ekb.eg/jufile?ar_sfile=142423
17. Drago, I., Mellia, M., Munafo, M., Sperotto, A., Sadre, R., Pras, A.: Inside dropbox: understanding personal cloud storage services. In: Proceedings of the 2012 Internet Measurement Conference, pp. 481–494. ACM, New York, NY (2012). https://doi.org/10.1145/2398776.2398827
18. Wang, Y.: Supporting synchronous distance language learning with desktop videoconferencing. Lang. Learn. Technol. **8**(3), 90–121 (2004). https://scholarspace.manoa.hawaii.edu/bitstream/10125/43997/08_03_wang.pdf
19. Wang, G., Zhang, Y., Zhao, J., Zhang, J., Jiang, F.: Mitigate the effects of home confinement on children during the COVID-19 outbreak. Lancet. **395**(10228), 945–947 (2020). https://www.thelancet.com/journals/lancet/article/PIIS0140-6736(20)30547-X/fulltext?fbclid=IwAR393Qg1UwsA8tLHX9xlJlwNzVqXbHtR1fBsTCMZ_pxBwVytKON2GzMv3KI
20. Al Musawi, A.S.: Redefining technology role in education. Creat. Educ. **2**(2), 130 (2011). https://www.scirp.org/html/5414.html

21. Osborne, M., Oberski, I.: University continuing education: the role of communications and information technology. J. Eur. Ind. Train. **28**(5), 414–428 (2004). https://www.ingentaconnect.com/content/mcb/003/2004/00000028/00000005/art00004
22. Hui, D.S., Azhar, E.I., Madani, T.A., Ntoumi, F., Kock, R., Dar, O., Ippolito, G., Mchugh, T.D., Memish, Z.A., Drosten, C., Zumla, A.: The continuing 2019-nCoV epidemic threat of novel coronaviruses to global health—the latest 2019 novel coronavirus outbreak in Wuhan, China. Int. J. Infect. Dis. **91**, 264–266 (2020). https://www.ijidonline.com/action/showPdf?pii=S1201-9712%2820%2930011-4
23. Humayun, M., Jhanjhi, N.Z., Alamri, M.Z.: Smart secure and energy efficient scheme for e-health applications using IoT: a review. Int. J. Comput. Sci. Netw. Secur. **20**(4), 55–74 (2020)
24. Jayakumar, P., Brohi, S.N., Zaman, N.: Top 7 lessons learned from COVID-19 pandemic. TechRxiv. (2020). https://doi.org/10.36227/techrxiv.12264722.v1
25. Khan, N.A., Brohi, S.N., Zaman, N.: Ten deadly cyber security threats amid COVID-19 pandemic. TechRxiv. (2020). https://doi.org/10.36227/techrxiv.12278792.v1
26. Brohi, S.N., Jhanjhi, N.Z., Brohi, N.N., Brohi, M.N.: Key applications of state-of-the-art technologies to mitigate and eliminate COVID-19. TechRxiv. (2020). https://doi.org/10.36227/techrxiv.12115596.v2
27. Bao, W.: COVID-19 and online teaching in higher education: a case study of Peking University. Hum. Behav. Emerg. Technol. **2**(2), 113–115 (2020). https://doi.org/10.1002/hbe2.191
28. Anandan, R., Suseendran, G., Zaman, N., Brohi, S.N., Balaganesh, S., Deepak, B.: Echinacea purpurea to treat novel coronavirus (2019-nCoV). TechRxiv. (2020). https://doi.org/10.36227/techrxiv.12241223.v1

Chapter 14
Mobile Technology Solutions for COVID-19

K. Rupabanta Singh, Sujata Dash, Bhupesh Deka, and Sitanath Biswas

Abstract The World Health Organization (WHO) has declared the outbreak of COVID-19 as a pandemic which has led to lockdowns of all sectors like primary education, higher education, industrial sector, logistics, etc. and a complete clamp down on sporting, cultural events, any form of social gathering, etc. The entire world is now striving to combat this pandemic with the aid of different technologies. Emerging technologies are being widely employed across the entire world to curb the outbreak of coronavirus. China has deployed robots for disinfecting hospitals and delivering medical supplies. In Singapore, the government database has enabled study of the outbreak, and in South Korea, the authorities are tracking the potential carriers by using mobile phone satellite technology. In India, drones are being used to monitor the lockdown and also to deliver essential commodities to the citizens. In addition, technology powered by artificial intelligence is enabling us to keep track of the outbreak, deliver supplies to hospitals, develop vaccines, etc. The development of mobile applications that suggest better solutions for personalized healthcare, disease management, flexible ways of communicating with physicians, and services to patients and caregivers has accelerated due to the advantages of wireless technology. In this chapter, the current Mobile Technology explores viable mobile big data solutions to combat this pandemic while adhering to principles of privacy and ethics. In addition to this study, a novel telehealth solution is proposed for combating the coronavirus.

Keywords Healthcare applications · Disease management · Telehealth solution · Surveillance · Diagnosis · Prevention · Treatment

---

K. R. Singh · S. Dash (✉) · S. Biswas
Department of Computer Science, North Orissa University, Baripada, India
e-mail: sujata.dash@nou.nic.in

B. Deka
Gandhi Institute for Technology, Bhubaneswar, India

© The Author(s), under exclusive license to Springer Nature Switzerland AG 2021

F. Al-Turjman et al. (eds.), *Emerging Technologies for Battling Covid-19*, Studies in Systems, Decision and Control 324,
https://doi.org/10.1007/978-3-030-60039-6_14

14.1 Introduction

COVID-19 pandemic affects almost all countries, and the number of COVID-19 patients is increasing day by day. It has made a significant effect into the healthcare sector on their available healthcare facilities and treatment system. Worldwide countries are responding differently to the virus outbreak. As the novel corona virus continues to spread and the number of infected patients increases continuously, all the government and the healthcare service providers have a challenging task. Social distancing, lockdown, case detection, isolation, contact tracing, and quarantine of individuals had revealed the most efficient actions to control the disease spreading [1].

Now the government and healthcare sector are giving interest on using Mobile Technology to fight against the COVID-19 pandemic. Many mobile applications are already launched for the purpose of tracking and tracing the COVID-19 patients in order to control the spreading of coronavirus [2].

Almost all cities got lockdowns; schools and colleges were closed to control the gathering of people and maintain social distancing. People who are suspected to be infected by coronavirus are kept in isolated places (quarantine center) or home quarantined. After doing all these exercises, coronavirus continues to spread. To control the spreading of coronavirus, the WHO advised some preventive measures like washing the hands frequently with soap and water or with sanitizers, maintaining social distancing, and practicing respiratory hygiene. Masks are also used for safeguarding people from COVID-19 patients. The most important preventive measure to control COVID-19 pandemic from spreading is by staying at home and avoiding social gathering (Fig. 14.1) [4].

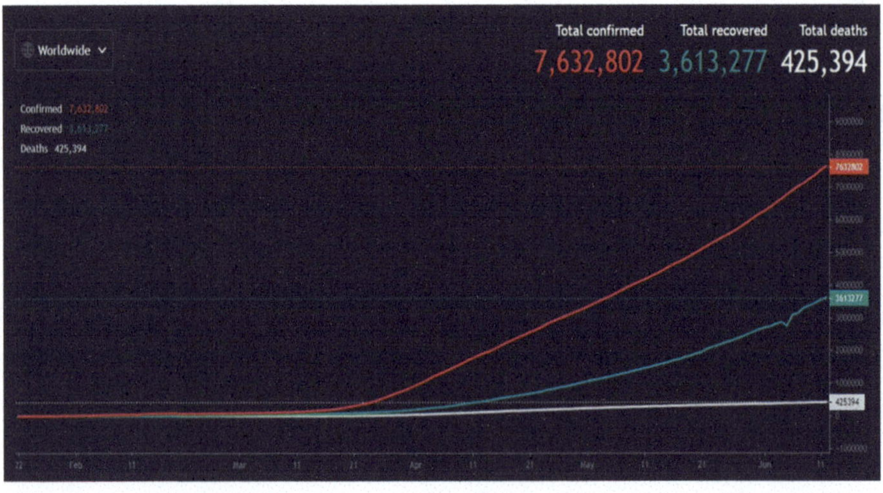

Fig. 14.1 Coronavirus (COVID-19) charts and stats [3]

Many countries preferred Mobile Technology in giving proper surveillance. GPS-based mobile applications are widely used around the world to track and trace the people for controlling the spread of coronavirus [5].

According to the present scenario, children and elderly are very risky to visit the hospital to do health check-up. Telemedicine service reduces the risk of infected people by giving healthcare services through online, [6, 7]. Using Telemedicine, people can consult doctors from home or their present location through video conferencing. It helps the healthcare service providers to give services to remote places where the health worker could not reach. It ensures to keep coronavirus-infected individuals out of the emergency care facilities or physician's offices.

Many tools are available for self-screening whether the coronavirus symptom is found in the user or not [8–11]. Using smartphones, everyone can do self-screening by staying at home or places where they feel comfortable. It helps to reduce the gathering of people at the hospital and the risk of people getting infected from other infected patients.

Healthcare workers who directly interact with COVID-19 patients need different types of training like how to care COVID-19 patients, what are the preventive measures they must follow, etc [12]. Many health organizations around the world conduct online training programs so that people from different geographical areas can participate in the training program by maintaining social distancing [13–17]. Some health organizations published webinar series to provide training to healthcare workers. Different video conferencing tools like Zoom, WebEx Meet, and Google Meet are used to give online training [18]. Hence, to fight against the novel coronavirus, it requires a combined effort from all the healthcare providers, government, and more importantly the public with the utilization of Mobile Technology.

The rest of the chapter is organized as follows: Sect. 14.2 defines the applications of Mobile Technology in healthcare, Sect. 14.3 explores Mobile Technology-based solutions for COVID-19 pandemic, Sect. 14.4 defines proposed Novel Telemedicine solution, and Sect. 14.5 concludes the chapter.

14.2 Mobile Technology in Healthcare

Mobile Technology becomes advanced, and the developer has been launching different applications that can be used in various areas where the healthcare sectors are giving importance to the application of Mobile Technology [19]. Today's healthcare environment using Mobile Technology and mobile devices has proven to be effective. Mobile application is widely recommended for asthma peak flow monitoring [20]. Mobile Technology can be used for recording and gathering asthma data. During asthma data, gathering an electronic peak flow meter can be use, and it is linked to a mobile phone that will record current asthma symptoms.

The facilities provided by the healthcare sector are leveraging Mobile Technology in new ways to decrease the costs and make their service affordable for any category of people. For the last 15 years, the healthcare sector has been trying for technological improvement. According to a 2015 report, 52% of smartphone users gather healthcare-related information on their phones [21]. People are demanding better connectivity between patients and their service providers. As of now, Mobile Technology is already changing the healthcare sectors. Healthcare sectors are interested more and more in mobile computing that enables doctors and nurses to access electronic health record (EHR) directly from the bedside as the patients demand better connectivity between healthcare service providers and the patients. With the help of EHR, patient and physician interaction increases as the EHR is updated regularly. Again using Mobile Technology, doctors can access a patient's imaging result, open files at the patient's bedside, and review the results together with the patient [21]. By doing so, it enhances the quality of care and improves outcomes by engaging the patient activity in their own care management. Today's Telemedicine service is widely used throughout the world and reduces the expenditure of the patients [22]. With the help of Telemedicine, service patients can get the care they need from home or where they are. It reduces many of the external costs that are associated with healthcare delivery, including the cost of transportation from nursing home to the providers, arranging elders care, and hours spent in the waiting room. Therefore, Telemedicine significantly reduces the cost of healthcare delivery for both the patient and the service provider (Fig. 14.2).

Many industries have launched Internet of Thing (IoT)-based wearable devices for healthcare and make it possible for remote monitoring of patients by the physicians [24]. These IoT-based healthcare devices enable the physician to send their patients home earlier, track their condition, and lower the overall cost of hospital visits. Therefore, it is just as if the healthcare service providers fully depend on Mobile Technology. Hospitals got an opportunity to introduce the application of Mobile Technology for reducing the costs with providing the same or better standards of patient care.

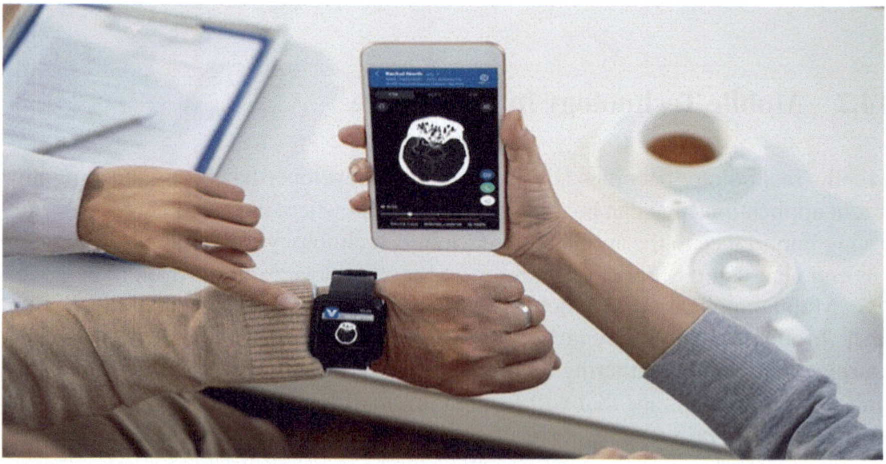

Fig. 14.2 Viz.ai—diagnosing anyone showing symptoms of stroke [23]

Now Mobile Technology plays one of the major roles in fighting against COVID-19 pandemic. Mobile Technology is used to track and trace the COVID-19 patients. It enhances COVID-19 surveillance to control the spreading of coronavirus. Many mobile applications are available to do self-screening for coronavirus symptoms from home [8–11]. It reduces the risk of the user getting infected by coronavirus from the infected patients at hospital. As the number of COVID-19 patients increases, healthcare service providers could not reach remote places. Telemedicine service helps the user to get healthcare services from home or from places where they are. Mobile Technology is also used for giving training to healthcare workers those who are directly interacting with COVID-19 patients by the health organization.

Mobile Technology is not a new technology to healthcare, and it can improve the healthcare in four different ways [25]:

1. Increase the conformity of the medication.
2. Enhance posttreatment perception.
3. Health information can be shared with the patient.
4. Aggregation of data enhances population healthcare.

14.3 Mobile Technology to Fight Coronavirus

Coronavirus is continuously increasing, and it has forced countries to use different technologies with new methods to control the spreading of coronavirus. Asian countries have used a range of technologies to fight against COVID-19 pandemic. All the healthcare system and the government are trying to use the better technology that helps in fighting against COVID-19 pandemic. Mobile Technology is used worldwide as a tool to fight against COVID-19 pandemic; AI technology is used for diagnosis of the patients, medical imaging process, disease tracking, and its prediction [3]. Many tools are available for tracking the COVID-19 patient, self-screening for coronavirus, and treating the COVID-19 patient. Some countries use electronic bracelets for tracking and tracing the patient, and the system alerts the monitoring station when the patient leaves the quarantined or isolated places [26]. It helps to control the spreading of coronavirus. Using a screening tool, everyone can do self-screening for coronavirus, and if it is found to have some symptoms, the system will give necessary steps to be taken [8, 9, 27]. Many healthcare sectors provide telehealth services. With this telehealth service, a patient can consult a physician through video conference. It reduces the risk of infection of coronavirus from other patients at the hospital. Many countries use drones for proper monitoring during curfew and total shutdown enforcing social distancing in public area. Mobile technology is also performing the major role in the spreading of information related to the preventive measures of the virus to the people.

14.3.1 Mobile Tracking and Study of Behavior Trends Using Google and Facebook

The role of public health experts for proper monitoring of the coronavirus patients is a mammoth task. Apart from providing treatment, the patient's history of traveling and further keeping track of the patients after recovery are essential. Location tracking is one of the best means to monitor the coronavirus patients, and it helps to control the spreading of the pandemic [28]. Google has launched COVID-19 Community Mobility Reports web tool to support health experts for monitoring the spread [29]. It also helps to identify large-scale behavior trends at public places. With the help of Google maps, it is easy to determine whether certain business or public places are busy at a particular time of day using location tracking data from mobile devices. Google provides downloadable Community Mobility Reports that highlight movement-trend differences at country, state, or regional levels [29]. These reports are intended to support public health officials and other major decision-makers as they work to control coronavirus spread. These reports maintain privacy protection by adding artificial noise to the dataset enabling high-quality results without identifying any individual person. In these reports, initially it covers 131 countries and regions as the urgent need of this information [30]. Still they are working to add additional countries and regions to ensure these reports remain helpful to public health officials across the globe looking to protect people from the spread of coronavirus. This information can be used to understand changes in daily essential trips that can define recommendations on business hours or inform delivery service offering. It also helps to indicate the requirement of additional buses or trains in order to allow people who need to travel with 1-m distance of maintaining social distancing.

Facebook offers mapping tools that show population movement and help the researchers and nonprofit organization to understand the crisis [31]. These mapping tools include disease prevention maps to help disease forecasting and protective measures (Fig. 14.3).

A voluntary survey has been designed to help health researchers to identify COVID-19 hotspots. The health researchers have used disease prevention maps to better understand how population dynamics influence the spread of coronavirus and its response to the pandemic. Facebook has launched three mapping tools which aimed at tracking the potential spread of the pandemic [31] as described as follows:

1. The first map is a co-location map which can define the probability that different Facebook users will come into contact with each other in person. This map can estimate the probability of different people coming in contact with each other [31]. Therefore, it can figure out the relationship among people in different places and can send an alert message if any people in those places got infected with Coronavirus. The blue lines in the Fig. 14.4 indicate people movements, based on location tracking on mobile devices. The more blue lines indicate more

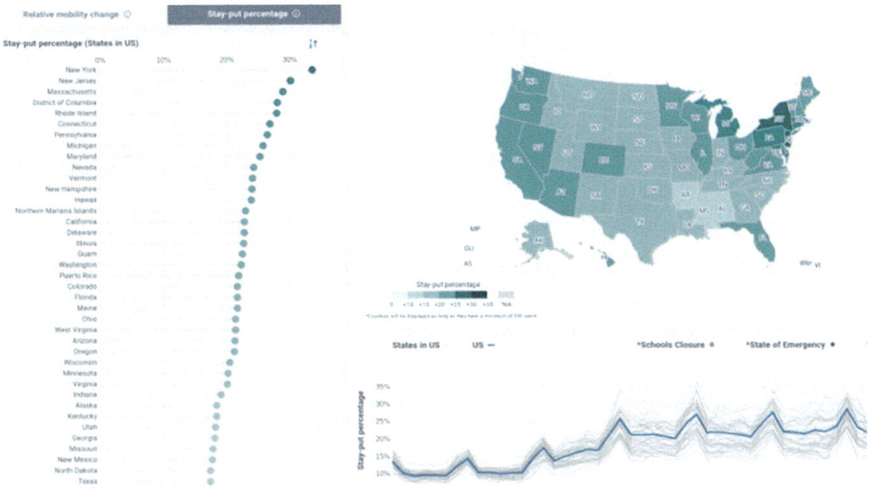

Fig. 14.3 COVID-19 mobility data network [4, 32]

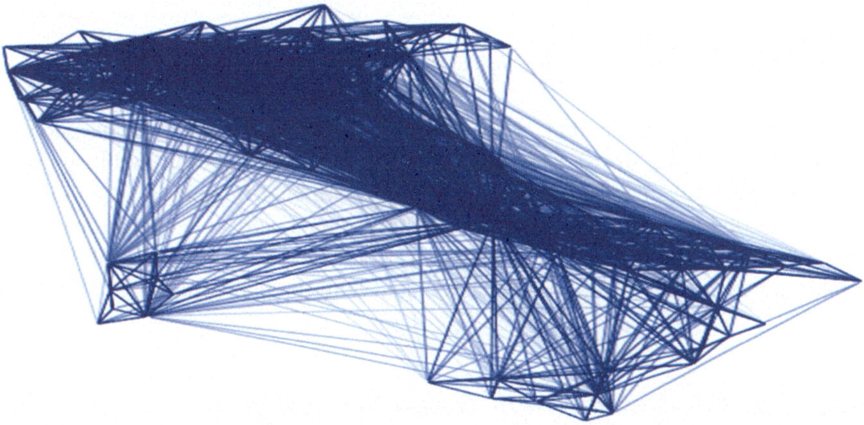

Fig. 14.4 A Facebook co-location map for Italy [31]

people are traveling between each region and showing the risk of spreading of the virus.

2. The second map is called a "movement range map." It shows the details of people staying at home or moving out a lot. This map helps us to understand about the people moving out for essential work and who has to travel long distances for pharmacy or grocery store (Fig. 14.5).
3. The third map is called "social connectedness map" which focused on insight around Facebook friends across geographic lines (Fig. 14.6).

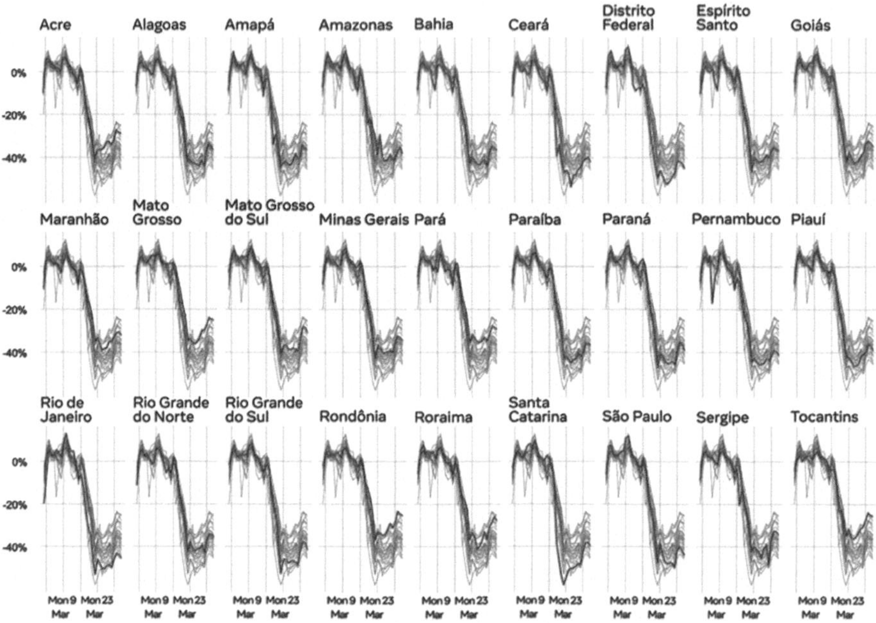

Fig. 14.5 A Facebook movement range map of Brazilian counties [31]

It has been since 3 years that "The Data for Good" is used by Facebook. Slowly, it is looking at natural disaster [31]. Facebook provides population mobility information, and it always needs to be contextualized with an arrangement of additional data sources on local demographics, infrastructure, and socioeconomic indicators in order to understand the underlying reasons for observed variations in mobility and can also aid us to understand the risk associated with the pandemic.

14.3.2 Mobile-Based Health Technology Solution for Coronavirus

With alarming cases arising daily, many countries started working on developing tools of Mobile Technology to control the virus. The digital health community monitoring the spread of the coronavirus is still trying to create more advance tools. The medical community tries for a better solution to curb the spread of coronavirus. Technology has also helped the medical industry track and treat viruses since the last decades. In 2018, Kinsa's smart-connected thermometers helped to a great extent during the severe flu season in the United States [33]. The uses of digital epidemiology tools, chatbot helper, EHR guidance tools, and rapid-response test kits are increasing. Mobile Technology is becoming one of the most helpful technologies to control coronavirus. Apple and Google announced that they have plans

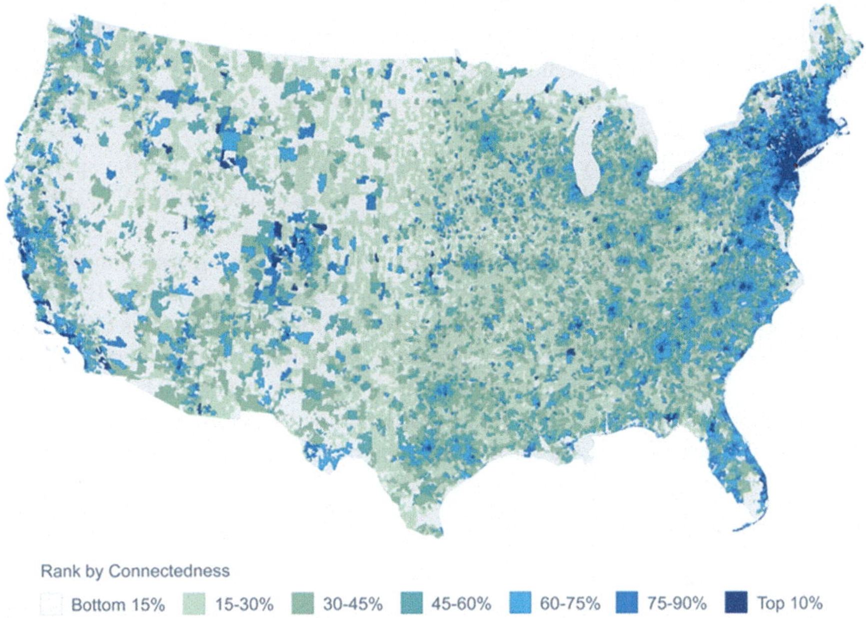

Fig. 14.6 A map of social connectedness between ZIP codes in the United States [31]

to launch an API that will enable interoperability between IOS and Android products to support the uses of Mobile Technology for the pandemic. Telehealth services started providing mental therapy by leading licensed mental health practitioners to deal with the stress and anxiety of the patients at free of cost. Walgreens has expanded their telehealth program to include a COVID-19 risk assessment, information of clinical trials, and a greater number of providers where they can connect with physicians [34].

Numerous people are also working to develop tools for tracking and tracing the COVID-19 patient. Few companies have already introduced the tracking and tracing device with the help of Mobile Technology and GPS service. In order to control the spread of coronavirus, many quarantine centers are available in every state or country for keeping the patients or persons who are suspected to be COVID-19 positive. Government needs to continuously monitor the suspected patients staying in the quarantined centers. However, the monitoring has not been successful, and as a result, patients got an opportunity to stay out of the quarantine center. Therefore, tracking and tracing device is one of the necessary devices to keep a track of the positive cases and thus control the spreading of coronavirus.

The Kingdom of Bahrain is using an app "Beware" for monitoring infected/suspected patient's unwanted activity. Any unwanted activity of these patients triggers an alert message. Based on this, the government can take necessary actions [26].

The wristbands must be always connected to the app via Bluetooth, with GPS enabled to track the patient movement. This technology ensures that the patient will not leave the quarantined center. Similarly, the device can track the self-isolated people by setting their location. Facebook started a program called "Data for Good" with the aim to trace the potential spreading of coronavirus [31]. It has used co-location maps to determine whether people are staying at home on a county-by-county level (Fig. 14.7).

Telemedicine technology and services also contribute to control the spread of coronavirus. Chatbots are also performing a major role to prevent COVID-19 pandemic by giving COVID-19 information to millions of people every day. Some chatbots use artificial intelligence (AI) and machine learning that can perform prescreening for coronavirus symptoms [35, 36]. Apple launched a COVID-19 app which gives services for both screening and information platforms. This COVID-19 app user needs to answer a couple of questions including symptoms, risk factors, and exposure. At the end, the user will get the possible next steps to be taken.

Telemedicine has been used by Japan to quarantined passengers of a cruise ship for a week. Drones having loud speaker are used by Chinese government to provide instructions to the people like "make social distance."

14.3.2.1 Solution for COVID-19 Surveillance

The spread of coronavirus is still a major issue even after there was complete lockdown. One of the important reasons is the lack of surveillance. During curfew and total shutdown, people are still roaming and doing social gathering. Government advised us to stay at home during lockdown, and curfew is not followed strictly. There is a need for better surveillance and monitoring systems. Today, Mobile Technology has become one of the important technologies in controlling the spreading of coronavirus. Many countries have already started using Mobile Technology as a solution of COVID-19 surveillance.

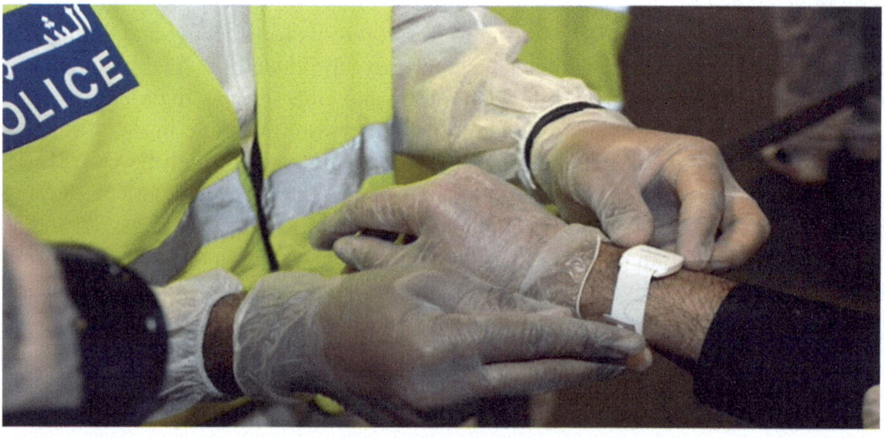

Fig. 14.7 Electronic bracelets to keep track of active COVID-19 cases [26]

China has currently in use of tracking system to deal with the COVID-19 outbreak. They are using Health Code Color system and tracking bracelets for proper COVID-19 surveillance [37]. These systems are deployed all over the main metropolitan areas of China. They are using the Health Code Color system: red color code is assigned for infected people, yellow color code is assigned for quarantined people, and green color code for healthy people for proper COVID-19 surveillance [37]. These systems are deployed all over the metropolitan areas of China, and it is also upgraded with facial recognition capabilities to track people moving without face masks. The system is capable of extracting the user's travel history thereby understanding whether he has come in contact with infected patients or quarantined people. For example, Mr. Chang is color green, but has come in contact with an infected person, then Mr. Chang becomes a potential threat for coronavirus.

In Hong Kong, they are using electronic wristbands to track the infected locals. Every infected person or self-quarantined at home is assigned a wristband, and they are compulsory to wear at all times [37]. This wristband is paired with a smartphone through Bluetooth. If the user left the isolated place, removed the bracelet, switched off the phone, or moved away far from the phone that is paired with the bracelet, the app on the device would send an alert signal to the Department of Health. New version of bracelet with built-in GPS tracker is also launched to quarantine people or infected locals. They are also using drones for surveillance, and the people are following COVID-19 safety guidance. All these drones have the loudspeaker to give instructions like "make social distance," "go home," or "use face mask regularly."

In Israel, the government passed emergency by granting access to the entire country's cell phone location data to police and the Shin Bet security service [37]. It is used to track down all those people who are in contact with an infected patient and then notifies them via SMS about the next steps they must take. The government also planned to use the cell phone surveillance system with Tel-Aviv to ensure the infected patient could not leave their isolated place.

Government of India also already launched the mobile app called "AarogyaSetu" for tracking coronavirus patients [38]. This will be one of the most important tools of India in fighting against coronavirus. When the users come near a COVID-19-infected patient, the user will get notification through this app. The AarogyaSetu may become the mother of all apps related to COVID-19 pandemic in India [39]. The government has also plan to make it a single point of access for food shelters, night shelters, and all the Suraksha retail stores that are being launched throughout the country. Many other apps like telemedicine platform may also be attached with AarogyaSetu app. The tracking of this app is done through Bluetooth and location-generated social graph which can notify the user interaction with anyone who has tested positive. The geo-fencing technology is used in Tamil Nadu to ensure that the persons who are in quarantine will stay inside the quarantined center [40]. In Delhi, the city police and civic agencies are using drones for proper monitoring during curfew and total shutdown enforcing social distancing in public areas and spraying disinfectants (Fig. 14.8).

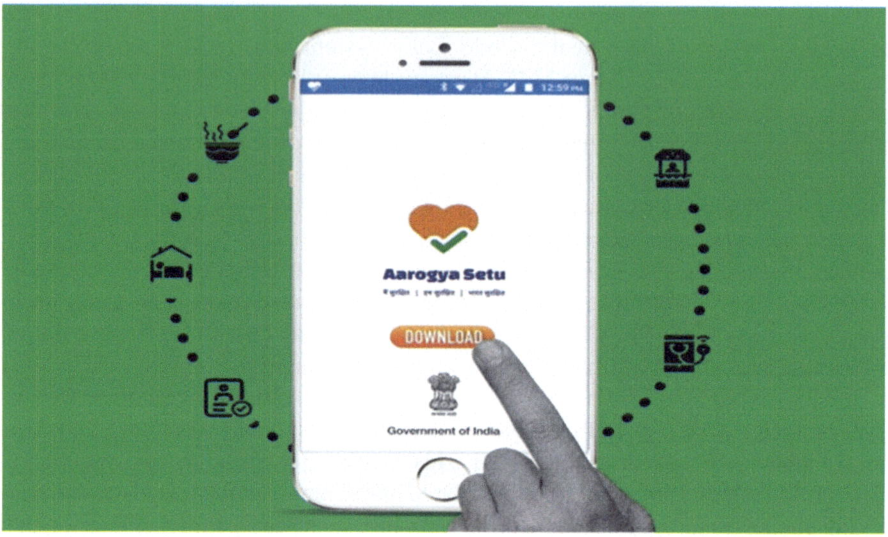

Fig. 14.8 AarogyaSetu app [41]

14.3.2.2 Solution for COVID-19 Prevention

The Mobile Technology performs a major role in the spread of information related to the preventive measures of coronavirus to the people. It helps to control the spread of coronavirus.

In South Africa, HealthAlert is implemented to give right information to the citizens through smart phones [42]. HealthAlert is a WhatsApp-based helpline to support users on health queries or concerns and helps them to direct the accurate information sources when they require [43]. The users will get all the necessary information related to the spread of coronavirus. They do not need to call the helpline and thus reduce the traffic at the call center helpline. An automated information response system is used in HealthAlert helpline that gives answers to the most frequently asked questions. HealthAlert ensures that the citizens will get the best possible health information during COVID-19 outbreak. This tool helps users self-assess their COVID-19 risk category based on their symptoms and their exposure history. Health Alert is straightforward, and questions of the users answered immediately.

Interactive radio is widely used in many countries to deliver coronavirus preventive measures to all the citizens of the countries [3]. It pairs AM and FM radio broadcasts with mobile phone responses. This is the best way for reaching rural and remote communities. The listener can give a response using a mobile phone for any clarification about COVID-19 outbreak. Interactive radio broadcasts in different languages so that all the citizens will understand the preventive measures of COVID-19 pandemic. This helps to increase knowledge and change attitudes and practice. Interactive radio answers listeners' questions, gives information, removes fear and false ideas, and surveys listeners' attitudes.

Inclusive E-learning program is widely used to support prevention efforts of COVID-19 pandemic by educating everyone on good hygiene practices and COVID-19 prevention strategies [3]. Many online programs are conducted for those people who directly interact with COVID-19-positive patients by giving procedures in order to prevent coronavirus. Many mobile apps are available at free of cost to conduct E-learning programs. Using these apps, people can easily attain an E-learning program from home or any places they are comfortable. The Government of India delivers COVID-19 prevention strategies to everyone with the help of Telecommunication and social media. Caller tunes of cell phones are widely used to deliver prevention strategies by the government. The Punjab government developed an app called "COVA" to spread awareness of COVID-19 prevention [44]. The users need to login with their mobile number, and then the user can get information like preventive care information and other government advisories. The Kerala government also launched a mobile app called "GoK Direct" aimed to give citizens' awareness over the COVID-19 pandemic and to check fake information on coronavirus being spread [45].

The World Health Organization (WHO) is leaving no stone unturned in publishing coronavirus-related prevention and control technical guidance to people. They have also exclaimed the importance of technology. Noora Health organization has a huge storage of COVID-19 health education resources. These are also available in different languages [46]. With the collaboration of the government of Bangladesh, they are attempting to deliver WHO-verified and accurate information using the WhatsApp platform. They also launched a training app called "Namaste Nurses" that gives training to nurses about COVID-19 prevention. In some places, COVID-19 doctors and other health professionals restrict the suspected patient from directly entering their room by giving a video call facility on mobile devices or tablets to interact with them. It helps to prevent the spread of coronavirus.

14.3.2.3 Solution for COVID-19 Diagnosis

People need to be diagnosed when they catch the flu or normal fever. In order to help these people, a self-testing app of coronavirus is available at free of cost. As of now, many tools for COVID-19 diagnosis are available in every country. Any time a user can do self-screening and testing by giving answers to the questions given on the app. Users will get advice about necessary steps to be taken if the testing system got some positive signs and symptoms from the user.

In India, Goa Ministry of Health introduces automated self-evaluation assessment mobile app to identify the risk patients for coronavirus. This app was India's first self-testing app for coronavirus. Goa Ministry of Health developed this app in collaboration with Innovaccer to self-diagnose COVID-19 symptoms [8]. The user needs to give their basic information, and then it performs a survey with basic questions that can be answered in either "Yes" or "No." These questions are related to present symptoms and the user's travel history. After giving all the answers, the user will get information whether the user has COVID-19 symptoms or not. The Puducherry government developed a similar app called "Test Yourself Puducherry" in collaboration with Innovaccer [9]. Reliance Jio, largest telecom operator, also upgraded MyJio app with self-testing facility for COVID-19 symptoms [10]. Apollo Hospitals Group has tied up with telecom operator Airtel and introduced a new feature in Airtel's existing app called "Airtel Thanks App," for self-testing of the user [11]. This new feature was developed through AI-based technologies that allow users to assess their COVID-19 risk profile by answering a few simple questions on any of the devices.

In Sri Lanka, the CommonWealth for Digital Health launched a mobile app called "COVID Shield" for combating COVID-19 [27]. It can help people keep track of health status and seek medical care early. It provides coronavirus-specific advice to the user following a self-health check, which includes an automated and AI-driven breathing assessment.

In the United Kingdom, self-test mobile app called "COVID-19 Tracker" is used to control the spread of coronavirus. This app allows user to self-report symptoms to help reduce the rate of spreading coronavirus. If the user has found COVID-19 symptoms, the app will alert with contacts so that the user can seek medical care to prevent the measure of the virus.

In United States, Pinterest CEO and a team of leading scientists launched a self-reporting coronavirus tracking app called "How We Feel." This app is available for both IOS and Android that everyone can download at free of cost. It was designed to make it easy to self-report about the symptoms the user has [47].

The Aga Khan University of Karachi has launched a self-testing app called "CoronaCheck" that enables users to easily check their symptoms at home and understand the next steps to follow [48]. This app uses an interactive chatbot, driven by AI, which allows users to understand their symptoms, recognize whether they may be COVID-19 positive, and seek help in a timely manner. It reduces the need for patients to visit for testing and also reduces the burden on the healthcare system.

Apple Company also released COVID-19 website and app with a self-screening tool and other information about the coronavirus pandemic [49]. The screening tool of this app will ask users to answer a series of questions around risk factors, recent exposure, and symptoms. Based on their responses, users will get CDC recommendations on the next steps, including guidance on social distancing and self-isolating, how to closely monitor symptoms, whether or not a test is recommended at this time, and when to contact a medical provider.

14.3.2.4 Solution for COVID Treatment

Providing proper treatment to home quarantine patients is one of the challenging tasks of the health organization. Digital health community to monitor the spread of the disease and facilitate better treatment of those patients who are home-quarantined has released new tools to reach out in rural areas. Many people use chatbot to figure out the right steps of their treatment. Healthcare sector has been using Mobile

Technology since many years. Many doctors and nurses use smartphones and ipads to aid hospital rounds communicate and guide the patients in treatment recommendations. It helps to improve posttreatment understanding and patient's access to health information using mobile health apps (Fig. 14.9).

A growing number of hospitals are turning to automated tools to help them manage the coronavirus pandemic. These automated tools are based on AI. The University of British Columbia (UBC) researcher applied a virtual care platform called "WelTel" to COVID-19 pandemic [51]. The WelTel was developed to improve the treatment of HIV in Kenya, and it was successfully implemented. The aim of WelTel is to improve patient engagement and personal care by connecting physicians and their patients through text messages. It allows physicians to send SMS text check-in to their patients. After the successful implementation and the effective outcomes in Kenya, expanded its scope and scale by automating check-ins and giving more features, it is used in several other African countries for HIV and tuberculosis. Now, the platform is modified so that it can be used for coronavirus, to provide daily check-ins for people in self-isolation. This platform can give response to people's questions very quickly and concerns while in home quarantined, as well as being able to more easily triage patients who need additional assistance.

Oracle has launched a Therapeutic Learning System app on 30th March 2020 to fight COVID-19 pandemic [52]. The goal of this app is to provide real-world data on which medication and dosages work against the coronavirus. This app has many functions like registration page of doctors to enter their credentials, records of their patients, and for practitioners and patients to update daily progress data, and the app provides real-time dashboards on patient status. There are also administrative screens that check authentication and credentials to guard activities against the database. This app is used to get the aggregated picture of what medicine is working, how, and under what scenarios and what medicine is not (Fig. 14.10).

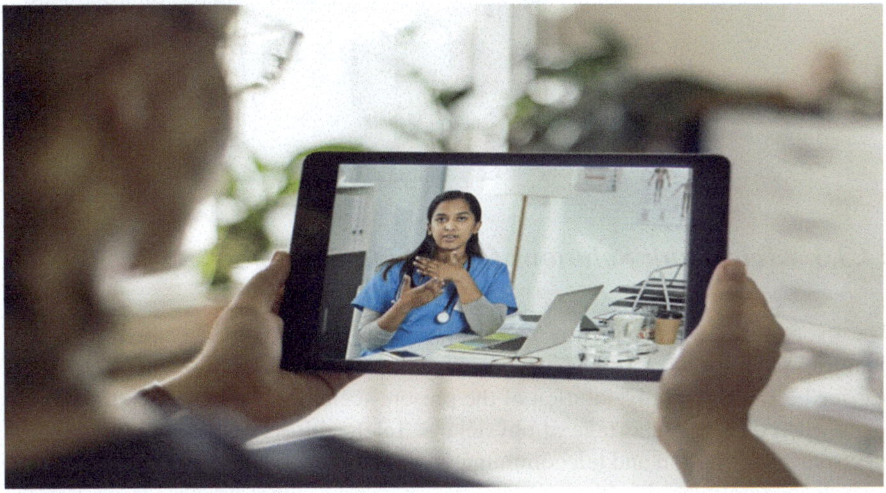

Fig. 14.9 Patient interaction with doctor using Telehealth service [50]

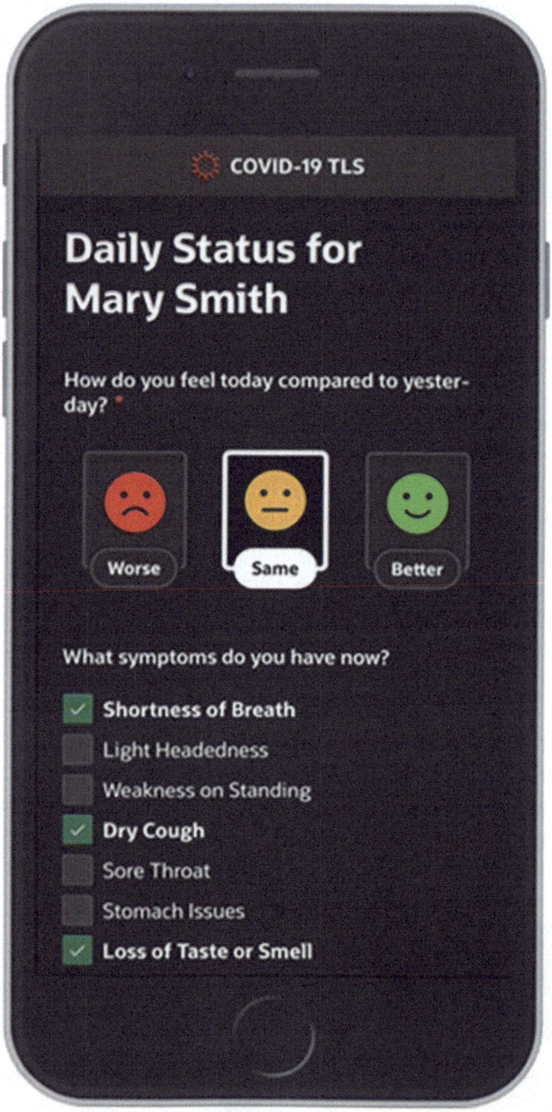
COVID-19 TLS
Daily Status for Mary Smith
How do you feel today compared to yester-day? *
Worse
Same
Better
What symptoms do you have now?
Shortness of Breath
Light Headedness
Weakness on Standing
Dry Cough
Sore Throat
Stomach Issues
Loss of Taste or Smell

Fig. 14.10 Oracle's COVID-19 therapeutic app [1]

14.3.3 Telehealth Solutions for Coronavirus

The overwhelming coronavirus pandemic makes some of the hospitals in many countries unable to give proper services due to the shortage of physicians. Telehealth service becomes the only solution of the present scenario to provide healthcare services when there is a shortage of physicians. Telehealth service is the utilization of electronic information and telecommunication technologies to support and promote long distance clinical healthcare, patients, and professional health administration.

Telehealth services can give health services to remote places where the physicians could not visit. Telehealth can connect those needy patients to the healthcare services through remote monitoring, video conferencing, electronic consultation, and wireless communication. It will reduce the spread of coronavirus. The patients do not need to visit the hospital for doctor consultation. It will also reduce the risk of other family members.

Since the last decades in the United States, almost all hospitals are providing telehealth service. According to a 2019 report from the American Hospital Association, 76% of US hospitals connect with patients at a distance through the use of video and other technology [7]. During coronavirus pandemic, they depend on telehealth service. The benefits of telehealth service are that patients and providers can overcome common barriers to healthcare like physical distance, limited access to reliable transportation, and lack of available healthcare providers [53]. The telehealth can provide service to those who are in medically not deserved or rural communities. It increases the relationship between doctor and patient by providing services through flexibility and convenience with the help of telehealth services to increase quality and affordable care. It reduces the gathering of patients in the hospitals and helps to reduce the spreading of coronavirus. It reduces hospital admission and readmission by allowing remote monitoring and consulting.

Telehealth services keep potentially infected individuals out of emergency care facilities or physician's offices. It reduces the risk of coronavirus transmission to other patients or healthcare staff. In the United States, it offers a free COVID-19 evaluation, screening, and escalation tool to all the hospitals. If the screening tool identifies the patient as being at high risk for the virus, they are directed to the appropriate facility and given instructions on how to manage the virus. This tool is also updated frequently with new recommendations and guidelines from the CDC.

One of the major problems in fighting against COVID-19 pandemic is the shortage of test kits to go around. With the help of telehealth, the healthcare service providers can safely evaluate and identify potentially infected patients whether through video conferencing or text-based communication [54]. If the patient has been diagnosed with it based on symptoms, they will most likely be advised to stay at home and self-quarantine. Using telehealth, the service provider can keep a watchful eye on disease progression, enabling them to treat and monitor patients with milder cases and know who is sick enough to refer to a hospital. When dealing with those patients who are living in urban areas, the service provider can provide proper healthcare services to the patients. However, rural towns are more isolated, so the service provider could not reach many places to give healthcare services. Many people in rural areas are not following COVID-19 pandemic prevention guidelines. This could lead to the increase of COVID-19-infected patients. Implementation of telehealth service is very necessary in rural areas to get them proper health service and to slow down the spreading of coronavirus. Some rural areas have limited Internet speed or no Internet; they can also use text messages service to consult with physicians.

Telehealth service is the ideal solution of dealing communicable diseases like COVID-19 pandemic. It helps those people who are at higher risk of being affected by coronavirus like older adults with preexisting medical conditions and by providing convenient access to routine care without the risk of exposure in a congested hospital or in a medical waiting room. Telehealth service has been used in many countries since the last decades.

The North Atlantic Treaty Alliance (NATO) developed a multinational telemedicine system in 2000 that has been deployed with their military forces during various crises. During the Acute Respiratory Syndrome (SARC) pandemic in 2003, China began working on telehealth service for use in the future when they are facing a similar situation [55]. The aim of telehealth service is to provide services in remote places and rural areas where the physicians could not reach. However, to fight against COVID-19 pandemic, telehealth service is also useful for people living in metropolitan areas since the population density is high in these places.

In Australia since 13th March 2020, many temporary Medicare Benefits Schedule (MBS) telehealth items are available for helping to reduce the risk of coronavirus transmission in hospitals and provide protection to patients and healthcare service providers [56]. These telehealth items are available to GPs, nurse practitioners, medical practitioners, participating midwives, and allied healthcare service providers. These items are for those people who are living in remote places and rural areas or who do not like to take risk of coronavirus transmission. These temporary MBS telehealth items help people to stay at home with essential Medicare-funded health service without the risk of coronavirus transmission within the community.

There are three major roles of telehealth to fight against coronavirus [57]:

1. Screening of patients remotely. People can get medical advices without going to the hospital for illness like cold and fever. This reduces the risk of spreading COVID-19 through social contacts, thus saving other patients and healthcare staff.
2. It provides unchanging care for those high-risk COVID-19 patients.
3. It aids in keeping the COVID-19 patients isolated in the quarantine center.

14.3.4 Mobile-Based Educational Technology Solutions for Coronavirus

The existing and new healthcare staff, those who directly interact with patients' needs, are upskilling to practice safely with the necessary skills and sufficient knowledge. It is required to teach them with reliable information. According to the present scenario, online teaching and training is the better solution to improve their skills. Many tools have been developed for both trainers and trainees. Using these tools, the healthcare staff can learn from experts without face-to-face delivery. Many video-conferencing tools are available at free of cost so that any expert can give training to other health workers and the other people also. Most commonly used video-conferencing tools are as follows [18]:

1. Cisco WebEx Meetings
2. Go to Meeting
3. Hangouts Meet
4. Skype
5. Zoom Cloud Meetings

Currently, all the countries are making all arrangenments to conduct training programs on COVID-19 for healthcare professionals. Experts can also share how to handle the COVID-19 patients in live video. An authorized health expert can also provide training throughout the world using video conferencing. Many SAARC countries conduct training programs on COVID-19 pandemic for healthcare professionals in different countries [15].

In India, many health organizations provide training programs for healthcare workers to handle coronavirus patients. On March 22, 2020, a training program was conducted nationwide for critical care management of COVID-19, at 1000 places through video conferencing [13]. Indian Nursing Council (INC) also plays a major role in India to fight against COVID-19 pandemic by giving training to healthcare workers who are dealing with COVID-19 patients through Webinar series [14]. On the first day of the INC, conduct a Webinar series on the topics "COVID-19 Facts and Myth and Preparedness, readiness and response for COVID-19." On the second day, conduct a Webinar series on "IPC-standard precautions and transmission based precautions and IPC-Hand Hygiene." Total number of participants was 12,000 healthcare workers in this Webinar series. It is not possible to provide training on 12,000 participants at a time without Mobile Technology. Till today, many Webinar series have been conducted, and thousands of healthcare workers have been trained by the INC to fight against COVID-19 pandemic. INC uses Zoom apps to provide online training through video conferencing. Zoom apps are available at free of cost, and every participant can easily download them from the Internet. Some Webinar series are helpful to those family members who provide care to COVID-19 patients. Like this normal people can also go through the Webinar series of INC, and it is freely available on YouTube. A Webinar on the topic "Response to COVID-19 in South Asia" was hosted by the Public Health Foundation of India in collaboration with the South Asia Institute Harvard University on April 15, 2020 [16]. They have used Zoom apps for video conferencing and giving knowledge to a huge amount of people without any registration. They have offered an overview of varied in-region responses to the coronavirus and their impact on the health system and social sector. Many employers in India are faced with a business continuity crisis due to lockdown and being challenged with the need to put in place new and possible models. Therefore, to help them, a Webinar was hosted by AZB and partners, in collaboration with Conventus law on March 26, 2020 to address common questions and concerns faced by Indian employers [17]. The World Health Organization (WHO) gives coronavirus disease training, and it is online for those people who are directly interacting with the patients [58].

All the countries are providing training to their healthcare workers through Webinars. All of these online trainings are conducted with the help of Mobile

Technology. Currently, all the schools, colleges, institutions, and universities are also affected because of COVID-19 pandemic. However, Mobile Technology helps to overcome these problems [59]. On 3rd March, UNESCO announced the impacts of COVID-19 on the shutting down of the schools and its effect on the students. By 10th March 2020, one of the five students are staying at home, and by 29th March 2020, 90% of the students are staying at home [60]. In India, the COVID-19 impact has been on the examination of the 10 + 2. Furthermore, the entrance examination for engineering, medical, law, fashion, etc. has been postponed, and the government is working for a model for conducting the same. The need for engaging the students had become a challenge, and all the educational institutions and teachers started opting for the online class mode. Technology has been playing a vital role during this pandemic. Many apps are available for video conferencing, and almost all are at free of cost. One of the most used apps is Zoom. Zoom was having ten million users till Dec 2019. By February, it reached 12.9 million, and by the end of April, it was 300 million users. The Zoom stock price has increased from $68.72 to $146.12 by 30 March [61]. In India, the adaption to online classes by students has increased. However, there are still many to be a part of the online class due to lack of awareness, knowledge, interest, and network connectivity issues. However, few of the higher education institutes/universities have successfully rolled out online classes and also conducted examinations through Zoom and Moodle (Open source Learning Platform). During this COVID-19, many of the MOOC's major players like Coursera, edX, Udemy, and Udacityetc are providing free online courses. Major companies like TCS and Tata Steel also have come up with free courses and internship for the students.

14.4 Proposed Novel Telemedicine Solution

Telemedicine solutions have become very popular during the pandemic. The utilization to the most effective way is the thought of the day. In this paper, we are proposing a cloud-based 24 × 7 Telemedicine solution using the Mobile Technology. As there are millions of users in Facebook, Twitter, Instagram, and YouTube accessing them, we proposed a 24 × 7 streaming of COVID-19 precaution, measures, and quantized methodology need to be followed. It also includes the answering of questions. Through an App, a user can put the relevant questions and see the time slot in which it will be answered. If the question is similar to one previously asked, it will tell the user about the already scheduled time in which the question will be answered. It will also provide the statistics of the number of users who has asked making the user satisfied that he is putting forward the right question. The doctor's schedule for the interaction was provided to the doctor before 24 h. Each doctor will be having a half an hour slot and will receive alert message before the commencement of the slot. The doctor can also find the statistics of people logging in the sessions, number of questions put, the diversity of the people, etc. The app will have an SOS module, which will be used for two purposes: first, you need to know the answer immediately and, second, get the help of a physical interaction with the doctor immediately. The doctors/staff for the immediate SoS will be scheduled daily, and each of the concerned will receive his duty information prior to 24 h. Furthermore, there will be slots for psychology doctors as there are many cases of depression observed during this pandemic. Depression is the second deadly disease after cancer. The app will also schedule interaction of famous personalities for different walks of life to provide an insight on their experience in COVID-19 followed by few activities like poem recitation, singing a song, etc. The app will also schedule the interaction of the recovery patients and their experience, will power, and faith. Through this Telemedicine solution, we will try to establish a connection and continuity with people to motivate them and ascertain the hope to live tomorrow, and each of us has an individual role to achieve it.

14.5 Conclusion

Mobile Technology is used by the government, health organization, healthcare workers, and the people for different purposes related to the pandemic. Without Mobile Technology, it will be very difficult to fight against the spread of coronavirus and deal with pandemic situations. Through Mobile Technology, the surveillance of coronavirus has been successful. It is the mobile which can be used to track the movement of the people thereby can be used to maintain social distance as much as possible, alert the alarming zone, provide up-to-date statistics of the active cases which are around the mobile user [62]. Self-quarantined people are getting full online support for their improvement. In online MOOCs, the teacher of the institution/university is using the Mobile Technology to get themselves connected with the students during the COVID-19 pandemic. This has helped the student community not to sit ideal during the pandemic and thus have a sound mental health. Our proposed Telemedicine solution is also focused to provide an ecosystem where each one of us get benefited by connecting to each other and knowing what is happening in and around us. Today, in this pandemic, Mobile Technology is a savior and courage to fight against this pandemic.

References

1. Khanna, R.C., Cicinelli, M.V., Gilbert, S.S., Honavar, S.G., Murthy, G.S.V.: COVID-19 pandemic: lessons learned and future directions. Indian J. Ophthalmol. **68**, 703–710 (2020)
2. 10 Educational technology solutions for COVID-19 out-of-school children. https://www.ictworks.org/educational-technology-solutions-covid19-response/#.XrftJmgzbIU
3. 10 Digital health technology solutions for global COVID-19 response. https://www.ictworks.org/digital-health-solutions-covid-response/#.Xt9pdjozbIU
4. Coronavirus disease (COVID-19) advice for the public. https://www.who.int/emergencies/diseases/novel-coronavirus-2019/advice-for-public

5. COVID-19 apps. https://en.wikipedia.org/wiki/COVID-19_apps
6. Kapoor, A., Guha, S., Das, M.K., Goswami, K.C., Yadav, R.: Digital healthcare: the only solution for better healthcare during COVID-19 pandemic? Indian Heart J. **72**, 61–64 (2020)
7. Combatting COVID-19 through use of telehealth and telemedicine. https://hub.appirio.com/cloud-powered-blog/combatting-covid-19-through-the-use-of-telehealth-and-telemedicine
8. Government of Goa launch the Self-Assessment App for COVID19. Express Computer. https://www.expresscomputer.in/news/government-of-goa-launch-the-self-assessment-app-for-covid19/51168/
9. Govt of Puducherry partners with Innovaccer to launch Self-Assessment App for COVID-19. https://www.expresscomputer.in/news/govt-of-puducherry-partners-with-innovaccer-to-launch-self-assessment-app-for-covid-19/51632/
10. Reliance MyJio App adds a coronavirus self-diagnostic tool that is available for everyone. https://www.news18.com/news/tech/reliance-myjio-app-adds-a-coronavirus-self-diagnostic-tool-that-is-available-for-everyone-2548619.html
11. Apollo 24|7 AI based COVID-19 test with Airtel Thanks app. https://www.technologyforyou.org/apollo-247-ai-based-covid-19-test-with-airtel-thanks-app/
12. Medical realities launches free online COVID-19 platform for medical workers. https://www.mobihealthnews.com/news/europe/medical-realities-launches-free-online-covid-19-platform-medical-workers
13. Coronavirus: health ministry undertakes training for critical care management through video conferencing. https://www.thehindu.com/news/national/coronavirus-health-ministry-undertakes-training-for-critical-care-management-through-video-conferencing/article31128972.ece
14. Webinars/publication. http://www.indiannursingcouncil.org/COVID-19.asp
15. ReAct Africa and Africa CDC: COVID-19 webinars. https://www.reactgroup.org/news-and-views/news-and-opinions/year-2020/react-africa-and-africa-cdc-covid-19-webinars/
16. INDIA - WEBINAR ALERT: the response to COVID-19 in South Asia. https://noharm-asia.org/articles/news/asia/india-webinar-alert-response-covid-19-south-asia
17. Webinar - India – responding to COVID-19 – guidance for Indian employers. http://www.conventuslaw.com/report/webinar-india-responding-to-covid-19-guidance-for/
18. 5 best video conferencing apps for Android. https://www.androidauthority.com/best-video-conferencing-apps-android-904757/
19. Rahman, A., Dash, S., Kamaleldin, M., Abed, A., Alshaikhhussain, A., Motawei, H., Amoudi, N.A., Abahussain, W.: A comprehensive study of mobile computing in telemedicine. In: Communications in Computer and Information Science, vol. 956, pp. 413–425. Springer, Singapore (2019)
20. Wu, A.C., Carpenter, J.F., Himes, B.E.: Mobile health applications for asthma. Clin. Commun. **3**, 446 (2015)
21. Mobile technology is changing the healthcare industry. https://www.healthitoutcomes.com/doc/how-mobile-technology-is-changing-the-healthcare-industry-0001
22. MBS online: COVID-19 temporary MBS telehealth services. http://www.mbsonline.gov.au/internet/mbsonline/publishing.nsf/Content/Factsheet-TempBB
23. All in the timing. https://richmondmagazine.com/life-style/health/all-in-the-timing/
24. Javaida, M., Haleema, A., Vaishyab, R., Bahlc, S., Sumand, R., Vaishe, A.: Industry 4.0 technologies and their applications in fighting COVID-19 pandemic. Diabetes Metab. Syndr. Clin. Res. Rev. **14**, 419–422 (2020)
25. 4 Ways mobile technology can improve care. https://www.beckershospitalreview.com/healthcare-information-technology/4-ways-mobile-technology-can-improve-care.html
26. Bahrain launches electronic bracelets to keep track of active COVID-19 cases. https://www.mobihealthnews.com/tag/tracking
27. COVID Shield App. https://covid.iq.lk/covid-shield-app.php
28. How countries are using technology to fight coronavirus. https://economictimes.indiatimes.com/tech/software/how-countries-are-using-technology-to-fight-coronavirus/articleshow/74867177.cms?from=md

29. Google mobilizes location tracking data to help public health experts monitor COVID-19 spread. https://www.mobihealthnews.com/news/google-mobilizes-location-tracking-data-help-public-health-experts-monitor-covid-19-spread
30. Helping public health officials combat COVID-19. https://www.blog.google/technology/health/covid-19-community-mobility-reports/
31. Data for good: new tools to help health researchers track and combat COVID-19. https://about.fb.com/news/2020/04/data-for-good/
32. COVID-19 mobility data network. https://visualization.covid19mobility.org/?date=2020-05-10&dates=2020-04-05_2020-05-10
33. Roundup: Tech's role in tracking, testing, treating COVID-19. https://www.mobihealthnews.com/news/roundup-techs-role-tracking-testing-treating-covid-19
34. Walgreens expands telehealth as COVID-19 demands social distancing. https://www.healthcare-financenews.com/news/walgreens-expands-telehealth-covid-19-demands-social-distancing
35. Chatbots provide millions with COVID-19 information every day. https://www.weforum.org/agenda/2020/04/chatbots-covid-19-governance-improved-here-s-how/
36. Kumar, A., Gupta, P.K., Srivasta, A.: A review of modern technologies for tackling COVID-19 pandemic. Diabetes Metab. Syndr. Clin. Res. Rev. **14**, 569–573 (2020)
37. US, Israel, South Korea, and China look at intrusive surveillance solutions for tracking COVID-19. https://www.zdnet.com/article/us-israel-south-korea-and-china-look-at-intrusive-surveillance-solutions-for-tracking-covid-19/
38. AarogyaSetu app crosses 75 million downloads. https://economictimes.indiatimes.com/tech/internet/aarogya-setu-app-crosses-75-million-downloads/articleshow/75359890.cms?from=mdr
39. AarogyaSetu app primed to take lead in COVID-19 war. The Economic Times. https://economictimes.indiatimes.com/news/economy/policy/aarogya-setu-app-primed-to-take-lead-in-covid-19-war/articleshow/75238590.cms
40. The Covid-19 pandemic is accelerating the adoption of emerging technologies in India. https://qz.com/india/1838195/edtech-telemedicine-drones-get-a-coronavirus-push-in-india/
41. Aarogya Setu app primed to take lead in Covid-19 war. https://tech.economictimes.indiatimes.com/news/mobile/aarogya-setu-app-primed-to-take-lead-in-covid-19-war/75240045
42. COVID-19 HealthAlert concept note. https://www.praekelt.org/covid-19-healthalert
43. Here'showAfricansareusingtechtocombatthecoronaviruspandemic.https://www.weforum.org/agenda/2020/04/africa-technology-coronavirus-covid19-innovation-mobile-tech-pandemic/
44. COVA app helps people of Punjab stay safe. https://www.outlookindia.com/newsscroll/cova-app-helps-people-of-punjab-stay-safe/1807666
45. Kerala Govt launches mobile app for details of COVID-19. https://english.mathrubhumi.com/technology/tech-news/kerala-govt-launches-mobile-app-for-details-of-covid-19-1.4608234
46. COVID-19 – innovations in healthcare. https://www.innovationsinhealthcare.org/covid-19-innovations-in-healthcare-responds/
47. Pinterest's CEO launched a free iPhone and Android app for self-reporting your symptoms to help experts track the spread of the coronavirus. https://www.businessinsider.in/science/news/pinterests-ceo-launched-a-free-iphone-and-android-app-for-self-reporting-your-symptoms-to-help-experts-track-the-spread-of-the-coronavirus/articleshow/74971008.cms
48. AKU launches coronavirus self-screening app. https://nation.com.pk/09-Apr-2020/aku-launches-coronavirus-self-screening-app
49. AppleReleases COVID-19 website and app with screening tool. https://www.news18.com/news/tech/apple-releases-covid-19-website-and-app-with-screening-tool-2554639.html/
50. Telemedicine is essential amid the covid-19 crisis and after it. https://www.economist.com/open-future/2020/03/31/telemedicine-is-essential-amid-the-covid-19-crisis-and-after-it
51. UBC researcher applying virtual care platform to COVID-19. https://www.ubyssey.ca/science/covid-19-virtual-care/
52. Launching Oracle's COVID-19 therapeutic app: the back story. https://www.zdnet.com/article/launching-oracles-covid-19-therapeutic-app-the-back-story/

53. Telemedicine during COVID-19–benefits, limitations, burdens, adaptation. https://www.healthcareitnews.com/news/telemedicine-during-covid-19-benefits-limitations-burdens-adaptation
54. COVID-19 and Telehealth_Technology can help us triage a nation in crisis. https://www.medicaleconomics.com/news/covid-19-and-telehealth-technology-can-help-us-triage-nation-crisis
55. Telemed, J.: Telehealth for global emergencies: implications for coronavirus disease 2019 (COVID-19). J. Telemed. Telecare. **26**(5), 309 (2020). https://doi.org/10.1177/1357633X20916567
56. COVID-19 temporary MBS telehealth services. http://www.mbsonline.gov.au/internet/mbsonline/publishing.nsf/Content/Factsheet-AmendedMentalHealth
57. When eHealth goes viral: the strengths and weaknesses of health tech during COVID-19. https://www.mobihealthnews.com/news/europe/when-ehealth-goes-viral-strengths-and-weaknesses-health-tech-during-covid-19
58. Coronavirus disease (COVID-19) training: online training. https://www.who.int/emergencies/diseases/novel-coronavirus-2019/training/online-training
59. How technological innovation in education is taking on COVID-19. https://www.forbes.com/sites/jeanneallen/2020/03/13/how-technological-innovation-in-education-is-taking-on-covid-19/#57b733f37bc7
60. Impact of the COVID-19 pandemic on education. https://en.wikipedia.org/wiki/Impact_of_the_COVID-19_pandemic_on_education
61. Zoom revenue and usage statistics (2020). https://www.businessofapps.com/data/zoom-statistics/
62. New cases over time. https://news.google.com/covid19/map?hl=en-IN&gl=IN&ceid=IN:en
63. Facebook provides location-tracking maps, new user surveys for COVID-19 research. https://www.socialmediatoday.com/news/facebook-provides-location-tracking-maps-new-user-surveys-for-covid-19-res/575572/
64. A general update on direct relief's Covid-19 response to date. https://www.directrelief.org/2020/05/coronavirus-response-live-updates-may/
65. Coronavirus (COVID-19) charts and stats. https://in.tradingview.com/covid19/

Chapter 15
Predictive Analysis of COVID-19 Transmission: Mathematical Modeling Study

K. Anitha

Abstract A novel COVID-19 caused by the virus SARS-CoV-2 was identified at China in December 2019, and it was declared as global pandemic on 11th March 2020 by the World Health Organization. In India on 30th January 2020, the first COVID-19 case was confirmed at Kerala. As of 6th June 2020, 6,702,662 cases have been reported in India even though stringent nationwide lockdown has been implemented. It is essential to identify the rate of disease transmission and its characterization. ICMR stated that 80% of COVID patients in India are without symptoms. In that case, we should focus on identifying the optimal attributes that will give the rate of transmission of this disease. Statistical machine learning is a powerful tool to fight against COVID-19 which gives the potential models for identifying the pattern of this disease, predictive analysis, and rate of transmission. This chapter aims to construct the predictive model to identify the severity of this disease transmission and also find the topographical spread of the contagion.

Keywords Predictive analysis · Parametric and nonparametric modeling · Estimation of parameters · Regression

Mathematics Review Subject Classification 92B05, 92B10, 97M60.

15.1 Introduction to Mathematical Epidemiology

In human history, communicable diseases play major revolution and drastic fatality rate. From Spanish flu to COVID-19, it is essential to identify the rate of transmission. In 1916, Greenwood JR stated that remarkable results have been to control the

K. Anitha (✉)
Department of Mathematics, SRM Institute of Science and Technology, Ramapuram, Chennai, India
e-mail: anithak1@srmist.edu.in

© The Author(s), under exclusive license to Springer Nature Switzerland AG 2021

F. Al-Turjman et al. (eds.), *Emerging Technologies for Battling Covid-19*, Studies in Systems, Decision and Control 324,
https://doi.org/10.1007/978-3-030-60039-6_15

disease with the help of mathematical methods in epidemics. Daniel Bernoulli first gave the mathematical analysis for small pox in 1760. Mathematical models incorporated with computational tools bring the new insight to key issues like drug discovery, vaccination, transmission rate based on the various parameters, and treatment methods. The process of constructing the mathematical model that will improve the optimality in prediction is known as predictive analysis. Global search engine Google, Netflix, and financial sectors handling credit cards are widely using this predictive analysis. Always communicable diseases play vital role in human history. One of the best incidents is the 1918 Spanish flu which created more than 50,000,000 deaths. In 1980, more than 2,600,000 were occurred by measles, but it was drastically reduced in 2011 with the help of measles vaccine. The efficient understanding of the particular disease is more important to develop the drug. For this understanding, mathematical modeling helps the epidemiologist to identify the various factors involving the disease like age, rate of transmission, rate of mortality, demographic structure, etc.

The first mathematical model was initiated by Daniel Bernoulli against smallpox in the year 1760. In his model, he focused the competitive risk about smallpox, and he focused on how to control the death rate. Another remarkable spatial model was introduced by John snow in the year 1855 for cholera (London). For constructing the mathematical model for communicable diseases, it is essential to maintain some basic assumptions about its rate of transmission. The transmission rate always depends on the number of susceptible and infective persons [10]. This idea is the building block for compartmental model. In 1911, Ross proposed the simple compartmental model for malaria transmission, and he stated that the population of mosquitoes below the critical level will minimize the infection. Kermack and Mckendrik consecutively published three papers for basic compartmental model in 1927, 1932, and 1933. The formation of their epidemic model is represented by the following equations:

$$v(t) = -s'(t)$$

$$s'(t) = -s(t)\left[\int_0^t N_1(u)\,v(t-u)\,\mathrm{d}u + N_1(t)K_0\right]$$

$$r'(t) = \int_0^t N_2(u)\,v(t-u)\,\mathrm{d}u + N_2(t)K_0$$

$$w(t) = \int_0^t N_3(u)\,v(t-u)\,\mathrm{d}u + N_3(t)K_0$$

where

$s(t)$ = No. of susceptibles,
$w(t)$ = No. of infected people,
$r(t)$ = No. of recovered people.

$$N_3(u) = e^{-\int_0^t \alpha(u)\mathrm{d}u}, \quad \alpha(u) \rightarrow \text{Rate of recovery at the infection age } u$$

$$N_1(u) = \beta(u) N_3(u), \quad \beta(u) \rightarrow \text{Rate of recovery when the infection age is } u$$

Simple mathematical model which describes the transmission level is being defined by individual compartments to capture the status of individual, and this model gives the significant result. SIR (Susceptible-infectious-recovered) frame is the basic structure for all disease modeling. In this model, any individual can be in single compartment based on impact of infection. Julie C. Blackwood analyzed the basic framework of SIR frame. Compartmental models first divide the population into different clusters or compartments in which each compartment has the same level. They can move from one compartment to another compartment over a time with respect to their level of infection. Number of Infectious, Number of susceptible individuals, rate of recovery and lifelong immunity are some of the variables used in this model.

Effects of control measures like social distancing in public places, patterns of outbreak, positive cases of local and foreign nationals, health history, age, and migration details have to be reported. Kiesha Prem et al. stated that mixing pattern of social distancing will reduce the number of infections and they addressed the limitations of quantifying the contact persons in public places. This chapter proposes biological waves of COVID-19 in Sect. 15.2, construction of SIRD model along with its analyzation in Sect. 15.3, testing and validation in Sect. 15.4, and followed by experimental results and conclusion in Sects. 15.5 and 15.6.

15.2 Biological Waves of COVID-19

Pandemics are framed by bacteria and viruses. The COVID-19 pandemic is new to humans and it attacks the respiratory system; hence human body needs strong immune system. The severe acute respiratory syndrome coronavirus 2 (SARS-CoV-2) has started its impact in India on 30th January 2020 at Kerala. It is a single-stranded enveloped RNA Virus-1 which has a spherical shape with glycoprotein projections. It has many subtypes like alpha-, beta-, gamma-, and delta-type coronavirus. It has been found in bats, mice, cats, pigs, and some bird family. Figure 15.1 describes the genome and structure of COVID-19.

As per the scientists point of view in India, COVID-19 may have plateaued and could fall after certain period of lockdown is lifted. So far, 6,702,662 positive cases, 393,210 deaths, and 3,045,695 recovered cases have been reported globally. In India, 226,770 positive cases, 6363 deaths, and 109,462 recovered cases have been reported as on first week of June 2020. The duration for peak will depend on the maintenance of social distancing even after the relaxation of lockdown. Once lockdown is lifted, the second wave of COVID-19 will start again. In that case, curve

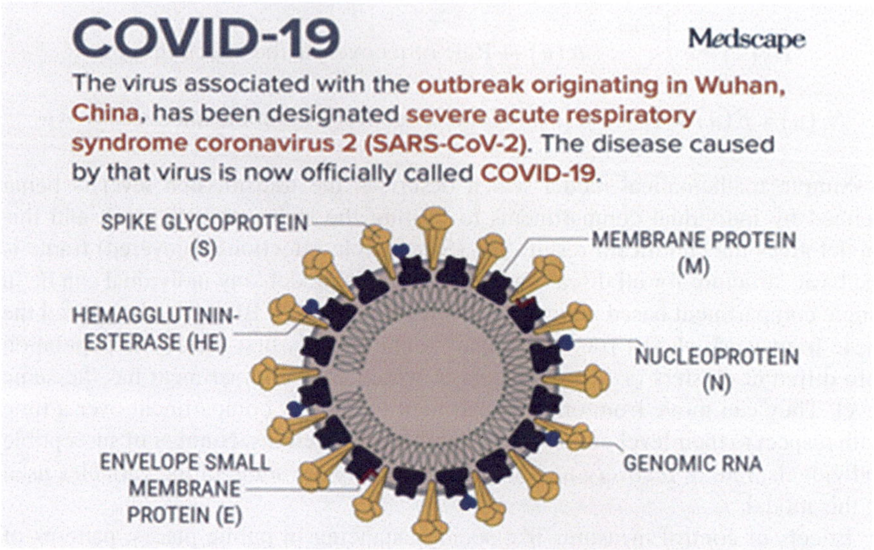

Fig. 15.1 Structure of COVID-19-SARS

will reach the peak based on social distancing. Before that, vaccine or drug has to be initiated. More numbers of mathematical models are being developed to forecast and control COVID-19 worldwide.

The pathogen defined the significant challenges for health, planning about the pandemic, and the healthcare systems. Until the identification of vaccine, some of the non-pharmaceutical measures have to be considered. Infective individual's contact tracing and isolation will minimize the level of outbreak. Epidemiological models should reduce the morbidity and mortality.

The following pictures show the data of COVID-19 status in India up to 16th May 2020 (Fig. 15.2).

15.3 Construction of Mathematical Model: SIRD

Let $N(t)$ be the population at a time t based on the status of infection. The population is categorized as Susceptible (S), Infected (I), Recovered (R), and Death (D). The following flow chart exhibits the working method of this model (Fig. 15.3).

Assume that the constant population of the state = ten million

$$N(t) = S + I + R - D$$

Then, the rate of change of population is considered as

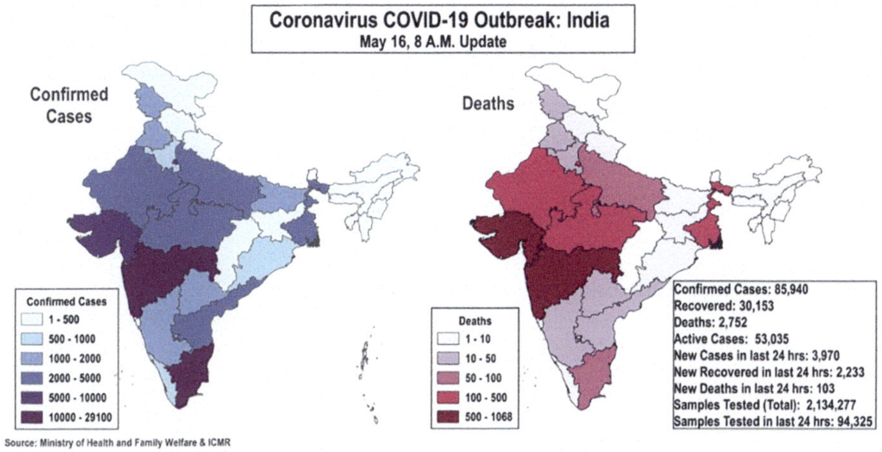

Fig. 15.2 COVID-19 outbreak in India

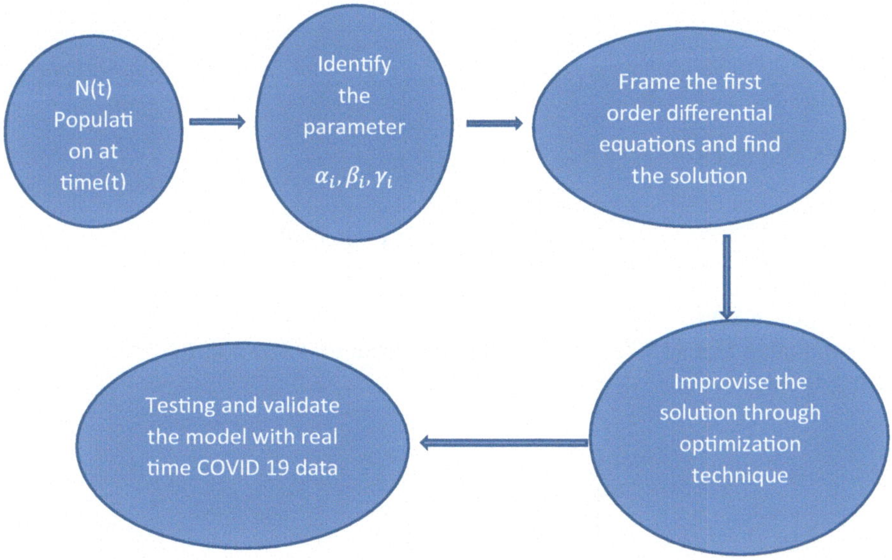

Fig. 15.3 Flow chart of SIRD model

$$\frac{\mathrm{d}N}{\mathrm{d}t} = (S + I + R)N - DN$$

$$N(t) = N_1 e^{(B-D)t} \tag{15.1}$$

where $B = S + I + R$, which is the exponential growth.

For the process of self-limiting, Eq. (15.1) can be modified as follows:

$\frac{dN}{dt} = r_i N\left(1 - N/F\right)$ (logistic growth)

The solution of the above equation is (Fig. 15.4)

$$N(t) = \frac{N_1 F e^{(r_i)t}}{\left[F + N_1 (e^{(r_i)t} - 1\right]} \rightarrow F \text{as} t \rightarrow \infty \tag{15.2}$$

The differential equation of susceptible population is given by

$$\frac{ds}{dt} = N(t) - \alpha_1 S - \alpha_2 S - \alpha_3 S - d_1 S \tag{15.3}$$

where α_1—quarantined individuals, α_2—recovered individuals, α_3—not confirmed, and d_1—natural death.

Similarly, the differential equations of infected and recovered population are defined by

$$\frac{dI}{dt} = N(t) - \beta_1 S - \beta_2 S - \beta_3 S - d_2 S - d_3 S \tag{15.4}$$

d_3—infected death

$$\frac{dR}{dt} = N(t) + \gamma_1 Q(t) + \gamma_2 I - d_1 S - d_2 S \tag{15.5}$$

$Q(t)$—quarantined

Combining Eqs. (15.2)–(15.4) with initial conditions $S(t) > 0$, $I(t) \geq 0$, $Q(t) \geq 0$, $R(t) \geq 0$, the solution is defined as

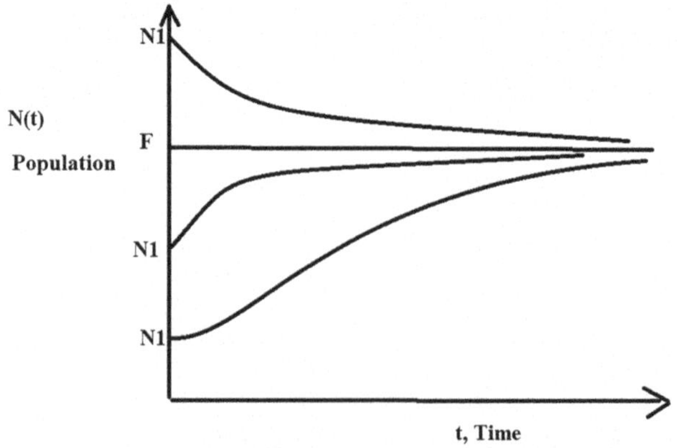

Fig. 15.4 Logistic growth of infected population

$$\frac{\mathrm{d}s}{\mathrm{d}t} \geq -\omega S(t) \qquad \omega = \alpha_1 + \beta_1 + d_1$$

$$\frac{\mathrm{d}I}{\mathrm{d}t} \geq -\varphi R(t) \qquad \varphi = \alpha_2 + \beta_2 + d_1$$

The SIRD model structure is locally asymptotically stable under the condition when $R(0) < 1$ and becomes unstable when $R(0) < 1$.

The Jacobian of the above system is given by

$$J(E) = \begin{bmatrix} -\omega & \frac{-\alpha_1 \omega}{S} & 0 & 0 \\ 0 & \frac{-\alpha_1 \omega}{S} - \varphi & 0 & 0 \\ \beta_1 & \beta_2 & 0 & 0 \\ 0 & \alpha_1 & \alpha_2 & -d_1 \end{bmatrix}$$

The characteristic Equation is $\det\left(J(E) - \lambda I\right) = 0$

where λ is the eigen value and the eigen values are $-\omega, \frac{-\alpha_1 \omega}{S}, \frac{-\alpha_1 \omega}{S} - \varphi, \alpha_2$.

15.3.1 Analysis and Optimization Process of SIRD

The process of constructing the mathematical model or the particular model which generates the accurate prediction is called predictive modeling. Splitting of data, data prediction, performance analysis, and comparative study are the key roles of predictive modeling. The software R—has the package named applied predictive model package. For the implementation of above set of equations, we need to analyze and optimize with some set of data. Data splitting is the initial process in modeling. We have to check how well the derived model extrapolates for different population. Furthermore, it is essential to find how much data should be considered for testing and validating. Scaling and centering the predictor variables is the most significant process in data transformation. The predictor variable has zero mean in centering, while each variable is divided by its standard deviation in scaling process. These values increase the numerical stability of the calculation. For the transformation process, Box and Cox proposed the following transformation function:

$$f(x) = \begin{cases} \frac{x^{\theta} - 1}{\theta} & \theta \neq 0 \\ \log(x) & \theta = 0 \end{cases} \tag{15.6}$$

The value of θ can be identified using the training data.

Principal component analysis (PCA) is one of the common methods to reduce the irrelevant information from the data. In this method, linear combination of predictor variables is considered as principal components. Mathematical formation of *i*th component of PC is written by

$$\mathrm{PC}_i = \sum_{j=1}^{P} a_{ij} P_j \qquad (15.7)$$

where P is the number of predictors.

The technical term collinearity is the technical term which is being used when the pair of predictor variables have correlated between them. Multiple correlations are also available between the variables. In this process, the first step is formation of correlation matrix between the predictor variables. Next select the pair of highly correlated variables. Let the pair be C_1 and C_2. Now calculate the average correlation between C_1 and other variables and similarly for C_2 and other variables. If C_1 has the larger correlated value, then remove the variable C_1; otherwise remove C_2. Continue the process until no absolute correlation is found.

15.4 Testing and Validation

COVID-19 statewise status of India has been taken from https://www.mohfw.gov.in/ which displays the COVID-19 affected people from all the states of India up to June 6, 2020, and the values are displayed here. Figures 15.5 and 15.6 give the numerical values of number of active cases, number of death, and total number of affected people.

The predictive model has been verified with this data. For implementation process, Weka classifier is being used for analyzation. The results are being displayed here.

15.5 Experimental Results (Fig. 15.7)

Test mode: Tenfold cross-validation	
Classifier model for full training set	
Locally weighted learning	
Using classifier: Decision tree, Linear Weighting Kernals and all Neighbour with Cross Validation	
Co-efficient of Correlation	0.7315
Mean absolute error	11,200.3906

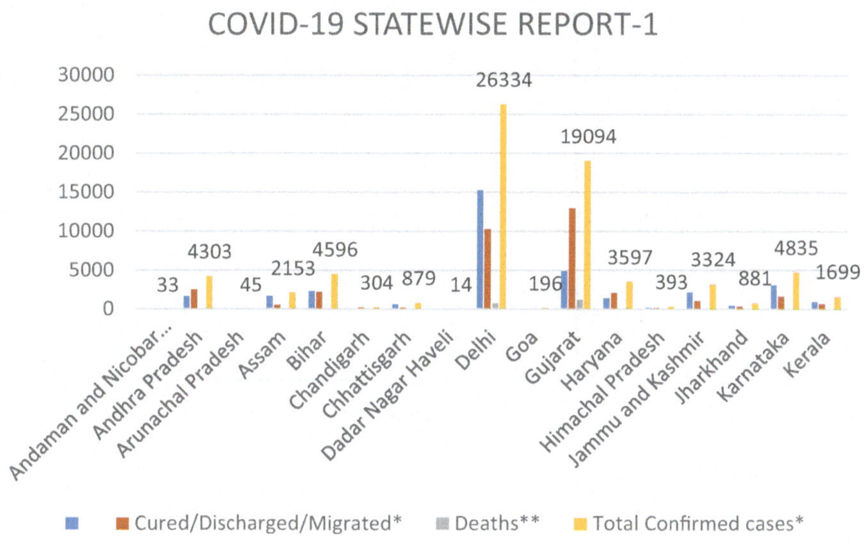

Fig. 15.5 COVID-19 statewise report-I

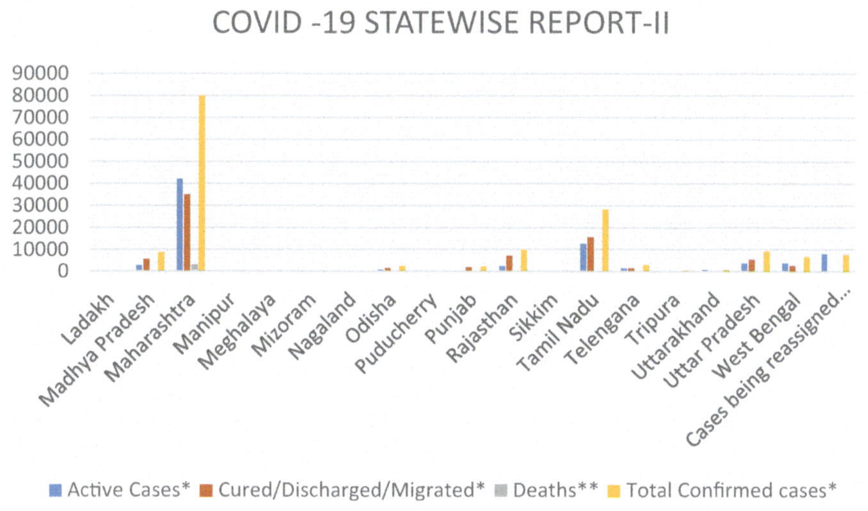

Fig. 15.6 COVID-19 statewise report-II

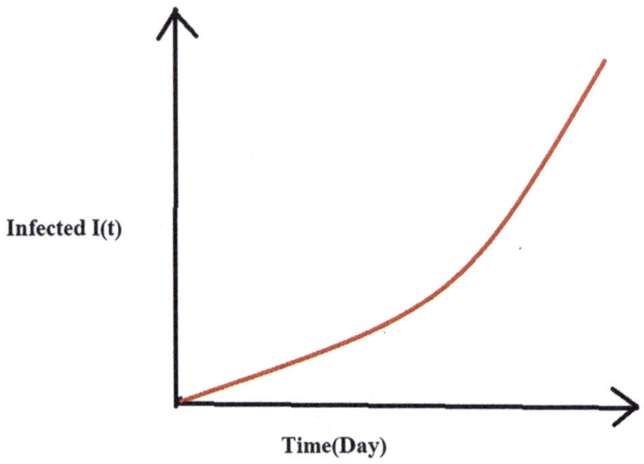

Fig. 15.7 Time series plot for infected people

Test mode: Tenfold cross-validation	
Classifier model for full training set	
Locally weighted learning	
Root mean squared error	36,790.2434
Relative absolute error	59.0362%
Root relative squared error	87.7999%
Total number of ınstances	37
Attributes: 6	
1. Number of hits	
2. Name of state/UT	
3. Active cases	
4. Cured/discharged/migrated	
5. Deaths	
6. Total confirmed cases	

Test mode: evaluate on training data
Simple K-Means—Euclidean Distant—R first lasst
@attribute 'Name of State / UT' {'Andaman and Nicobar Islands','Andhra Pradesh','Arunachal Pradesh',Assam,Bihar,Chandigarh,Chhattisgarh,'Dadar Nagar Haveli',Delhi,Goa,Gujarat,Haryan a,'Himachal Pradesh','Jammu and Kashmir',Jharkhand,Karnataka,Kerala,Ladakh,'Madhya Prade sh',Maharashtra,Manipur,Meghalaya,Mizoram,Nagaland,Odisha,Puducherry,Punjab,Rajasthan,S ikkim,'Tamil Nadu',Telengana,Tripura,Uttarakhand,'Uttar Pradesh','West Bengal','Cases being reassigned to states',Total#}
@attribute 'Active Cases*' numeric
@attribute Cured/Discharged/Migrated* numeric
@attribute Deaths** numeric
@attribute 'Total Confirmed cases*' numeric
Number of iterations: 3

(continued)

Test mode: evaluate on training data	
Within cluster sum of squared errors: 40.04935720953203	
Initial starting points (random):	
Cluster 0: 12, Haryana, 1439, 2134, 24, 3597	
Cluster 1: 25, Odisha, 996, 1604, 8, 2608	
Correlation coefficient	0.7534
Mean absolute error	10,527.7943
Root mean squared error	35,716.3567
Relative absolute error	55.491%
Root relative squared error	85.2371%
Total number of ınstances	37

Parameters for five states

Parameters	Maharashtra	Tamil Nadu	Gujarat	Uttar Pradesh	Kerala
$S(t)$	25,600	17,000	12,000	10,000	5389
Death due to COVID-19	0.36	0.24	0.37	0.33	0.12

15.5.1 Age-Parameter Compartmental Model

Equations (15.2)–(15.5) can be reframed for age-related model. From https://www.kaggle.com/covid19-in-india, age group data is taken. This data contains ten unique values which represent the age group from 0 to 9, 10–19, … up to ≥80 along with missing data, and the percentage of cases affected in the age group (Figs. 15.8 and 15.9).

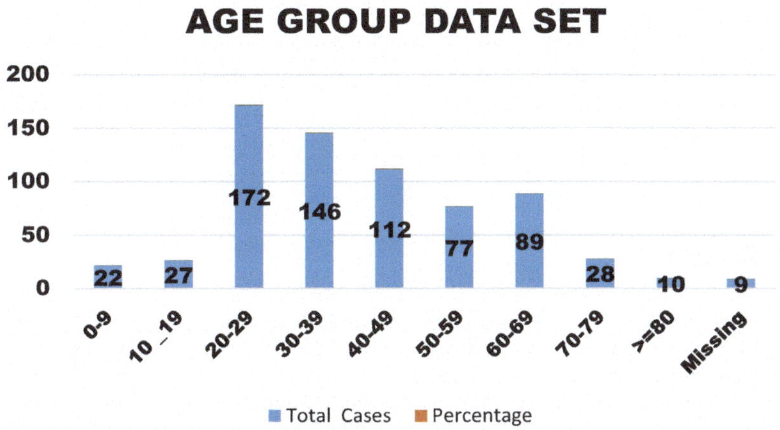

Fig. 15.8 Age group data

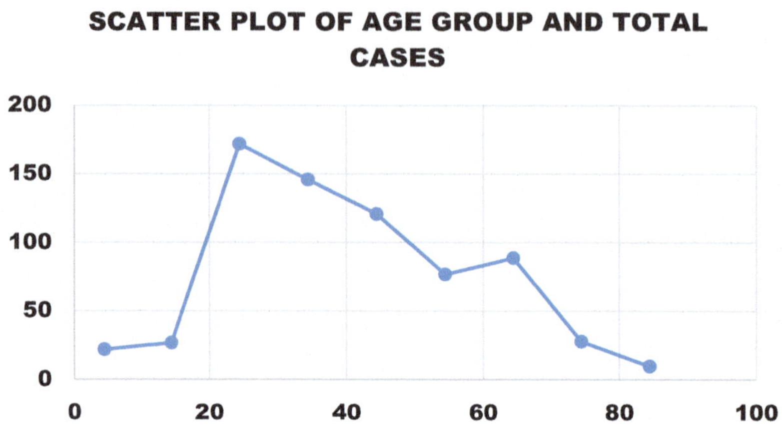

Fig. 15.9 Scatter plot

Regression equations for the above data are $y = -0.475x + 98.026$.
Correlation coefficient between age group and affected people is −0.214.

15.6 Conclusion

In this chapter, predictive epidemic model of COVID-19 has been framed. The confirmation cases are increasing rapidly for each and every day. The prediction factor of every infected individual is more important to avoid the transmission. The various parameters like age, health factors, respiratory syndrome level, and density of the population should be focused properly. It has been observed that when the value of $R(0) < 1$, then the system is locally stable. Based on the numerical results, it has been shown that there is the correlation between infected and susceptible individual. Hence, social distancing and invention of drug are more important. In future, the predict model can be extended to Bayesian network model which gives the result based on categorical responses. It is the acyclic graph which analyzes the various factors and constructs the network which will give the optimal result in decision-making.

Bibliography

1. Ahmed, F., Zviedrite, N., Uzicanin, A.: Effectiveness of workplace social distancing measures in reducing influenza transmission: a systematic review. BMC Public Health. **18**, 518 (2018). https://doi.org/10.1186/s12889-018-5446-1
2. Tuite, A.R., Fisman, D.N., Greer, A.L.: Mathematical MODELLING of COVID-19 transmission and mitigation strategies in the population of Ontario, Canada. CMAJ. **192**, E497 (2020)

3. Andreasen, V.: The final size of an epidemic and its relation to the basic reproduction number. Bull. Math. Biol. **73**(2011), 2305–2232 (2011)
4. Bernoulli, D.: Reflexions sur les avantges de l'inoculation. Merc. France, 173 (1760)
5. Bichara, D., Kang, Y., Castillo-Chavez, C., Horan, R., Perringa, C.: *SIS* and *SIR* epidemic models under virtual dispersal. Bull. Math. Biol. **77**, 2004–2034 (2015)
6. Castillo-Chavez, C.: Mathematical and statistical approaches to AIDS epidemiology. In: Lecture Notes in Biomathematics, vol. 83, pp. 289–300. Springer, Berlin (1989)
7. Breuer, F.: Mathematical epidemiology: past, present and future. Infect. Dis. Model. **2**(2), 113–127 (2017)
8. Fong, M.W., Gao, H., Wong, J.Y., et al.: No pharmaceutical measures for pandemic influenza in no healthcare settings—social distancing measures. Emerg. Infect. Dis. **26**, 976 (2020). https://doi.org/10.3201/eid2605.190995
9. Greenwood Jr., M.: The application of mathematics to epidemiology. Nature. **97**, 243–244 (1916)
10. Hamer, W.H.: Epidemic disease in England - the evidence of variability and of persistence. Lancet. **167**, 733–738 (1906)
11. Blackwood, J.C., Childs, L.M.: An introduction to compartmental MODELLING for the budding infectious disease modeler. Lett. Biomath. **5**(1), 195–221 (2018). https://doi.org/10.1080/23737867.2018.1509026
12. Kermack, W.O., McKendrick, A.G.: A contribution to the mathematical theory of epidemics. Proc. R. Soc. Lond. A Math. Phys. Eng. Sci. **115**, 700–721 (1927)
13. Prem, K., Liu, Y., Russell, T.W., Kucharski, A.J., Eggo, R.M., Davies, N.: The effect of control strategies that reduce social mixing on outcomes of the COVID-19 epidemic in Wuhan, China. Lancet Public Health. **5**, e261 (2020)
14. Kermack, W.O., McKendrick, A.G.: Contributions to the mathematical theory of epidemics, Part II. Proc. R. Soc. Lond. **138**, 55–83 (1932)
15. Kermack, W.O., McKendrick, A.G.: Contributions to the mathematical theory of epidemics, Part III. Proc. R. Soc. Lond. **141**, 94–112 (1933)
16. Abraham, P., Aggarwal, N., Babu, G.R., Barani, S., Bhargava, B., Bhatnagar, T., Dhama, A.S., Gangakhedkar, R.R., Giri, S., Gupta, N., Kurup, K.K., Manickam, P., Murhekar, M., Potdar, V., Prahara, I., Kiran, R., Reddy, D.C.S., Saravanakumar, V., Shah, N., Singh, H., Thangaraj, J.W.V., Yadav, N.: Laboratory surveillance for SARS-CoV-2 in India: performance of testing & descriptive epidemiology of detected COVID-19, January 22 - April 30, 2020. Indian J. Med. Res. **151**, 424 (2020). https://doi.org/10.4103/ijmr.IJMR_1896_20044
17. Ross, R.A.: The Prevention of Malaria (with Addendum). John Murray, London (1911)
18. Stehlé, J., Voirin, N., Barrat, A., et al.: Simulation of an SEIR infectious disease model on the dynamic contact network of conference attendees. BMC Med. **9**, 87 (2011)
19. Kim, S., Seo, Y.B., Jung, E.: Prediction of COVID-19 transmission dynamics using a mathematical model considering behavior changes in Korea. Epidemiol. Health. **42**, e2020026 (2020)
20. Wallinga, J., Teunis, P., Kretzschmar, M.: Using data on social contacts to estimate age-specific transmission parameters for respiratory-spread infectious agents. Am. J. Epidemiol. **164**, 936–944 (2006)
21. Woelfel, R., Corman, V., Guggemos, W., Seilmaier, M., Zange, S., Mueller, M., et al.: Clinical presentation and virological assessment of hospitalized cases of coronavirus disease 2019 in a travel-associated transmission cluster. medRxiv. (2020). https://doi.org/10.1101/2020030520030502
22. Wang, D., Hu, B., Hu, C., Zhu, F., Liu, X., Zhang, J., et al.: Clinical characteristics of 138 hospitalized patients with 2019 novel coronavirus-infected pneumonia in Wuhan, China. JAMA. **323**, 1061 (2020)
23. Li, Y., Wang, B., Peng, R., Zhou, C., Zhan, Y., Liu, Z., Jiang, X., Zhao, B.: Mathematical MODELLING and epidemic prediction of COVID-19 and its significance to epidemic prevention and control measures. Ann. Infect. Dis. Epidemiol. **5**(1), 1–9 (2020)
24. Zhang, J., Klepac, P., Read, J.M., et al.: Patterns of human social contact and contact with animals in Shanghai, China. Sci. Rep. **9**, 1–11 (2019)

Chapter 16
Analyzing the Economic Depression Post-COVID-19 Using Big Data Analytics

Bandana Mahapatra and Kumarsanjay K. Bhorekar

Abstract Various industries like technology, food, agriculture, and education are predicted to suffer major financial and production depreciation. The economic crisis suffered by the major large-scale industry on the other hand is predicted to effect the other economic enterprises effecting the world on a major scale. The lockdown incurred upon the general public is implemented all over the world in order to control the widespread of this pandemic. Coronavirus has hit the worldwide economy tremendously all over the world. Various countries have suffered life loss, temporary stop gap in various industries, economic growth, loss in revenues collected, etc. Though after a span the lockdown was made open, certain extra policies and rules were implemented such as social distancing and no gathering of people more than two or three in a close proximity. Restriction over number of people who can board at the same time over any public places like shops malls have effected the cash inflow to a huge extent. This chapter aims at analyzing the depression suffered by various sectors post-COVID-19 as a result of the lockdown along with various recent policies implemented. It also covers visualizing these issues with big data analytics perspective and how the concept of AI and other technologies is working across in order to solve these issues. It covers in brief how these upcoming technologies have been able to contribute in the healthcare sector while fighting against COVID-19 or uplifting the economy by helping the industry to build and design new models or plans to regain the cash inflow.

Keywords Economic deflation · Production crisis · Big data analytics · Post-COVID crisis · AI-based analysis for economic deflation · Market movement due to COVID-19

B. Mahapatra (✉) · K. K. Bhorekar
Symbiosis Skills and Professional University, Pimpri-Chinchwad, India
e-mail: bandana.mahapatra@sspu.ac.in

© The Author(s), under exclusive license to Springer Nature Switzerland AG 2021

F. Al-Turjman et al. (eds.), *Emerging Technologies for Battling Covid-19*, Studies in Systems, Decision and Control 324,
https://doi.org/10.1007/978-3-030-60039-6_16

16.1 Introduction

Deflation is the decline in the price of goods or services due to falling aggregated demand and lower costs of production.

The world has changed recently in the last few months with the inception of COVID-19 pandemic disease [1, 2]. As all counties have mandate a proper quarantine and lockdown, therefore the day-to-day, essential activities have got stacked. This pandemic situation has shown a huge impact over small and big sector like automobile, marketing, education, financial, agriculture, healthcare, etc. The situation has made every country suffer from economical deflation. Regular activities are suffering a huge collapse, where the current crises surpass every crises seen in the past many decades giving rise to apprehensions regarding its impact over people's lives and livelihoods [3].

Multiple countries are currently facing various kinds of crises with respect to health, financial, economic, and social and a severe collapse in commodity prices, which interacts in a complex manner [4]. Policymakers are formulating various methods of providing support to households, firms, and financial markets, which is currently vital for a robust recovery, but it is quite an apprehension about what the economic landscape will appear post lockdown [5, 6].

The estimates have indicated that the virus could trim global economic growth by 3.0–6.0% in 2020, with a partial recovery in 2021, assuming there is not a second wave of infections as depicted in Fig. 16.1.

The economic fallout from the pandemic raises the risks of a global economic recession with levels of unemployment. The human costs in terms of lives lost have permanently affect global economic process. In addition to the cost of rising levels of poverty, lives upended, careers derailed, and increased social unrest have also

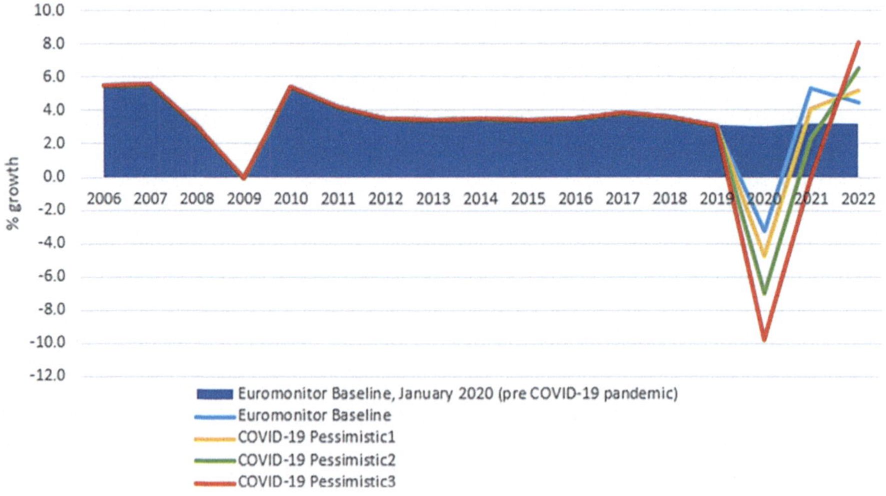

Fig. 16.1 Economic growth rate post-COVID-19 [7]

impacted the humans socially, economically, and physiologically. Global trade could also fall by 13–32%, counting on the depth and extent of the global economic downturn, exacting an especially heavy economic toll on trade-dependent developing and emerging economies [7].

Considering the fact that both the pandemic and needed containment are at its peak during the second quarter for almost many countries, and it recedes within the last half of this year, during April the World Economic Outlook projected a global growth fall up to −3% and a downgrade of 6.3 percentage points. This makes the good lockdown the worst recession since the good Depression and much worse than the worldwide financial crisis. Considering the spread of the virus within almost all countries during the end of March 2020, the global growth forecast has assumed that all countries undergo disruptions with respect to economic activity [7, 8] The world has shown a drastic change within a span of 3 months since the inception of coronavirus as updated by the *World Economic Outlook* in January [7]. A highly rare disease named as COVID-19, a coronavirus pandemic, resulted in tragic death of large number of human lives. As countries implement procedures of quarantines and social distancing practice and policies in order to control the spread of infection, the world has undergone a great lockdown which was the first experience of its own accord faced by various industries. The magnitude and speed of decline in activity that has followed is unlike anything experienced in lifetimes [8, 9].

This has been tagged as an unmatched crisis that has substantial uncertainty regarding its overall impact on human life and livelihood.

The epidemiology of the virus has a major role to play where the impact of measures undertaken to cure via development of therapeutics, vaccines, etc. is hard to predict. Multiple countries are currently facing crises with respect to health, finance, major fall in commodity prices, and interaction in complex ways [10].

Nevertheless, policymakers are currently offering support to various households, firms, and financial markets. Though it is important for a strong recovery, it has been observed that it does involves quite an uncertainty about what the economic landscape would appear as once lockdown is over. This chapter aims at projecting the impact of COVID-19 on various industry sectors and its effect over the economics of the country. The paper comprises of global crises caused due to the COVID-19 pandemic situation in Sect. 16.2, Sect. 16.3 is about the issues faced by the country due to the lockdown, and Sect. 16.4 is regarding how AI and big data analytics can be used to overcome this crisis situation as discussed in details in Sect. 16.6.

16.2 Global Crisis Due to COVID-19

The COVID-19 situation has shown a drastic effect over both emerging and advanced economies resulting in a market undergoing huge recession. It is predicted that post-COVID-19, the world economy will experience the worst recession since the great depression. Figure 16.1 shows the GDP growth post-COVID-19 of the international monetary fund [10, 11].

Hoping the pandemic to suppress within the second half of 2020, various policy actions have been undertaken in order to save the major countries in the world from suffering bankruptcy, with an extension to unemployment, as well as system-wide financial strains. A recent study undertaken by economic times has projected a global growth in 2021 to rebound to 5.8% [12].

The assumed recovery claimed in the article for year 2021 is partially portrayed since the level of economic activity stays below the extent that has been projected for 2021, before the virus hit the economy. The cumulative loss to global GDP over 2020 and 2021 due to the pandemic crisis is assumed to be approximately around 9 trillion dollars. Figure 16.2 shows the cumulative output loss over 2020 and 2021 [13, 14].

As shown in Fig. 16.3, we can consider the current economy indicating to undergo a real global crisis where no country will be spared from being affected. The various countries whose economy relies over tourism, travels, hospitality, and entertainment for their economic growth and upliftmen will suffer major disruption. The countries having various emerging markets and developing economy would suffer various challenges due to the unprecedented reversal of cash flows due to issues such as global risk appetite wanes, currency pressures, coping with weaker health systems, and more limited fiscal space to provide support. Several countries have currently entered the crisis state suffering a sluggish growth and huge debts [13, 14].

It was commented globally by major economists of the world that "for the first time since the Great Depression both advanced economies and emerging market and developing economies are in recession." The current economy has projected a growth of −6.1%. Various emerging market and developing economies having normal growth levels were also projected as showing a negative growth rate of −1.0% in 2020, as well as −2.2% excluding China. It was further shown that the income per

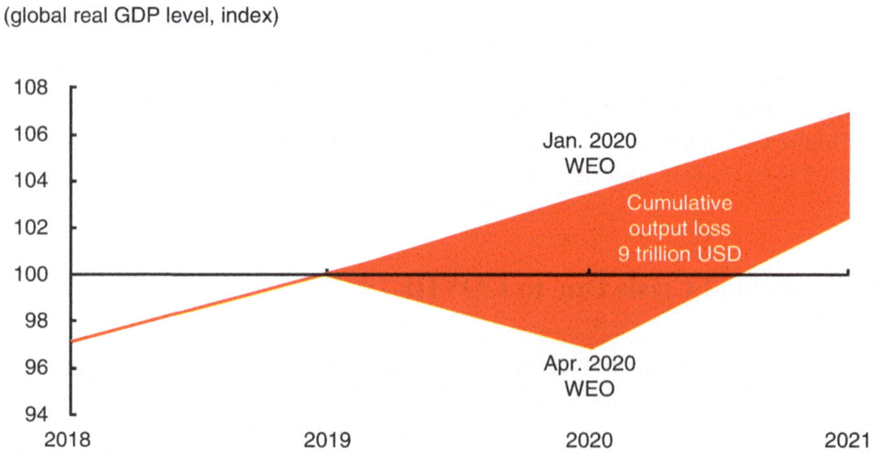

Fig. 16.2 Global real GDP level index [12]

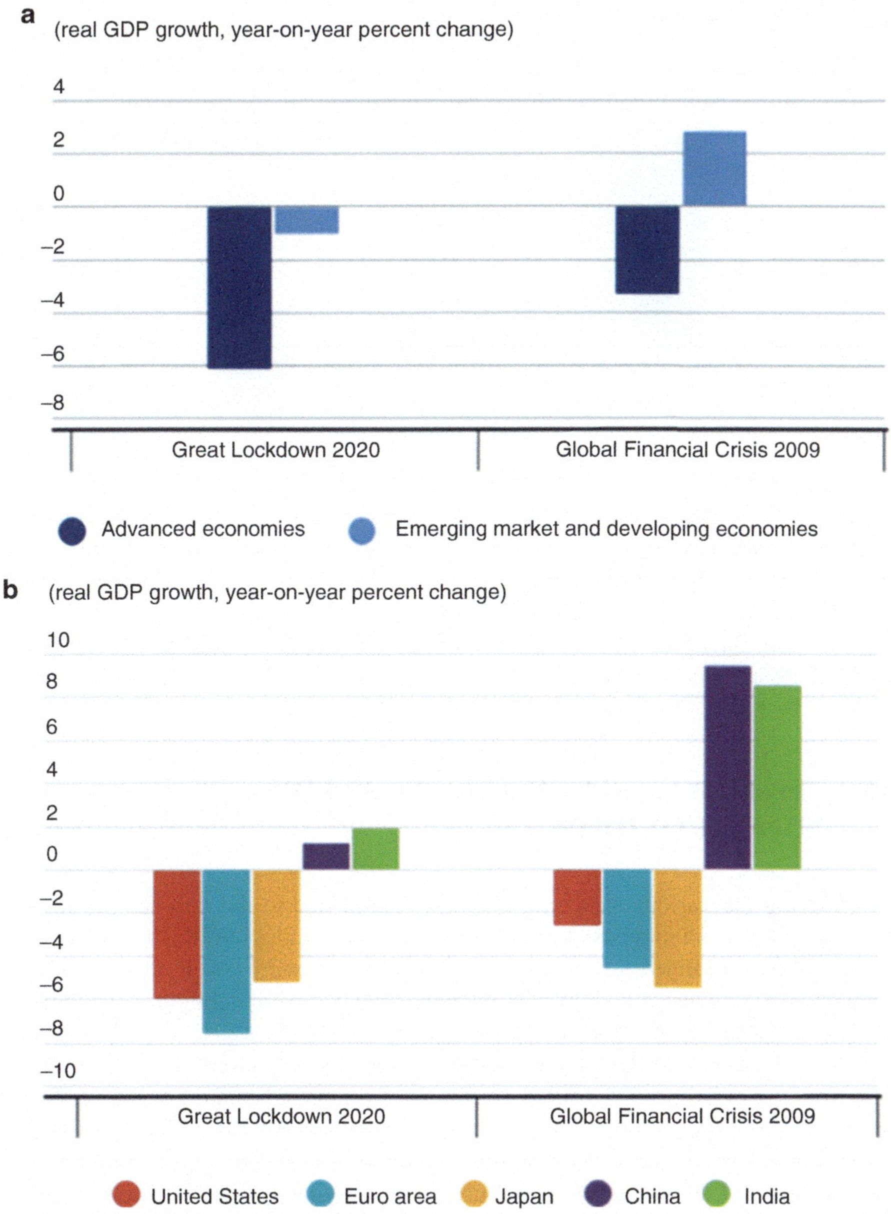

Fig. 16.3 (**a**) Real GDP growth of advanced companies and developing companies for year 2020 vs. 2009 (source: https://blogs.imf.org/2020/04/14/the-great-lockdown-worst-economic-downturn-since-the-great-depression/). (**b**) Depicts the detailed GDP growth of various countries. (**c**) World economy since great depression

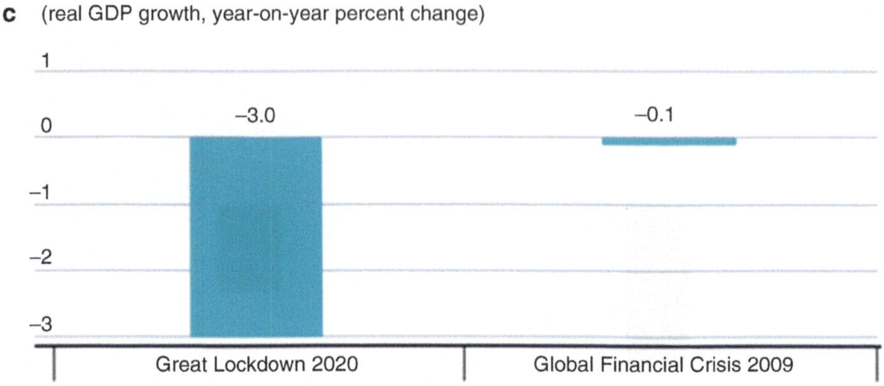

Fig. 16.3 (continued)

capita was supposed to shrink over 170 countries and advanced economies, emerging market, and developing economies are expected to overcome the depreciation partially by year 2021. Figure 16.3a shows the degradation of world major economies [15].

Figure 16.3a–c shows the GDP growth effecting the world economy post-COVID-19 situation [15].

16.3 Problem Faced by Country Locked Down Due to COVID-19

Considering the various structural changes caused due to the coronavirus in our lives, we have faced immense loss in various means, e.g., loss of life due to increase in mortality, prolonged social distance due to lockdown as well as government implemented policies, etc.; however, the pandemic has even highlighted the vulnerabilities existing in our current technological infrastructure [16, 17]. Few of the technical issues raised during the course of pandemic situation are outdated business systems, existing analog mode of communication, and existing nondigital payment infrastructure followed by small town laborers and farmers. The challenges thrown up at us to face were something never heard or can be stated as beyond imagination and the requirement of a privacy preserving system for the purpose of contact tracing. Figure 16.4 shows the impact of the pandemic over the world economy as a whole [18–20].

Such numerous major technical lacunas have triggered us with the thought to think about measures that can be undertaken to bridge them and undergo digital transformation in the coming years [9].

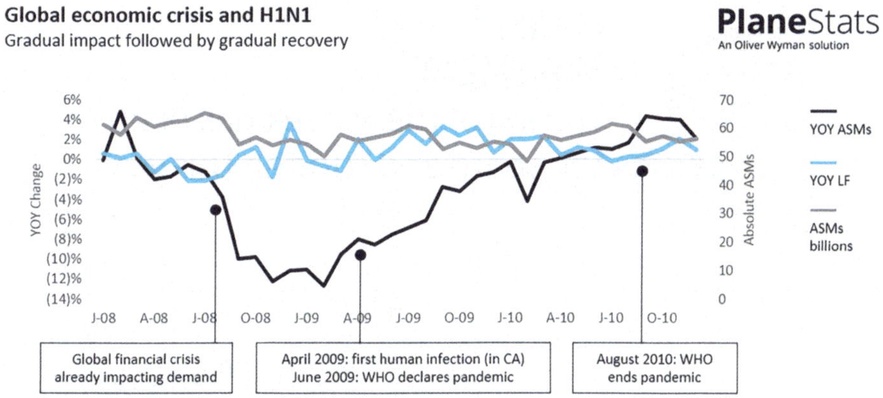

Fig. 16.4 Global economic crises due to lockdown [15]

16.3.1 Change Is a Market Scenario

The healthcare sector can be considered as one of the most affected areas that has faced the brunt of this COVID-19 pandemic in terms of life loss as well as health deterioration. The senior government officials are currently working on planning various strategies so as to cope up with the economic deflation caused by post-COVID-19. As a result, it becomes all the more important for us to navigate through the post-peak environment scenario [10, 11]. The general public health tools include at-scale testing, sophisticated real-time surveillance, rigorous contact tracing, and targeted quarantine in order to isolate cases and contacts. Likewise, insurance companies have a major role to play at crucial times of economic stress so as to help companies and households into managing risks and prepare cushion against losses (Fig. 16.5) [14].

The heavy trends in economic have been heavily augmented by the shocking wave of COVID-19. The impact of COVID-19 has reduced the global interest rates extremely low in the current economic cycle. As a result, the banks have extended the loans for the hard hit borrowers as well as renegotiating the credit terms. In the meantime, members of congress are calling over digital dollar in order to reignite COVID-19 stimulus [14].

16.3.1.1 Problem #1: Supply Chain Disruptions

The COVID-19 lockdown has completely disrupted multiple manufacturing units and supply chains across the globe. Many strategic planners of companies are still working over policies to be implemented that can deal with this pandemic situation, which includes overcoming fear or apprehensions around shortage or gauging overall impact of COVID-19 over the trends of supply chain or logistics monitoring. This has triggered the companies to adopt immediate measures in order to meet

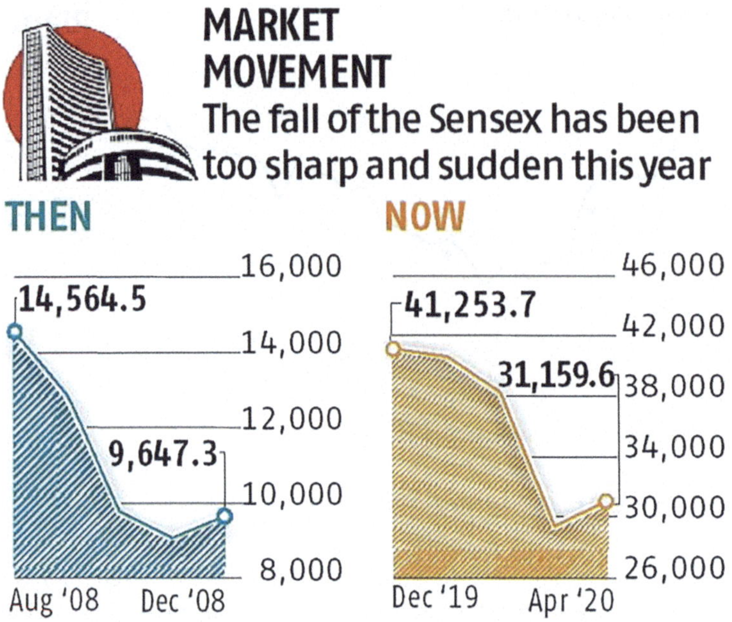

Fig. 16.5 Shows the market scenario due to COVID-19 pandemic [16]

supply and the customers need. This indicates the need of analyzing current plans for future disruptions which is quite a challenging task to undertake.

Artificial intelligence and various other emerging technologies have had an intense contribution into maintaining business continuity and uncertainty. Organizations can see through the huge amount of data storage and extract useful insights that can help predict disruptions and vulnerabilities and provide long-term visibility.

For example, IBM developed a cognitive control capability model in order to maintain its own supply chain, which can point out early warnings derived out of external data or social media. It helps the supply chain experts to have relevant as well as actionable information at their disposal. These information help them into quickly responding and focusing attention over higher activities, like communication with customers, suppliers, as well as other impacted stakeholders.

Though we live in the world of uncertainty where future is unpredictable, Ai and such technologies can make us smart and enhance the strength of global supply chain which helps these business sectors in various ways.

As quoted in IBM Institute for Business Value report, "COVID-19 and Shattered Supply Chains," supply chains is expected to be dynamic, responsive, and interconnected to an organization's ecosystem and processes which requires end-to-end visibility, real-time insights, and decisive actions, particularly in escalating situations [15, 16].

16.3.1.2 Problem #2: Manufacturing in a Safe Environment

As we know huge amount of product assembling operation is done by humans with their hands who are working at a gap of 0.6 m interval. As predicted by the WHO, increasing the space among the individual by 1 or 2 m raises both the assembly line length as well as manufacturing cost of the given product. The outfitting factory workers may also generate additional cost that can drastically reduce the finger dexterity that is needed in order to assemble small components.

16.3.1.3 Problem #3: Limited Movement of People

With restrictions imposed over the movement of people like laborer and workers the can be achieved by keeping the electronic products at a distance of around 1000 miles away from each other. This makes traveling a mandate component while undergoing production of new products.

The restrictions regarding maintaining social distance imposed over movement of people all over the globe are expected to continue for roughly about 18–24 months. It is therefore well quoted as "necessitating a new way to develop products remotely."

16.3.1.4 Problem #4: Limited Remote Oversight

In order to attain the mature products and process quickly, various multinational companies delegate mechanical manufacturing engineers to factory site during the period of development building. These engineers work in process in order to fix various issues as possible while going through a series of building which gradually improves the product maturity. For example, running experiments and highlighting specifications regarding applications like glue or grease, measuring improvements during real-time with respect to the factory partners.

Though the factory-related data and reports provide useful insights by providing context, misaligned incentive along with human error existing in the spreadsheet depicting data may end up in error.

Since early production of data trend was the dominating factor, hence the spreadsheet lacked hugely in portraying the critical elements existing in the data that are present in the physical world. This lacunae forced the companies to search multiple methods into extract factory data. The task is possible only with the support of the appropriate technology. Under the current COVID-19 situation, it is well commented that, "without trustworthy real-time, aggregated data," companies are undergoing product development process being built in the dark [14, 16].

16.3.1.5 Prioritization Pitfalls

Keeping in account a long list of problems to be addressed such as limited team resources and completely diverse condition of working enjoinment like complete sanitization and social distancing, multiple companies have followed the path of Maslow's pyramid of needs which ended in making the production process all the more slow and challenging to attain desired goals. This problem was solved by empowering the manufacturing teams and individuals the skillset of acting immediately during urgency of removing the bureaucracy factor. Clear mission alignments help to enable the teams to take over the ownership while acting urgently to address during emergency situation, e.g., ventilator refurbishment efforts undertaken by bloom energy [17].

The speed of putting the solutions in place, the lesser is the disruption caused to overall business. Various leaders looking up to reduction of bottlenecks for adopting it in their organizations must look to expedite overall decision-making process as well as streamline procurement, legal, and security review processes.

The issue surfaced during the pandemic COVID-19 is expected to witness fast adoption of innovative technologies at huge scale. The rate at which progress in innovation is taking place currently would be apt to state, "necessity is truly the mother of invention."

16.3.2 Education Industry

The education industry since pandemic lockdown is seen to undergo huge struggle to meet out the academic schedules and the predefined dates for the commencement of academic activity. Though majority of the classes have moved into online mode of delivering education, the universities are still unable to deliver certain specific skillset in terms of practical classes with respect to highly technical field. Moreover, there are multiple areas existing in the world which are yet to attain a good Internet connectivity and bandwidth.

16.4 Understanding the COVID-19 Pandemic as a Big Data Analytics Issue

The current global trade can be stated as undergoing a sudden shock due to the ways companies have been transacting cash in the last few months. Various industry related problems such as supply chain disruptions, enforcement of refocus round track, and tracing solution so as to gain popularity and visibility. In the meantime, certain financial intuitions such as bank or trade finance are looking forward toward implementation of paperless transaction in order to avoid contacts. Coming down to many large popular industries such as Teleco, acute disruptions are quite visible as a result of threats imposed due to human physical contact. For example, COVID-19 has currently stalled the rollout of 5G networks further to add on the network capacity is resilient to providing huge consumer demand of growing video conferencing or cloud and data service [12, 15].

The current new erupting era of digitalization has enormous growth and advantages due to which majority of top economic performers are shifting their business models to digital mode. The Software vendors here play a key role into modernizing the technology stacks of companies that range from almost every industry or geographical location. Due to the sudden booming of prevalence and accessibility data during this pandemic situation, software vendors may harness upon this opportunity toward implementing a new platform-based business models extracted from collaboration among customers providing a control over various ways, and methods data can be shared and transactions are implemented (Fig. 16.6).

Apart from the vendors, various other emerging technologies such as blockchain and Corda can also have a part to play where blockchain provides foundational technology to enable certain characteristics such as multiparty transparency, and Corda can accelerate the process of digital transformation with more promising and collaborative solutions. While addressing the requirements of an enterprise IT environments, such as privacy, scalability, and settlement finality. Such software firms that leverage latest technologies or other digital solutions have an extra opportunity to come up with wave of solutions that are not only during this COVID-19 pandemic crisis but also as a critical step undertaken in order to connect as well as future-proof industries for years to come.

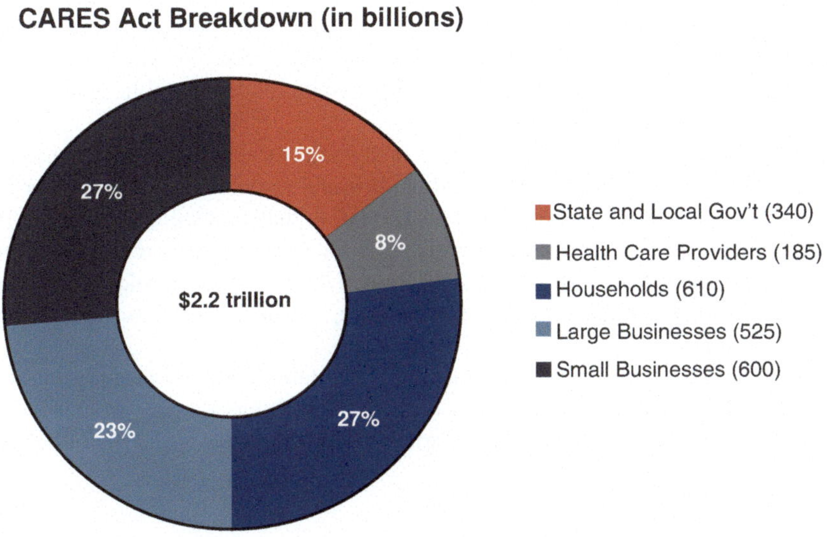

Fig. 16.6 COVID-19 causes unprecedented response as analyzed by Big Data analytics [12]

While manufacturing sectors are typically slow, COVID-19 has imposed a sequence of challenges for them to overcome, for example, disruptions in supply chain management, social distance being practiced at high touch assemble line, limited ability to travel, or restricted movement permitted. For electronics manufacturing industry, the urgency of handling the situation is even more demanded where such challenges could pose further issues of delayed launch schedules effecting the entire cash flow, lower financial returns, and quality issues that can damage the brand reputation [10, 14].

The current researchers and developers have started to use AI machine learning, and natural language processing vigorously is now **increasingly used** in order to keep track of coronavirus and gaining a more clear understanding of the overall disease.

In the last couple of months, researchers are trying hard at work in order to uncover and comprehend the nature, features, as well as traits of the virus. There are multiple related questions to be addressed such as why it has effected humans much more than any other virus giving birth to worldwide pandemic situation. What measures are supposed to be undertaken that can help reduce the spread and where the disease likely would go next [17, 18]?

Putting these factual aside, the bottom line of all these efforts is the information it generates which is currently the essence of a big data problem. Recently, professor James Hendler stated that they are currently working over tracking the spread of COVID-19 disease around the world. He further stated that he is currently collaborated with various organizations over modeling and dealing with the corona via supercomputer. He has further created websites in order to contribute into various organizations for conducting research over COVID-19 by providing the open data and documents.

The researchers in RPI use big data and analytics to improve the understanding and study the novel coronavirus with the perspective of various facets. Various organizations have recently broadcasted the news regarding supports provided by government entities, research organizations, and industry access for various innovative AI tools, in collaboration with various experts in data related to public health sector to fight against COVID-19 [19, 20].

These projects conduct a study over analyzing various signs and symptoms, tracking virus, monitoring the availability of hospital resources, etc. Researchers are currently dealing with huge amounts of information that are extensively impossible for any humans to comprehend and analyze on their own. There are currently multiple big data components that have incorporated AI to play a big role.

AI technology can also work over developing vaccines or drugs that can fight against COVID-19.

These projects typically require molecular modeling, where currently many of them use AI and machine learning in order to map things ranging from what we know about the virus into things in pharmacological databases and genomic databases" [21, 22].

Many huge companies have launched major projects such as **"Amazon Web Services"** and **"Google Cloud"** . Multiple other companies have offered free access to open datasets and analytic tools in order to support the building of COVID-19 solution faster. The concept of AI has the capacity to eliminate false tracts while enabling the inclusion of identification of various potential targets.

- Various researchers also are observed to exploit various attributes of AI so as to identify and test the effects of COVID-19 interventions over the human kind across various countries.
- Another major component is natural language processing and social media where various text is processed from various sources and analyzed to extract important information.
- AI is currently being considered as a promising tool since it is contributed at various kinds of multifactor learning. Recently, the UT Health team has developed an AI tool which can **highlight** the need for stricter, immediate interventions at Greater Houston area. Likely, researchers at Stanford University have launched a **data-driven model** which can predict possible outcomes of various intervention strategies.
- Another area where AI can make an impact is in mining scientific literature.

16.5 Contribution of AI and Data Analytics in Healthcare to Fight COVID-19

Since the inception of COVID-19, the world's radar seems to undergo huge global health crisis, where the virus has proved itself to be both challenging and deadly.

The field of AI and data analytics recent emerged immensely in various fields of healthcare industries as line of defense against COVID-19. Few researchers have gripped over the various tools in order to do everything ranging from **"tracking hospital capacity"** to identifying high-risk patients [23].

Concepts like "machine learning and data analytics have a major role to play in understanding the reason and traits for spread of disease, as well as understanding the effectiveness of our various responses to disease, as stated by Joe Corkery, MD, director of product management at Google Cloud, told *Health IT Analytics*.

Currently, the concept of AI and machine learning is playing a major role over drug discovery at scale, along with studying the effect of data analytics in real time. This kind of research highlights the fact that there are quite new things that can be done in order to make data analytics more easily repeatable as well as specific to "healthcare use cases" [22, 23].

While COVID-19 has disrupted the settled and finalized state of affairs, it has contributed in giving a background for the industry players into coming together and upskilling data analytics capabilities (Fig. 16.7).

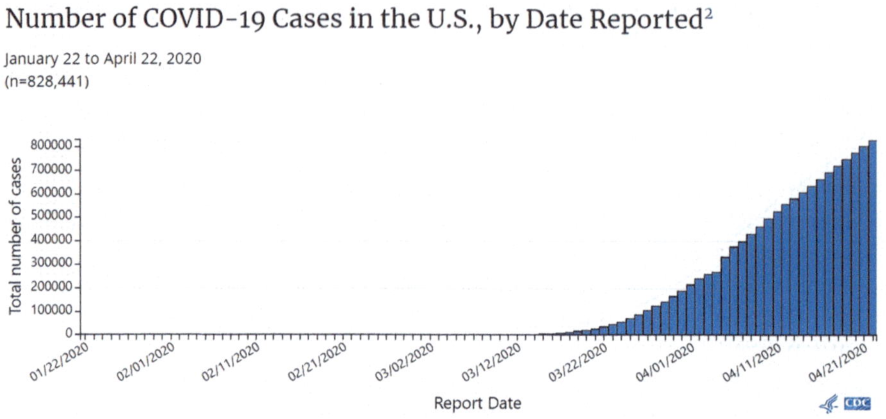

Fig. 16.7 COVID-19 cases reported in the United States [24]

16.5.1 Importance of Over Gathering and Accessing Quality Data

The requirement of a good quality, up-to-date data has always been foremost important in various sectors to achieve accuracy in data analysis. Moreover, it is even treated with high importance in various significant sectors such as healthcare. Moreover, the volatile nature of corona virus has made data accuracy all the more necessary [22].

The researchers are cautiously working over identification of various aspects of COVID-19, but any analysis undertaken and conclusion drawn is at a very nascent stage where the future is still unexplored. Corkery has stated in their article about new data being added and quite lot of information being evolved. These factors have triggered the great deal of research which is being undertaken in order to understand how accurately the disease can be addressed [23].

To ensure the good quality and updated information, researchers aim at collecting **real-world data** during the pandemic. The data collected from various primary and secondary sources may help stakeholders to extract patterns in order to make critical decisions [21].

As now most of the healthcare systems are encouraging individuals to stay home in order to protect themselves from being exposed to the deadly coronavirus leaves the government with the only option of conducting a survey over the population in order to identify the people who have symptoms. This motivated Dixon to carry out project that can allow individuals to report on their symptoms from their mobile or web browsers, giving insight to the researchers with a comprehensive picture of disease trends and hotspots.

Similarly, the Regenstrief and his team are conducting a survey that seeks to find new, viable ways of collecting data that can be used in the future [23, 25].

In addition to real-world data, researchers have shown inclination toward opening **publicly available datasets** in order to ensure reaching out to accessing quality

COVID-19 information. Using these datasets, teams can develop artificial intelligence and data analytics algorithms in order to have a clear understanding over the virus and its impact. It has been wisely commented that, "algorithms are the algorithms, but having that quality underlying data is what makes them work." Lack of refined content supporting the algorithm has successfully proved the importance of data collection.

16.5.2 Recent Collaborations Undertaken by Various Research Organization to Contribute During COVID-19

As the healthcare industry is working toward building its defense against coronavirus, various organizations from different sectors and individuals belonging to various geographical regions of the world have started to **work together** to find solutions to various problems surfacing related to multiple issues.

The unanticipated nature of the breakthrough of corona infection coupled with various other problems arising due to the preventive measures adopted has united all segments under a common goal to defeat and wipe out corona as well as its side effects [26, 27].

Assistant professor at Harvard Medical School and Dana Farber Cancer Institute have commented that, "the situation has opened up doors that we would have never thought to knock on." Not only in the field of medicine and healthcare but also technology has also come with collaborative efforts such as Harvard Medical School and Dana Farber Cancer Institute recently **joint hands** with Google Cloud to leverage advanced cloud and analytics technologies to accelerate the discovery of potential therapies.

The concept of open-source virtual drug discovery platform has enabled the researchers to able to reach out to billions of drug compounds against COVID-19, drastically reducing the time it would naturally take to analyze possible treatments [28].

The researchers have further commented that the partnership has helped them in order to reach the finish line in a time much lower than that it would have naturally taken.

16.5.3 Envisioning the Healthcare Industry in a Post-COVID-19 World

Considering with all positive hopes that the dust would be settled and the pandemic will be over, no matter when, there is a clear indication that the status quo of the world post-pandemic will be quite different from what we once knew. These changes can be of various measures ranging from huge to subtle based on the industry. For example, the effect in the healthcare, technology will be drastic and more evident with new ways of collecting, sharing, and evaluating data that will hopefully extend into life after COVID-19, leading to new technological advancements that have previously eluded the industry [29, 30].

With better data, increased collaboration, and faster analysis, researchers are looking forward to revolutionize the entire healthcare system providing a robust patient care facilities while preparing for any future emergencies.

As commented recently by researchers [30], "we did not know how to face this crisis, but the tools that we're developing could be very helpful for future drug discoveries, future pandemics, or other diseases that don't generate much pharmaceutical interest because they don't impact people in developed countries," which makes it quite evident that the combined efforts from stakeholders across the healthcare industry will facilitate more opportunities for researchers in all areas [31, 32].

16.6 Conclusion

This chapter has discussed various aspects of economic deflation post-COVID-19 across different industry sectors in the world. It covers the economic changes faced in the market across the world, then it moves into analyzing these problems using the current big data technology for analysis and various contributions of AI and big data analysis in areas pertaining to healthcare for fighting against COVID-19. The chapter also explained the importance of data collection for undergoing various analysis and how it can impact the results. Further, it throws light on various collaborative research work undertaken by various sectors, institutes, and organization, both technical and healthcare in order to fight COVID-19 pandemic situation which has given rise to various developments under all sectors that have come into existence for all time to come.

References

1. Vyas, M.: Unemployment rate touches 26%. Centre for Monitoring Indian Economy (CMIE) (2020). Accessed 24 Apr 2020
2. Sharma, Y.S.: Unemployment rate falls to pre-lockdown level: CMIE. The Economic Times (2020). Accessed 24 Jun 2020
3. Goyal, M.: Covid-19: how the deadly virus hints at a looming financial crisis. The Economic Times (2020). Accessed 23 Mar 2020
4. Research, Centre for Policy. Podcast: how has India's lockdown impacted unemployment rates and income levels?. Scroll.in. Accessed 24 Apr 2020
5. Covid-19 lockdown estimated to cost India $4.5 billion a day: Acuité Ratings. Business Line (2020). Accessed 11 Apr 2020
6. PTI: Experts peg India's cost of coronavirus lockdown at USD 120 bn. The Hindu @businessline (2020). Accessed 25 Mar 2020

7. Economics times: https://economictimes.indiatimes.com/tech/ites/covid-19-crisis-has-accelerated-importance-of-ai-hybrid-cloud-ibm-ceo-arvind-krishna/articleshow/75562060.cms. Accessed 27 May 2020
8. Biman.Mukherji: Coronavirus impact: Indian industry seeks relief measures to aid economy. Livemint. Accessed 23 Mar 2020
9. Chaudhry, S.A.: Covid-19 puts India's food supply chain to a stress-test. The Hindu @businessline (2020). Accessed 26 Mar 2020
10. Das, G.: 136 million jobs at risk in post-corona India. Livemint (2020). Accessed 2 Apr 2020
11. Young Indian startups hit as investors get cautious. Outlook India. IANS (2020). Accessed 1 Apr 2020
12. Singh, S.: Covid-19 Pandemic Spoils Indian Startup Funding Party, Growth Stage Worst Hit in Q1 2020. Inc42 Media (2020). Accessed 1 Apr 2020
13. Stock markets post worst losses in history; Sensex crashes 3,935 points amid coronavirus lockdown. The Indian Express (2020). Accessed 23 Mar 2020
14. Shah, A.: Sensex posts biggest gain in 11 years: investors richer by Rs 4.7 lakh crore. The Economic Times (2020). Accessed 25 Mar 2020
15. World Bank Fast-Tracks $1 Billion COVID-19 (Coronavirus) Support for India. World Bank (2020). Accessed 3 Apr 2020
16. RBI Governor Highlights: Shaktikanta Das cuts reverse repo; pumps in money, liquidity; eases rules for banks, NBFCs. The Financial Express (2020). Accessed 17 Apr 2020.
17. Economic cost of lockdown is nothing compared to people's lives: PM Modi. Business Standard. ANI (2020). Accessed 14 Apr 2020
18. Lockdown hurts economy but saving life is more important: PM Modi. India Today (2020). Accessed 14 Apr 2020
19. John, M.: How is the world dealing with lockdown? This poll has captured the public's mood. World Economic Forum (2020). Accessed 11 May 2020
20. https://www.wikizero.com/en/Economic_impact_of_the_COVID-19_pandemic_in_India. Accessed Apr 2020
21. Khanna, U.B., Anuja, P.: Modi says 'jaan bhi jahaan bhi', signals a shift in India's coronavirus playbook. Livemint (2020). Accessed 16 Apr 2020
22. Padmanabhan, A.: Opinion | New Delhi revisits the lives versus livelihood debate. Livemint (2020). Accessed 16 Apr 2020
23. Sharma, A.: Prime Minister Narendra Modi bats for unlocking economy, CMs divided. The Economic Times (2020). Accessed 12 May 2020
24. https://www.statista.com/statistics/1102816/coronavirus-covid19-cases-number-us-americans-by-day/
25. Gayan Varma, A.: PM Modi's meeting with chief ministers: five things to watch out for. Livemint (2020). Accessed 16 Apr 2020
26. Yadav, Y.: No matter how you look at it, India's lockdown-2 can cost as many lives as it will save. ThePrint (2020). Accessed 16 Apr 2020
27. Slowly increase public activities, PM throws challenge to CMs (Ld). Outlook India. IANS (2020). Accessed 12 May 2020
28. Coronavirus Global Economic Outlook: https://blog.euromonitor.com/coronavirus-global-economic-outlook-april-2020/ (2020)
29. COVID-19 crisis has accelerated importance of AI, hybrid cloud: IBM CEO Arvind Krishna
30. https://economictimes.indiatimes.com//tech/ites/covid-19-crisis-has-accelerated-importance-of-ai-hybrid-cloud-ibm-ceo-arvind-krishna/articleshow/75562060.cms?utm_source=contentofinterest&utm_medium=text&utm_campaign=cppst
31. https://www.business-standard.com/article/markets/how-economic-crisis-due-to-covid-19-is-different-from-2008-meltdown-120041200015_1.html
32. Ropes, Gray LLP.: COVID-19, data analytics & the FCA: big response, big data, big risk

Chapter 17
Intrinsic and Extrinsic Motivation for Online Teaching in COVID-19: Applications, Issues, and Solution

Kavisha Duggal, Parminder Singh, and Lovi Raj Gupta

Abstract Covid-19 has brought a challenging situation for the present education system. Online teaching adopted at various schools and colleges as a means to impart education to pupils has received a lot of confrontations not only by the students and parents who are at receiving end but also by the faculty who have utilized this method to continue the education program to enhance the learning of students. Adaptive analysis has been conducted on the present online education teaching involving various parameters. Regular teaching practices followed through online classes are not able to engage students to the best of their abilities so they need to incorporate fun-based learning methods. The online gamified education system is proposed to enhance the various intrinsic and extrinsic motivational factors which are directly proportional to high student engagement. Gamification acts as a strategy for the uplift contribution of members involved in online social communities. Gamified online learning is completely different from game-based learning. Gamified online education involves various elements of games, but the concepts of gamified learning include game-based learning, point-based system, virtual rewards, and high interaction among students by involving various gamified elements and mechanics.

Keywords Intrinsic motivation · Extrinsic motivation · Engagement · Game · Gamification · Online education system

---

K. Duggal · P. Singh (✉) · L. R. Gupta
Lovely Professional University, Phagwara, India
e-mail: parminder.16479@lpu.co.in

© The Author(s), under exclusive license to Springer Nature Switzerland AG 2021

F. Al-Turjman et al. (eds.), *Emerging Technologies for Battling Covid-19*, Studies in Systems, Decision and Control 324,
https://doi.org/10.1007/978-3-030-60039-6_17

17.1 Introduction

From March 2020 onwards according to UNESCO, 16,777 million students and children from 100 different countries are not attending their educational institutes due to the pandemic caused by COVID-19 [1]. It has been decided to close schools, colleges, and educational institutes nationwide, and University Grants Commission (UGC) has advised teachers and students to utilize this time to generate productive learning outcomes through online classes. The online education system is presently being adopted on a large scale by schools colleges and universities in India. Today's generation students are very much well versed with the latest technology, and the online teaching method is not new to them, but more hands-on experience related to software or technology at the beginning of any course can make them feel more persistent in the course [2]. Firstly, there should be structured online teaching in which the first-course instructor should make the students comfortable with various modes of platforms that will be used to provide the information, and secondly, there should be the existence of technical assistant to handle online technical issues to help the instructor as well as students if they face any technical issues during the session.

Problem identification It is a great matter of concern to enhance the student engagement and learning outcomes when the gamified online education system is implemented. While attending online classes if there is a lack of interest, trivial discussions, and low participation rate, it all leads to low student engagement. Self-determination theory plays a very important role which includes various intrinsic and extrinsic levels of motivation that are concerning student engagement for online classes [3].

Motivation To enhance the various factors of motivation, the concept of gamified online learning is introduced [4]. The gamified framework for the online education system involves the various mechanics, dynamics, and components that focus on augmenting student overall learning. Gamification acts as a strategy for the uplift contribution of members involved in online social communities. Gamification is defined as changing the non-gaming environment into the gaming environment. A situation where the whole world is struggling with unwanted pandemic, there needs to have intrinsic motivation among students to engage themselves maximum in the online classes scheduled for students. Regular teaching practices followed through online classes are not able to engage students to the best of their abilities so they need to incorporate fun-based learning methods.

Critical survey-based contribution In this chapter, we discussed various elements of teaching that should be implemented in e-learning to make the online classroom more interactive and inquiry-based; students should be allowed to explore by giving adequate tasks and assignments. Online classes not only will act as a medium of imparting education but also will lead to many more explorations in terms of modern teaching. The concept of gamified online education can bring new excitement among the students to explore various activities. In my previous research related to the gamified education system, remarkable results were shown by the students in terms of engagement and enhancement in learning in comparison to regular teaching. The involvement of various game design elements like points, badges, levels, challenges, feedback, leader boards, and avatars enriches user motivation, engagement, and learning experience. The major objective of gamified online learning is making monotonous online sessions more interesting and interactive. The concept of flipped classroom learning can make the online education system a new outlook in which the complete session will be based on discussion rather than a lecture-oriented session. Gamified online learning is completely different from game-based learning. Gamified online education involves various elements of games, but the concepts of gamified learning are completely designed to create a sense of gratification and comfort of learning through the new medium by exploring new methodologies involved to make the student more engaged. To make the learning goal-oriented and enhance student engagement through online teaching, there is a need to emphasize various activities which include planning, monitoring, and implementation of well-defined levels or strategies [2]. There is a need to identify various motivational beliefs and student's direct, behavioral attitudes toward online learning [5].

Article Structure This structure of the article is as follows: Some of the imperative work related to gamification, that is, game-based learning, is mentioned in Sect. 17.2. The online learning system and various motivational factors are discussed in Sect. 17.3. Section 17.4 consists of a gamified online education system that is different from the present online education system. At last, Sect. 17.5 consists of an analysis report in which various parameters of present online education are analyzed.

17.2 Literature Review

Gamification is defined as "simple gameplay to support productive interaction for the expected type of learners and instructors." In this heuristic definition, gamification is proposed as gamification of learning to assist gameful design. Gamification should upkeep creative interaction for expected instructors and learners [6]. With the use of gamification, the learning environment becomes more active, and it certifies that present users are doing, not merely watching. The concept of designing an interactive learning environment in the form of a generic virtual lab is a new concept used to enhance engagement. With the help of generic virtual lab architecture, instructors can work on experiments in their field. This is based on a fixed set of concepts related to the machine. The finite set machine is defined as a behavior model that is composed of a fixed number of states and transitions [7]. Internet-based learning is considered as a promising factor with qualitative learning outcomes. Electronic media and information available online are a fairly new approach to be used in health professions. The concept of gamification is implemented within

Internet-based learning to promote engagement and motivation for better learning experiences in health professions [8]. It is important that while providing a gamified solution to a problem, maximum user engagement must be achieved. This can be measured with game analytics. Designers must understand what motivates users and how different game elements may be combined to achieve this result [9]. Grades are emerged as valued contributors to rate student's performance in class. It has been analyzed the fact that they are negative contributors to students' engagement and behavior in class. So instead of assigning grades to the students, they have proposed to assign experience points. Students earn points for several activities related to ethical analysis. Students have the freedom to earn extra points also by performing extra activities. Freedom to earn extra points has also helped to gain their scoring momentum back as this was not available with the traditional grading system [10]. E-learning requires students to be more active, passionate, and motivated to grasp things easily. The author has tried to analyze the fact that does gamification increase engagement and learning capability for Internet-based content. Students' quantitative interaction was also considered an important part of this evaluation, and it was found that gamification played a significant role when it was introduced in e-learning [11]. Emotions contribute significantly to the learning process. The intensity and role of emotions are analyzed when players from different backgrounds are involved in-game. It was observed that traditional games have a strong impact on the emotions of players. Psychomotor, cooperative, opposition, and cooperative opposition games were used for identifying the emotional intensity of users [12]. To increase the engagement and motivation of students in game playing, one should determine the interest of students by taking their preferences based on different parameters [13]. Didactic and pedagogical concepts are preferred among a wide range of various well-developed fields of game applications. Like teachers, parents are also trying to identify good educational games for interactive learning; the authors also state that a three-level metadata format may be developed for the elaboration of serious gaming [14]. Computer games help in developing problem-solving and logical thinking in players. Games are also considered as a prime factor of motivation and user engagement. They also constitute rules as per gaming constraints. Games can be used as a valuable contributor to gaining extensive learning during educational deployments [15]. Table 17.1 demonstrates the difference between games and gamification. Games are always considered as motivational factors for all age groups. Various scenarios have been explored where gamification may take lead in early childhood education. In early childhood education, a firm definition of play may carry certain descriptors like intrinsic motivation, process-based focus, etc. The analysis of motivational factors done by them has resulted in positive outcomes after considering them for an early childhood education environment [17]. The framework has been created for examining the effects of gamification by identifying motivational affordances associated with it. It was identified that the effect of gamification lies in the fact which is based on the users using it and on the environment in which it is being used.

The gamification concept can be formulated with the help of motivational affordance, psychological outcomes, and behavioral outcomes. Measurement of the

Table 17.1 Comparison between game and gamification

Game	Gamification
In games, predefined rules and objectives are used	May just be a collection of tasks associated with points/levels/badges or some form of reward
There exists a probability of losing	The concept of gamification is directly related to motivation so losing may or may not be the outcome [16]
Sometimes just playing the game is intrinsically rewarding	Being intrinsically rewarding is optional
The implementation of games is normally hard and expensive to build	Gamification is usually cheaper and easy to implement
The morphing of content takes place to fit the story and scenes of the game	Usually, a game like topographies is included without making too many changes to your content

effectiveness of gamification was also varied from motivational to psychological outcomes [18]. The gamified learning system called reflex is developed. It presents a 3D virtual world in a browser that helps the user to enhance his learning and give his feedback. Based on the concept of gamification design, reflex can predict learner behavior during interaction [19]. Cloud computing has been used to share resources to reduce the operational costs, but it requires engaged users. The gamification is a method to ehnance the motivation and positive attitude toward the routine activities. Gamification may be considered a potential means to achieve this mechanism. The study has been done to bind the relationship between game mechanics and cloud computing volunteers so that it can be used more generically [20]. Learn2Mine supports a cloud-based environment for teaching purposes. Its architecture can be effectively used in teaching as well as in taking a formative assessment of data mining concepts. Student feedback was also taken on the completion of course. It was observed that students were very positive in using Learn2Mine for the teaching of data mining concepts. Constructive feedback was also collected to improvise the proposed system [21]. User involvement is a very critical element of e-learning systems. Less user involvement signifies the fact that the traffic is being diverted on another system. Autonomy, competence, and relatedness are considered as mandatory social needs to be fulfilled to support user engagement. Identification of the main objective and deployment of game mechanics must be done for increasing the effectiveness of the gamified learning process. It can be used as a tool to reach user experience goals for increased user engagements [22]. Web technologies are playing an important role in improving learning methodologies, whereas motivation and engagement are primary for the completion of any task [23]. Intrinsic motivation comes from within it is more self-determining and self-competent, whereas extrinsic motivation is surrounded by various factors like results, rewards, punishment, to meet someone else expectations, etc. [3]. There are several ramifications in terms of online instructors, researchers, and course designers for the successful implementation of online courses [2]. One of the innovative online assessment methods which got the attention of educators is online peer assessment. Intrinsic motivation engages the student in online assessment to increase its self-efficiency, whereas in extrinsic motivation, student involves himself in online assessment to get good grades and appreciation from faculty or to avoid any negative feedback [24].

17.3 Online Education Systems

As there is a rapid growth in terms of information and communication technology, even academic institutions are revolutionized, and there is a need to teach through different online platforms. Education has gone beyond classroom teaching, and the latest tools used for information technology help to provide education to school students, institutions, and universities in any part of the world. One of the best innovations in terms of communication technology and information is the Internet [25]. During this pandemic of COVID-19, online education is only possible due to the availability of the Internet. One of the major concerns in online education is online technology experience because it is very important to estimate how experienced are you with the latest technologies in terms of web browsers, installing various online applications used for online teaching platforms, surfing the Internet, and many more [5]. Online learning involves relatively more commitment, self-regulation, and willingness to learn a particular course or topic. Online teaching can only be successful where there are lively contribution and involvement of students [26]. The increased use of online learning strategy incorporating various interesting methodologies can surely help to achieve better results and enhance student satisfaction and can witness good progress in terms of engagement [27]. For effective online learning, the primary component is student engagement which is directly proportional to student's academic performance [16]. Student engagement is a construct of several subsets; each subset has its indicators. The online learning environment is highly autonomous, but it creates a hindrance for those who lack self-regulated and motivational skills [5]. Self-regulated learners are the active participants who effectively utilize all the possible resources and establish a productive work environment to enhance their learning skills. Web technologies are playing an important role in improving learning methodologies, whereas motivation and engagement are primary for the completion of any task. Any deficiency in any of the above properties may lead to distraction. The collaborative platform based on smartphone application for the preparation of official examinations helps students to test their knowledge and also users send their feedback [23].

The complete model of online education is represented in Fig. 17.1 which demonstrates the relationship as *n* ratio 1 (students–teacher) which is connected through the cloud and is using various adaptive learning and style acquisition to perform the teaching successfully. Various applications like Zoom, Google meet, LPU live, and specific school/university management systems are acting as lecture delivery platforms to overcome the gap of physical classrooms. These various learning environments help to connect with students and provide them all the necessary learnings in the form of lectures, online materials, and e-books to keep the students engaged. Students are connected to the interface by using various hardware mediums such as

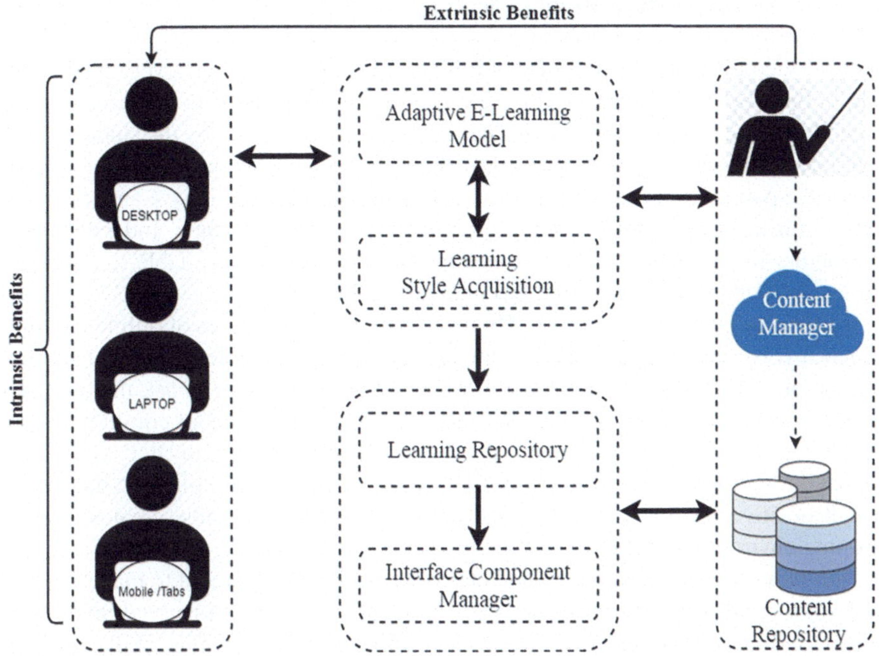

Fig. 17.1 Online education system

mobiles, laptops, desktops, etc. In the traditional education system, smartphones/tabs were never part of our learning, but the current situation is completely reverse, and various mobile applications are involved in the classroom learning to make the lectures more user interactive and effective.

17.3.1 Motivational Factors

Students need to focus on three parameters which include curiosity to achieve the goal, self-efficacy, and self-regulation [2]. Intrinsic or extrinsic motivation influences student engagement in a particular task [2]. The factors which include curiosity or interest can be termed under intrinsic motivation. The student wants to explore its capabilities and adopts the natural tendency to perform the challenges and achieve the best results without any external incentives. On the contrary, if we talk about extrinsic motivation, the students tend to perform to achieve its end-stage and along with its results, grades, appreciation, or punishment are attached to the task [2]. The high motivational level of students directly leads to an increase in engagement, and enhancement in learning takes place [28]. Low motivational levels presented by students degrade the student learning capabilities and result in a lack of interest [27].

17.3.1.1 Intrinsic Motivational Factors

Online video tutorials: Availability of online video tutorials plays a very prominent role in the world of education; this new learning method helps to improve student capabilities and competencies [25]. These videos can be viewed by the student at his own pace of time and can be viewed as many times as necessary until the student grasps the particular topic. This helps a lot of students who might have any technical issues during classroom learning or want to revise the topic independently. Instructors should make full use of vast multimedia material available to make the student learning more innovative and understandable.

Feedbacks/interactive learning: There exist four key principles of online learning which involve encouraging student interaction, understandable topic explanation, collaborative learning, and feedback [25]. If the student is free to ask the question through online chat or during the class, then there exists a sense of community and collaboration among students, and also they feel inherently motivated to be connected through virtual environment [26]. Emotional engagement plays a vital role in which positive feedback from an instructor, as well as students, creates a good learning environment [16].

Fun-based learning: Various game elements can be incorporated to make the lecture more interesting and fun-based [16]. Students can be also involved in a multiplayer online game-based task which can enhance their learning skills through collaborative learning behavior; collective enjoyment can be achieved by completing the task as a team [29]. To attain common goal, students can share common applications, that is, content resources which enhance informal learning abilities.

17.3.1.2 Extrinsic Motivational Factors

Attendance: In the education system, the accountability of teachers and students is always considered very important. Students are supposed to maintain a specific percentage of attendance depending upon their school/university regulations. Based on good attendance percentage, they are assigned a few bonus marks and regular attendance badges, nominated for class representatives, etc. The students who have low attendance are not allowed to appear in final exams or maybe not promoted to their next semester or grade.

Rewards: Students feel motivated by receiving rewards; it may be in terms of good marks, grades, or virtual gifts [30]. It is believed that extrinsic rewards act as the important motivational factor which is much liked by the students [31].

Fulfilling the expectations of parents/teachers: Expectations of parents and teachers play a very critical role in the student's academic performance. It has been analyzed when parents/teachers hold high expectations from students they perform better and get higher grades; it provides them with a positive and challenging environment to prove their ability [32].

17.4 Gamified Online Education System

The gamified approach has a high prospective to enhance learning and engagement among the students [28]. Gamification elements should be used extensively to increase user engagement and user participation in assigned tasks. Gamification primarily focuses on extrinsic motivation. Commonly used game elements include achievement, behavioral contrast, fixed interval reward schedules, and loyalty. Gamification is being used in almost all areas these days. Gamification provides motivational playful experiences through the use of interactive technologies. They have been applied commonly in operational tasks [33]. Student response systems are becoming popular these days. It is of immense benefit that instructors can get instant feedback from students which may not be available with traditional systems. The use of gamification to improve student learning in class results in improved user engagement and motivation. The game elements involved in the process of gamified online learning should be meaningful and interesting for students to achieve their learning goals [28]. The implementation of the online gamified forum was more fun and interesting in comparison to the traditional online discussion platform [16]. It was indicated by students that leader boards act as a motivational component and influence to perform with the best of the abilities and capabilities to sustain the name as top achievers [16]. The concept of gamification does not require a full-fledged game design platform, but it works on simple gameplay methodology which can be implemented without any major constraints [6]. To implement gamified learning, no specific tool is required on critical system thinking, and adequate use of game mechanics/elements can lead to a high level of engagement (Table 17.2).

17.4.1 Online Education Gamified Framework

Target behavior Intrinsically motivated students showed the active participation during the online classes. The framework designed to enhance intrinsic motivation among students comprises various factors such as prompt availability of information [34], compassionate learning environment, social engagement of students, and instructor. Having the right set of educational online platform, educators, teachers, etc. can streamline online teaching to be more effective and engaged.

Players Students, teachers, parents, technical support system

Game elements Points, virtual rewards, badges, leader boards, positive feedback

Points Points are assigned to the completion of a particular task [30]. In online education, system faculty can assign points to students on completing the assignment on time, creative tasks, answering questions while having online classroom discussions, and many more according to the subject and faculty requirements. This

Table 17.2 Comparison between online classes and gamified online classes

Comparison points	Online classes	Gamified online classes
Environment	Structured environment	Game-based learning environment
Teaching methodology	One way the teaching process	Two-way teaching process (point-based interactive learning)
Challenges	Assignments, online quiz	Game-based activities, group discussions, creative tasks allotted to students, open-book tests
Rewards	Students are assessed through marks/grades	Reward mechanism, assign weekly badges, leader board performance meter

makes the students more engaged, and interactive point-based learning can enhance student participation during online classes which seems to be low according to the analysis done. Normally, students' performance is only judged through exams that are also on a weekly or monthly basis, but to involve students on regular basis, the point-based system can enhance their productivity and also improve their monthly test performance.

Badges On completion of specific tasks, the weekly or monthly badges can be assigned to students [35]. We can assign badges through credly.com to students for the best performer, keen observer, best attendance, creative task, etc. Also, we can design our badges and assign them to students which motivate them to perform with their best capability and ability. Badges assigned to students are used as status symbols or credentials to display on various social networking platforms.

Leader board A leader board acts as a medium used for featuring a comparison of students and displaying their credibility and performance to the whole class daily [34]. The names displayed online screen will vary daily with the presence of virtual points, badges, and marks gained by students in their respective tasks.

17.5 Research Methodology

To have a clear outlook on the present online education system during the COVID-19 situation, a survey is conducted through Google forms. The survey is used to collect data on various parameters which include the intention to understand whether online classes are useful for students, analyze various motivational factors, and can deal with all technical challenges. Analysis of data can help us to find loop pools in the present online education system and suggest better engaged, motivated, and creative online classroom learning.

17.5.1 Data Collection and Respondents

The survey form is shared with various school faculties to share with students and parents to give their reviews on online classroom teaching. In this situation, parents are also playing an important role in helping their students to deal with online classes so the survey is not only to be filled by students but even parents can fill the survey form. The public platform like Facebook and Instagram is for the collection of data.

17.5.2 Research Questions

It is necessary to understand fissures in the present online education system to understand where our system lacks and what newly proposed mechanism can be designed to have more effective, motivated, and engaged online teaching. The corresponding questions cover the wide aspect of intrinsic and extrinsic factors that are part of effecting learning and teaching parameters.

Research questions	
RQ1	Online classes are a good way of imparting education to students
RQ2	Teaching approach followed during online classes is interactive
RQ3	During online classes, do you feel comfortable in asking doubts?
RQ4	Online classroom teaching motivates you to learn new concepts
RQ5	Do you face any technical issues during online classes related to software, laptop/desktop issues?
RQ6	Is there a need to improve the present online education system?
RQ7	Does school/college authorities help you deal with technical issues?
RQ8	Are you able to create a classroom bonding with your peer mates and faculties?
RQ9	Do you think online classes should continue even after school reopens?
RQ10	Are the students comfortable to take classes without the subscribed books?
RQ11	Which online education learning source is considered as the easiest to use?
RQ12	During online classes, have you faced any issues with the Internet connections?
RQ13	Do video lectures prepared by teachers easily comprehended by the students?
RQ14	Rate the present online education system
RQ15	Do you think the moral values which are an important part of student education can be imparted through the online education system?
RQ16	Is there a need to motivate students to enhance their learning through online classes?
RQ17	Sufficient online material in the form of PPTs or video lectures is provided to students
RQ18	Are you involved in any fun-based activity or game-based quizzes during online learning?
RQ19	Students are awarded with any virtual rewards or badges to enhance motivation levels
RQ20	Students attend online classes to fulfill attendance constraints

(continued)

17.5.3 Performance Analysis

A total of 166 responses have been received in the survey done for the online education system. In addition to responses, 15% of students belong to primary section (class 1–5), 42.5% of students belong to secondary section (class 6–10), 24% of students belong to senior secondary (class 11–12), and 18% of students belong to college/university level. The participation percentage of girls is 53.9% and boys 46.1%.

17.5.3.1 Reliability Test on Data Set

The method used to check the reliability of data is Cronbach's alpha method; it helps in the validation of data which is collected through the survey. The data consistency and acceptance of data are checked through this method. The spss software is used, and steps applied are demonstrated in Fig. 17.2.

Table 17.3 exhibits the data collected is valid and no inconsistent value is found. Table 17.4 defines the Cronbach's alpha value which is and if it is greater than 6 which demonstrates the collected data has good internal consistency.

17.5.3.2 Results of the Questionnaire

A primary survey has been conducted concerning the online education system; on behalf of inputs given by parents and students, the results are represented in the form of graphs. The inputs are taken on linear scale 1 = "Strongly disagree," 2 = "Disagree," 3 = "Neutral," 4 = "Agree," and 5 = "Strongly Agree."

During this pandemic situation, educational settings should continue, and students should be provided with the opportunity to learn, grow, and increase their knowledge under a safe and caring community. As the lockdown situation exists, students cannot go out. Rather, they need to have a fixed routine in which they are well-disciplined and engaged. Students and parents have widely accepted the online education system as in Fig. 17.3 around 21% of people result in disagree or strongly disagree rest, whereas 46.4% of students and parents agree that online education is a good way of imparting education to students and keeping them engaged through classroom learning. However, Figs. 17.4 and 17.5 demonstrate that there is a need to bring a few modifications in the present online education system. As this situation was so unpredictable that schools/universities, teachers, and students were not prepared, there exists a wide scope of improvement. Nearly 79% of students/parents

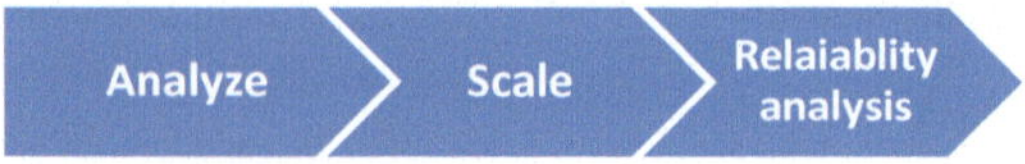

Fig. 17.2 Steps followed to check data reliability in spss software

Table 17.3 Case processing summary

Cases	*N*	%
Valid	166	100.0
Excluded[a]	0	0.0
Total	166	100.0

[a]Listwise deletion based on all variables in the procedure

Table 17.4 Reliability statistics

Cronbach's alpha	*N* of items
0.878	17

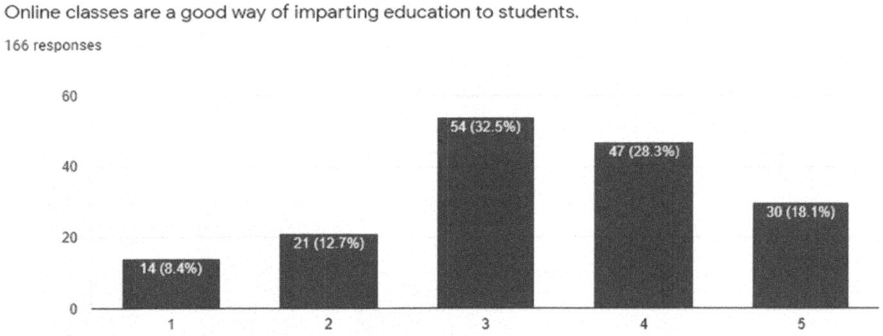

Fig. 17.3 Survey result of imparting education

believe that in this era of technology online education system should make the students more engaged, and enticement factors should be improved.

Figures 17.6 and 17.7 inculcate there exist interaction and doubt clearing sessions during online classes. To enhance learning, there is a need for maximum participation and student interaction that is most desirable and sensible to solve any particular problem. As in online classes, the eye-to-eye contact between student and teacher does not exist; thus, it is difficult at the faculty end to identify the students who have understood the concept or not. Hence, students need to interact and formulate collaborative learning. Faculties need to opt for various gamified methods to enhance the student–teacher interaction for high productive results.

Various activities can help the students gain moral values, respect, hard work, compassion, and cooperation; forgiveness does not require any specific platform; these ethics can be taught to students through different home-based practical assignments. Figure 17.8 shows more than 50% of students do not agree that moral education can be imparted through online classes. There is a need to enhance collaborative learning which indirectly also inculcates moral values like listening to your friends and group work, managing time, dividing tasks, etc. As Fig. 17.9 clearly states, there is less collaboration among students during online classroom learning so there is a need to involve students in various group activities and fun-based learning

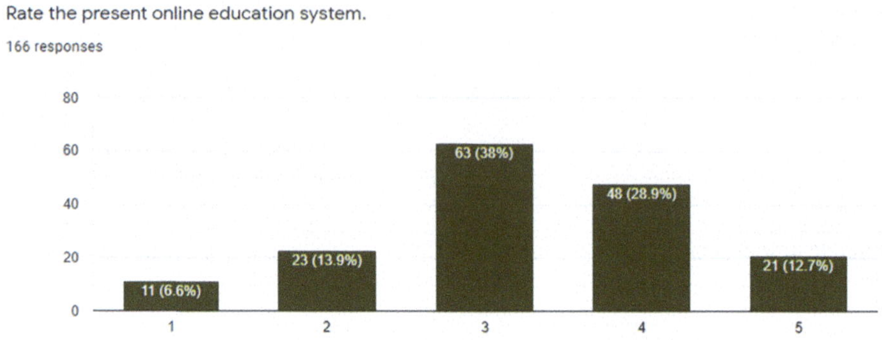

Fig. 17.4 Rating of the online education system

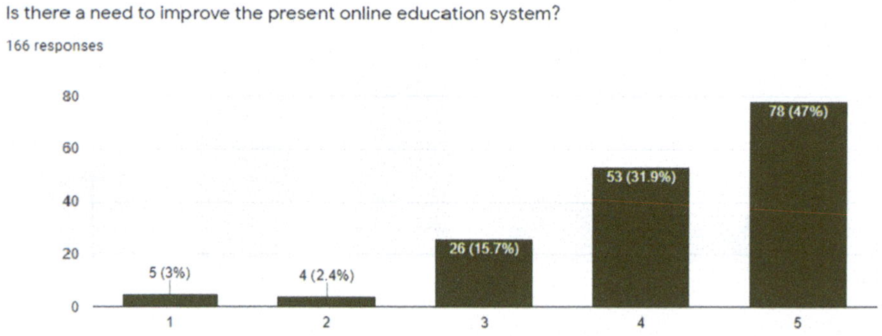

Fig. 17.5 Graph depicting the need to improve the online education system

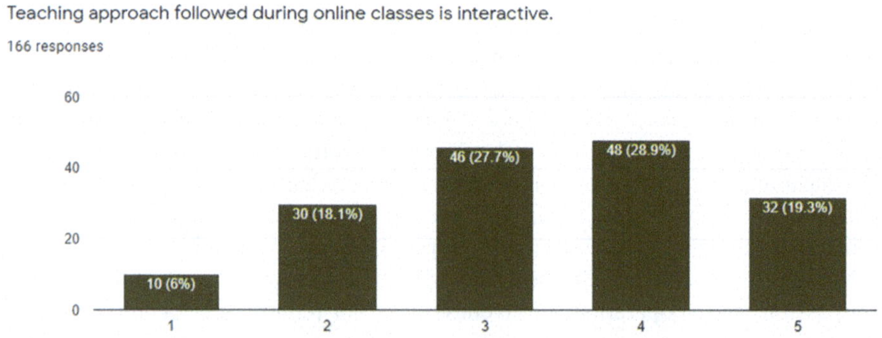

Fig. 17.6 Graph depicting the student–teacher interaction during online classes

sessions. Collaboration among the students will directly lead to imparting various moral values among students.

Various digital platforms are used to conduct online classes, and Fig. 17.10 depicts more than 50% of students are using smartphones which are being used as

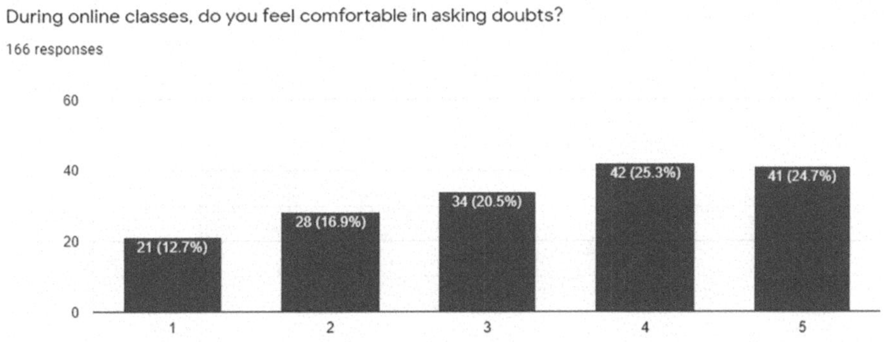

Fig. 17.7 Students comfortable in asking doubts during online sessions

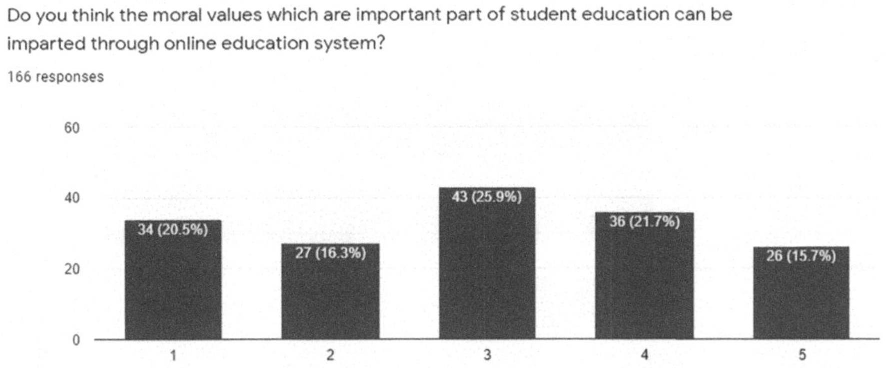

Fig. 17.8 Graph depicting response related to imparting moral values

an effective learning tool; it provides the opportunity to learners to access various online learning platforms and interact digitally. Many drastic changes have taken place in the education sector in the last 2 months: mobiles were never part of classroom learning, but now learning is only possible with the help of smartphones/tabs/laptops.

The transition from traditional classroom learning to virtual classroom creates a lot of challenges in technical aspects which include issues related to software, hardware, and connectivity issues. Figures 17.11 and 17.12 demonstrate that more than 50% of students have faced high technical issues and 72.9% of students have faced the Internet connectivity issues. For online learning, there is a requirement of high bandwidth and a strong Internet connection and one of the major constraints is nothing was well-planned. For the smooth conduct of online learning, technological proficiency is a must to both ends: the student and the teacher. Technical support provided by schools as mentioned in Fig. 17.13 has helped the students to participate in online learning with fewer interruptions. Sessions can be conducted with students or parents to deal with technical, software, and hardware issues for effective online learning.

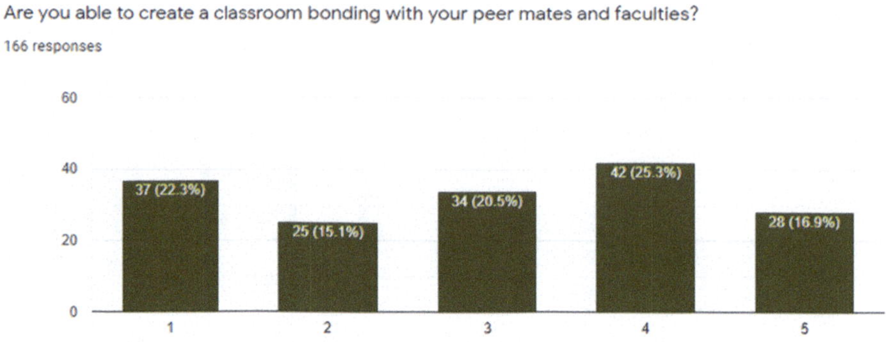

Fig. 17.9 Collaboration among students

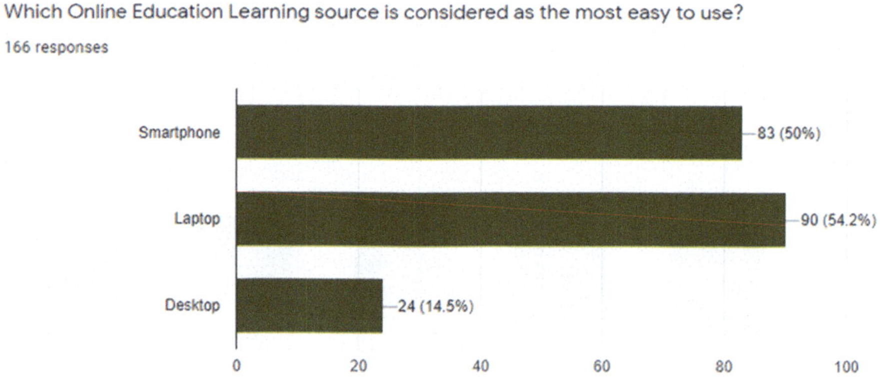

Fig. 17.10 Learning sources

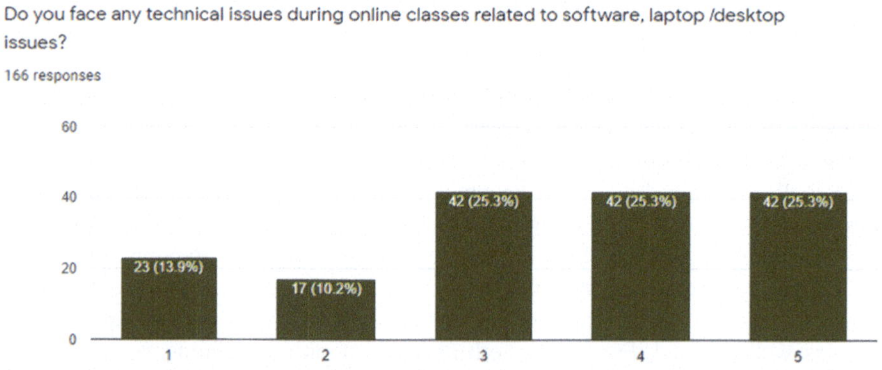

Fig. 17.11 Technical issues related to hardware and software

Books have been an integral part of our education system as the new session in schools starts in April school students are deprived of their textbooks. Figures 17.14 and 17.15 show a high percentage of students who agree that online material

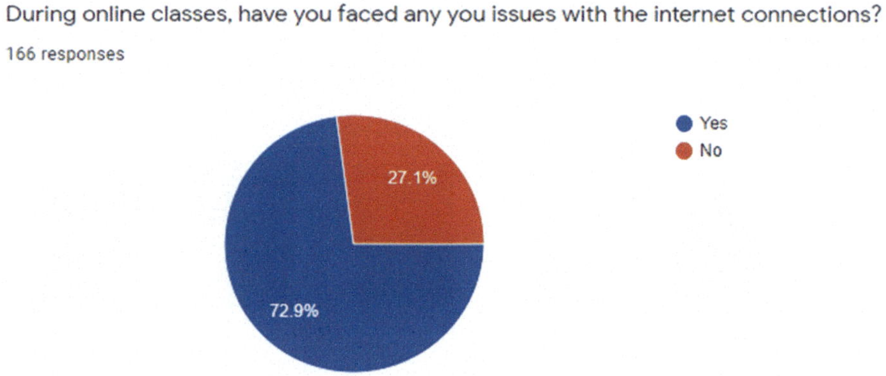

Fig. 17.12 Internet connectivity issues

provided to students in the form of ppt, video lectures, and etc. is readily understandable and effective. However, Fig. 17.16 depicts around 42% of students/parents believe students are not comfortable with the availability of manual textbooks.

Due to drastic changes in the education system, student and teachers have involved the technology tools to make sure learning remains a continuous process. Students have adopted online classes; Fig. 17.17 states around 50% of students are motivated to learn through virtual classes. However, there is a major requirement to boost and motivate students and make a shift from 50% to 100% by enhancing motivation among students for online classes. Figure 17.18 shows a matter of concern that more than 60% of parents/students feel that there is a need to enhance the motivation factors among the students. Motivation among students can be enhanced intrinsic and extrinsic factors discussed in Sect. 17.3. Game-based activities act as one of the important factors of intrinsic motivation. Various methodologies can be incorporated to make the classes more interesting and engaged. Still, the percentage of game-based learning is less than 45 as shown in Fig. 17.19; it should be enhanced which directly leads to high motivation among students. Rewards, virtual gifts, and badges act as high motivational factors that need to be embedded in the present teaching environment to enhance student motivation and engagement during online classes. As is evident in Fig. 17.20, only 30% of students are involved in any such mechanism. The new teaching mechanism surely needs new teaching motivational factors to make students feel enticed through virtual classes. Forced attendance is one of the constraints for students to attend the classes; as in Fig. 17.21, more than 50% of students/parents believe in this. Forced attendance system can make students log in to the virtual class but with zero interest and low engagement among students. In Fig. 17.22, there are 38% of parents/students who strongly disagree to promote online classes once the situation of COVID-19 is under control. The system needs to be gamified and bring a revolutionary change in the education system so that even after the school reopens students should be connected with an online platform for one particular subject to know the latest technologies and explore in a versatile manner.

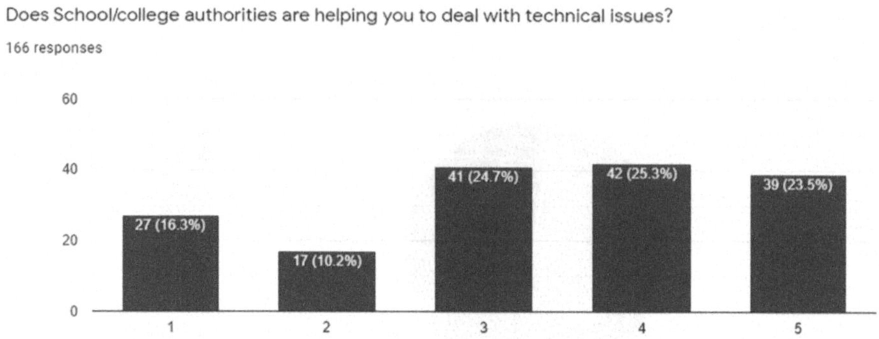

Fig. 17.13 Technical assistance

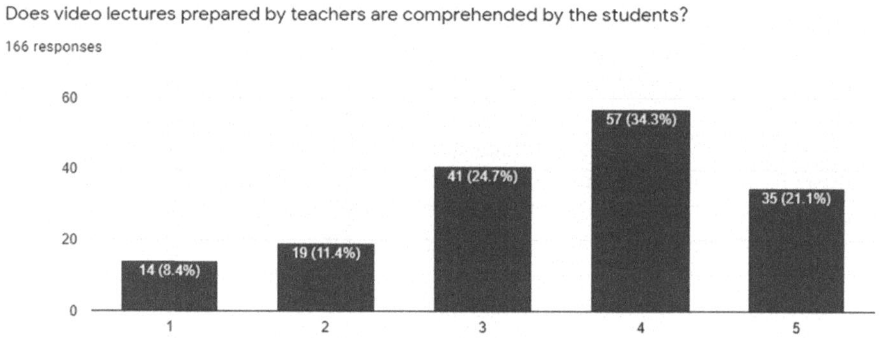

Fig. 17.14 Understanding of video lectures prepared by teachers

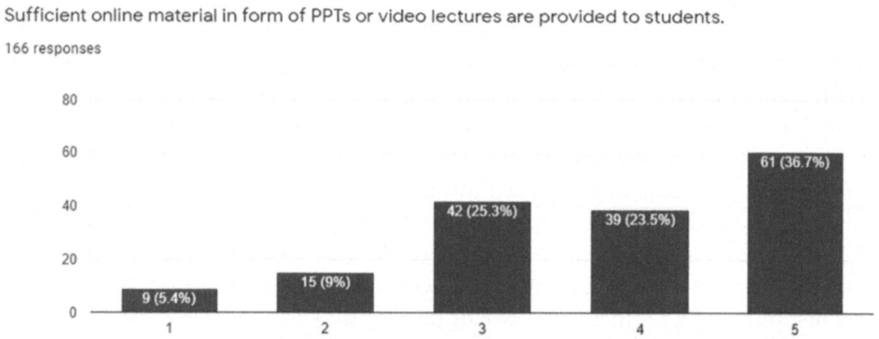

Fig. 17.15 Online material provided to students

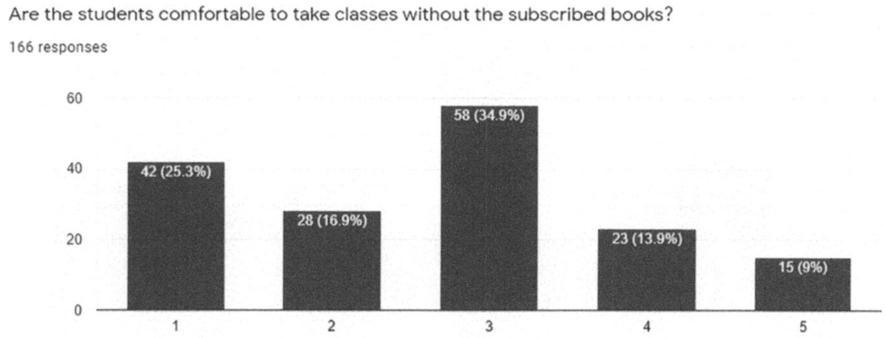

Fig. 17.16 Online classes without the availability of books

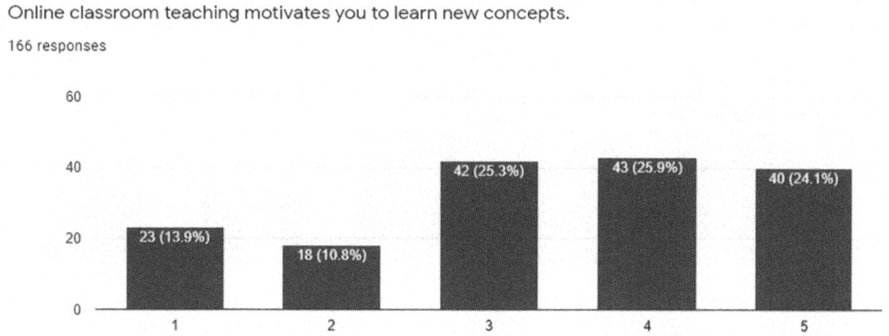

Fig. 17.17 Online classes motivate students to learn new concepts

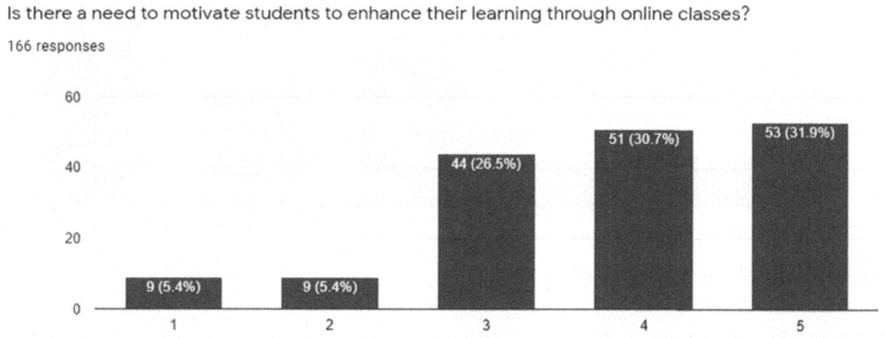

Fig. 17.18 Need to enhance motivation among students

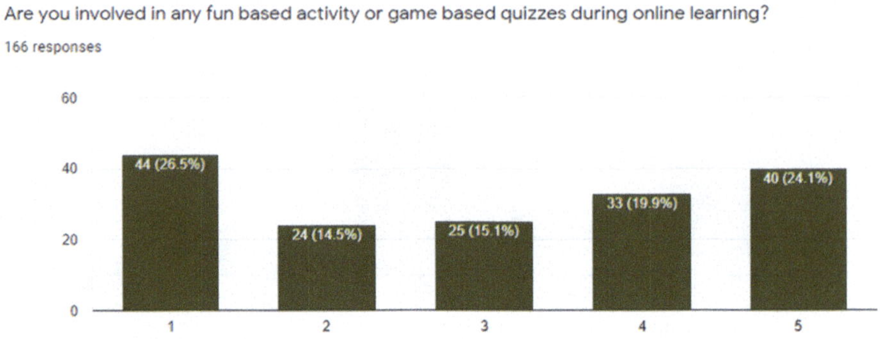

Fig. 17.19 Fun-based learning

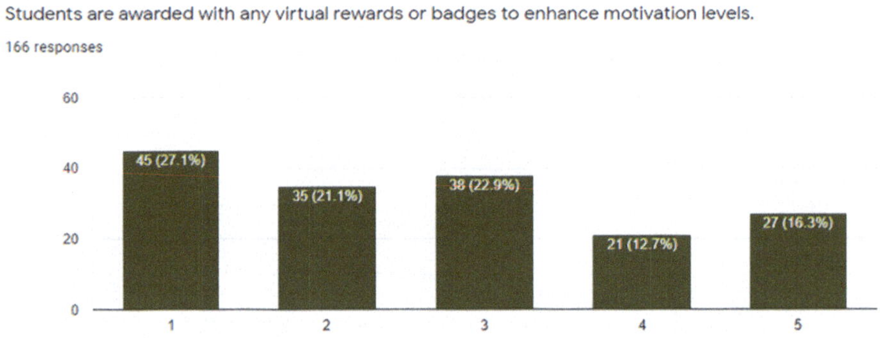

Fig. 17.20 Reward-based learning

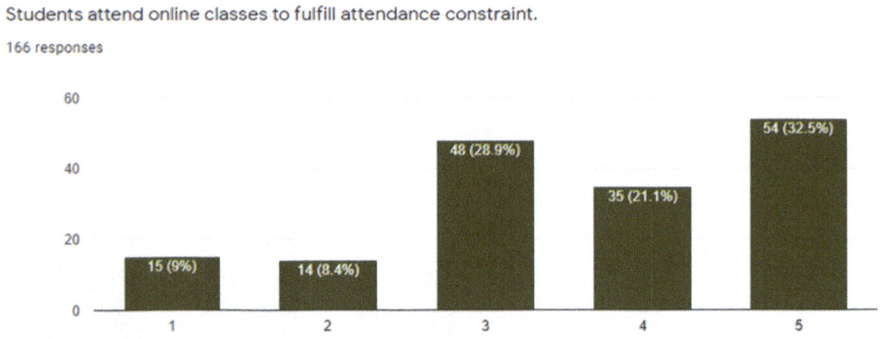

Fig. 17.21 Attendance constraints

17.6 Conclusion

Due to the pandemic COVID-19, transition has taken place form traditional learning to virtual learning. Learning environments help to connect with students and provide them all the necessary learnings in the form of lectures, online materials, and e-books

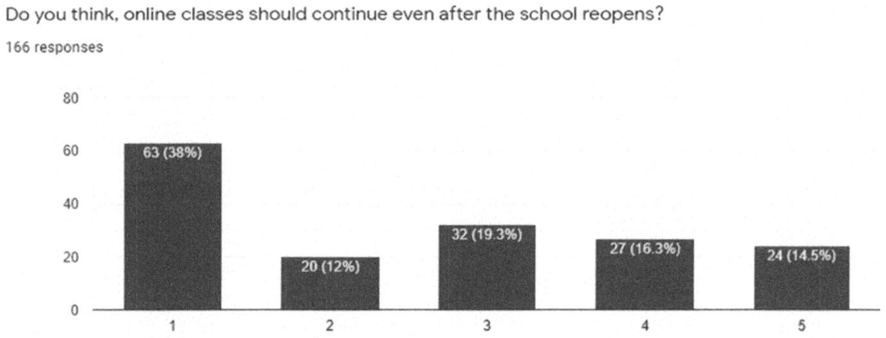

Fig. 17.22 Continuation of online classes

to keep the students engaged. According to our analysis, students have widely accepted the construct of the online education system, but there is a need to enhance various motivation levels to make the student more engaged and enticed. Mobile-based learning has become an important part of online learning and has a remarkable future to be part of our traditional education system in the future. To avail the maximum benefit of the online education system, there is a need to create a properly structured environment that is beyond the video lectures or replication of physical class. Furthermore, there is a need to incorporate new engagement methodologies that promote student involvement and high interaction among online classes and increases their knowledge. Implementation of gamified online education can bring a revolutionary change in the education systems. The various game elements which include point bases systems, rewards in the form of badges, and virtual gifts can have a high prospective to enhance learning and engagement among the students. In the future, mobile-based learning can be considered as an important component.

17.7 Future Scope

E-learning surely has a bright future in the education system. Enhancing the engagement factors and including various concepts of virtual reality, augmented reality solutions, and skill-based learning can bring a revolutionary shift from traditional learning to the online education system. Once this pandemic situation of COVID-19 is over, then also school universities should continue with online classes at least once a week to make the students aware of various technological assets and allow them to explore various parameters involved in the online education system.

References

1. van Fleet, J.W.: Opinion: education in the time of COVID-19. https://www.devex.com/news/opinion-education-in-the-time-of-covid-19-96765 (2020). Accessed 1 Jun 2020
2. Miltiadou, M., Savenye, W.C.: Applying social cognitive constructs of motivation to enhance student success in online distance education. AACE J. **11**(1), 78–95 (2003)
3. Hartnett, M., St George, A., Dron, J.: Examining motivation in online distance learning environments: complex, multifaceted, and situation-dependent. Int. Rev. Res. Open Dist. Learn. **12**(6), 20–38 (2011)
4. Gooch, D., Vasalou, A., Benton, L.: Exploring the use of a gamification platform to support students with dyslexia. In: 2015 6th International Conference on Information, Intelligence, Systems and Applications (IISA), pp. 1–6. IEEE, Washington, DC (2015)
5. Artino, A.R.: Motivational beliefs and perceptions of instructional quality: predicting satisfaction with online training. J. Comput. Assist. Learn. **24**(3), 260–270 (2008)
6. Rughiniş, R.: Gamification for productive interaction
7. Gaber, A., Naseef, O.A., Abdelbaki, N.: Creating an innovative generic virtual learning lab. In: 2013 World Congress on Computer and Information Technology (WCCIT), pp. 1–6. IEEE, Washington, DC (2013)
8. Rojas, D., Kapralos, B., Dubrowski, A.: Gamification for internet based learning in health professions education. In: 2014 IEEE 14th International Conference on Advanced Learning Technologies, pp. 281–282. IEEE, Washington, DC (2014)
9. Codish, D., Ravid, G.: Adaptive approach for gamification optimization. In: 2014 IEEE/ACM 7th International Conference on Utility and Cloud Computing, pp. 609–610. IEEE, Washington, DC (2014)
10. Gehringer, E., Peddycord, B.: Grading by experience points: an example from computer ethics. In: 2013 IEEE Frontiers in Education Conference (FIE), pp. 1545–1550. IEEE, Washington, DC (2013)
11. Amriani, A., Aji, A.F., Utomo, A.Y., Junus, K.M.: An empirical study of gamification impact on e-Learning environment. In: Proceedings of 2013 3rd International Conference on Computer Science and Network Technology, pp. 265–269. IEEE, Washington, DC (2013)
12. Lavega, P., Alonso, J.I., Etxebeste, J., Lagardera, F., March, J.: Relationship between traditional games and the intensity of emotions experienced by participants. Res. Q. Exerc. Sport. **85**(4), 457–467 (2014)
13. Ayan, S.: Games and sports preferences of children. Educ. Res. Rev. **8**(8), 396–404 (2013)
14. Göbel, S., Gutjahr, M., Steinmetz, R.: What makes a good serious game—conceptual approach towards a metadata format for the description and evaluation of serious games. In: Proceedings of the European Conference on Games Based Learning, pp. 202–210. Academic Conferences, Ltd., Reading (2011)
15. Lekka, A., Sakellariou, M.: Computer games and ethical issues. In: 2014 International Conference on Interactive Mobile Communication Technologies and Learning (IMCL2014), pp. 342–343. IEEE, Washington, DC (2014)
16. Ding, L., Er, E., Orey, M.: An exploratory study of student engagement in gamified online discussions. Comput. Educ. **120**, 213–226 (2018)
17. Tootell, H., Freeman, M., Freeman, A.: Generation alpha at the intersection of technology, play and motivation. In: 2014 47th Hawaii International Conference on System Sciences, pp. 82–90. IEEE, Washington, DC (2014)
18. Hamari, J., Koivisto, J., Sarsa, H.: Does gamification work?--a literature review of empirical studies on gamification. In: 2014 47th Hawaii International Conference on System Sciences, pp. 3025–3034. IEEE, Washington, DC (2014)
19. Herbert, B., Charles, D., Moore, A., Charles, T.: An investigation of gamification typologies for enhancing learner motivation. In: 2014 International Conference on Interactive Technologies and Games, pp. 71–78. IEEE, Washington, DC (2014)

20. Shahri, A., Hosseini, M., Ali, R., Dalpiaz, F.: Gamification for volunteer cloud computing. In: 2014 IEEE/ACM 7th International Conference on Utility and Cloud Computing, pp. 616–617. IEEE, Washington, DC (2014)
21. Anderson, P.E., Turner, C., Dierksheide, J., McCauley, R.: An extensible online environment for teaching data science concepts through gamification. In: 2014 IEEE Frontiers in Education Conference (FIE) Proceedings, pp. 1–8. IEEE, Washington, DC (2014)
22. Lubis, F.F., Rosmansyah, Y., Supangkat, S.H.: Math workout series: enhancing learning application with gamification. In: 2014 International Conference on Information Technology Systems and Innovation (ICITSI), pp. 290–294. IEEE, Washington, DC (2014)
23. López, J.P., Cerezo, A., Menéndez, J.M., Ballesteros, J.P.: Usage of mobile devices as collaborative tools for education and preparation of official exams. In: 2015 International Symposium on Consumer Electronics (ISCE), pp. 1–2. IEEE, Washington, DC (2015)
24. Tseng, S.C., Tsai, C.C.: Taiwan college students' self-efficacy and motivation of learning in online peer assessment environments. Internet High. Educ. **13**(3), 164–169 (2010)
25. Bondoc, C.M.D., Malawit, T.G.: Classifying relevant video tutorials for the school's learning management system using support vector machine algorithm. Glob. J. Eng. Technol. Adv. **2**(3), 001–009 (2020)
26. Lee, M.K., Cheung, C.M., Chen, Z.: Acceptance of Internet-based learning medium: the role of extrinsic and intrinsic motivation. Inf. Manag. **42**(8), 1095–1104 (2005)
27. Lin, C.H., Zhang, Y., Zheng, B.: The roles of learning strategies and motivation in online language learning: a structural equation modeling analysis. Comput. Educ. **113**, 75–85 (2017)
28. Ding, L., Kim, C., Orey, M.: Studies of student engagement in gamified online discussions. Comput. Educ. **115**, 126–142 (2017)
29. Kong, J.S.L., Kwok, R.C.W., Fang, Y.: The effects of peer intrinsic and extrinsic motivation on MMOG game-based collaborative learning. Inf. Manag. **49**(1), 1–9 (2012)
30. Jayasinghe, U., Dharmaratne, A.: Game based learning vs. gamification from the higher education students' perspective. In: Proceedings of 2013 IEEE International Conference on Teaching, Assessment and Learning for Engineering (TALE), pp. 683–688. IEEE, Washington, DC (2013)
31. Papp, T.A., Theresa, A.: Gamification effects on motivation and learning: application to primary and college students. Int. J. Cross Discip. Subj. Educ. **8**(3), 3193–3201 (2017)
32. Yamamoto, Y., Holloway, S.D.: Parental expectations and children's academic performance in sociocultural context. Educ. Psychol. Rev. **22**(3), 189–214 (2010)
33. Shreenath, V.M., Kornevs, M., Raghothama, J., Meijer, S.: A feasibility study for gamification in transport maintenance: requirements to implement gamification in heterogeneous organizations. In: 2015 7th International Conference on Games and Virtual Worlds for Serious Applications (VS-Games), pp. 1–7. IEEE, Washington, DC (2015)
34. Seaborn, K., Fels, D.I.: Gamification in theory and action: a survey. Int. J. Hum. Comput. Stud. **74**, 14–31 (2015)
35. Kiryakova, G., Angelova, N., Yordanova, L.: Gamification in education. In: Proceedings of 9th International Balkan Education and Science Conference (2014)

Index

© The Author(s), under exclusive license to Springer Nature Switzerland AG 2021
F. Al-Turjman et al. (eds.), *Emerging Technologies for Battling Covid-19*, Studies in Systems, Decision and Control 324,
https://doi.org/10.1007/978-3-030-60039-6

E

F

X

The manufacturer's authorised representative in the EU is Springer Nature Customer Service Centre GmbH, Europaplatz 3, 69115 Heidelberg, Germany. If you have any concerns regarding our products, please contact ProductSafety@springernature.com

Printed and bound by CPI Group (UK) Ltd, Croydon, CR0 4YY
30/09/2026
02225687-0006